Angiogenesis and Cardiovascular Disease

ANGIOGENESIS AND CARDIOVASCULAR DISEASE

Edited by

J. ANTHONY WARE

Sidney L. and Miriam K. Olson Professor of Cardiology
Professor of Molecular Pharmacology
Albert Einstein College of Medicine
Montefiore Medical Center
Bronx, New York

MICHAEL SIMONS

Associate Professor of Medicine
Harvard Medical School
Beth Israel Deaconess Medical Center
Boston, Massachusetts

New York Oxford
OXFORD UNIVERSITY PRESS
1999

Oxford University Press

Oxford New York
Athens Auckland Bangkok Bogotá Buenos Aires Calcutta
Cape Town Chennai Dar es Salaam Delhi Florence Hong Kong Istanbul
Karachi Kuala Lumpur Madrid Melbourne Mexico City Mumbai
Nairobi Paris São Paulo Singapore Taipei Tokyo Toronto Warsaw

and associated companies in
Berlin Ibadan

Published by Oxford University Press, Inc.
198 Madison Avenue, New York, New York 10016

Oxford is a registered trademark of Oxford University Press

Library of Congress Cataloging-in-Publication Data
Angiogenesis and cardiovascular disease /
edited by J. Anthony Ware, Michael Simons.
p. cm. Includes bibliographical references and index.
ISBN 0-19-511235-0
1. Cardiovascular system—Diseases—Treatment.
2. Neovascularization. 3. Growth factors—Therapeutic use.
I. Ware, J. Anthony. II. Simons, Michael.
[DNLM: 1. Cardiovascular Diseases—therapy.
2. Angiogenesis Factor—therapeutic use.
WG 166 A588 1999] RC671.A54 1999 616.1'06—dc21
DNLM/DLC for Library of Congress 98-22176

9 8 7 6 5 4 3 2 1

Printed in the United States of America
on acid-free paper

This book is dedicated to our families,
for their patience, support,
and understanding.

J.A.W.
M.S.

Preface

The concept of using therapeutic agents to induce the formation of new vessels to treat patients with vascular disease is relatively recent. The attractiveness of this concept has encouraged many clinicians and scientists to become interested in angiogenesis and the attendant principles of vascular cell and molecular biology that are its foundation, leading to the generation of a great number of innovative clinical and experimental observations. These observations have been fueled in part by an explosion of information available on the role of angiogenesis in cancer and the pioneering work of Judah Folkman, and in part by frustration at the lack of treatment alternatives available for patients with severe vascular disease.

Angiogenesis at both the clinical and fundamental scientific levels has emerged as an important area of study that exemplifies the importance of rapid translation of information learned at the laboratory bench to the bedside. There are compelling reasons to discuss the growth of new blood vessels, in both a clinical and mechanistic context, in a single book. Besides the wealth of recent information available on the biology of endothelial cells, growth factors, and developing vessels, recent technological developments have allowed the application of these advances to preclinical models of vascular disease, and to patients. The original inspiration for this book came from the students and trainees in our research laboratories, who joined us to explore fundamental questions about the growth of new blood vessels, but had no single resource to which to turn to acquire a contemporary understanding of the fundamental biology of this process or of its clinical implications for the patient with cardiovascular disease. It later became clear to us that this was an opportune time to summarize the current state of knowledge for the benefit of clinicians who wish to understand the potential role of therapeutic angiogenesis in their patients.

Angiogenesis and Cardiovascular Disease was written to integrate the current understanding of basic mechanisms in vascular cell and molecular biology with the experimental and clinical implications of these advances. Our goal was not to provide an exhaustively referenced compendium of the many topics that touch upon angiogenesis. Instead, we sought to create a practical and concise summary that would be equally useful for those first entering the field and for those with expertise in one facet of angiogenesis wishing to learn more about others. Part I, entitled Developmental and Normal Biology of the Vasculature, summarizes the current state of knowledge in developmental vascular biology, intracellular mechanisms for endothelial cell adhesion, migration, and proliferation, and angiogenic growth factors and their receptors. Part II, Angiogenesis in the Pathophysiology and Treatment of Ischemic Vascular Disease, reviews topics of practical, experimental, and clinical relevance, including the role of new vessel formation in the pathogenesis of atherosclerosis, the importance of collateral and new vessel formation in both experimental models and in nonischemic diseases, methods of drug delivery, and preclinical and clinical evidence of efficacy of angiogenic agents in treating myocardial and peripheral limb ischemia.

We believe that this book will solidify the concept that therapeutic angiogenesis is a dynamic, vibrant field with clear implications for understanding the pathogenesis of cardiovascular disease and for the treatment of patients. We hope that it will serve as a useful resource, not only for those involved in education and in the pursuit of new research programs, but also for those caring for patients with vascular disease.

Bronx, New York J.A.W.
Boston, Massachusetts M.S.
October 1998

Contents

Contributors

TAKAYUKI ASAHARA, M.D.
Department of Medicine (Cardiology)
St. Elizabeth's Medical Center
Tufts University School of Medicine
Boston, MA

RICHARD BLAIR, M.D.
Department of Medicine (Cardiology)
St. Elizabeth's Medical Center
Tufts University School of Medicine
Boston, MA

COLIN M. BLOOR, M.D.
Department of Pathology
University of California, San Diego School of Medicine
La Jolla, CA

LAURENCE L. BRUNTON, M.D.
Department of Pathology
University of California, San Diego School of Medicine
La Jolla, CA

THOMAS F. DEUEL, M.D.
Division of Growth Regulation
Beth Israel Deacones Medical Center
Boston, MA

ELAZER R. EDELMAN, M.D. PH.D.
Harvard-MIT Division of Health Sciences and Technology
Massachusetts Institute of Technology
Cambridge, MA
and
Cardiovascular Division
Brigham and Women's Hospital and Harvard Medical School
Boston, MA

KURT A. ENGLEKA, PH.D.
Department of Physiology
Jefferson Medical College
Thomas Jefferson University
Philadelphia, PA

ANTHONY ENGLISH, PH.D.
Harvard-MIT Division of Health Sciences and Technology
Massachusetts Institute of Technology
Cambridge, MA

NAPOLEONE FERRARA, PH.D.
Department of Cardiovascular Research
Genentech
South San Francisco, CA

HANS PETER GERBER, M.D.
Department of Cardiovascular Research
Genentech
South San Francisco, CA

LAURA HALEY
Department of Medicine (Cardiology)
St. Elizabeth's Medical Center
Tufts University School of Medicine
Boston, MA

DAVID HARRISON, M.D.
Department of Medicine
Emory University School of Medicine
Atlanta, GA

ANTONIS HATZOPOULOS, PH.D.
GSF Research Center
Institute for Clinical Molecular Biology and Tumor Genetics
Munich, Germany

JEFFREY ISNER, M.D.
Departments of Medicine (Cardiology) and Biomedical Research
St. Elizabeth's Medical Center
Tufts University School of Medicine
Boston, MA

WULF ITO
Department of Experimental Cardiology
Max-Planck-Institute
Bad Nauheim, Germany

ROGER J. LAHAM, M.D.
Angiogenesis Research Center
Beth Israel Deaconess Medical Center
Boston, MA

THOMAS MACIAG, PH.D.
Center for Molecular Medicine
Maine Medical Center Research Institute
South Portland, ME

J. GARY MESZAROS, PH.D.
Departments of Pharmacology and Pathology
University of California, San Diego School of Medicine
La Jolla, CA

RAMON MUNOZ-CHAPULI
Department of Animal Biology
Faculty of Science
University of Malaga
Malaga, Spain

ANN PIECZEK, R.N.
Department of Medicine (Cardiology)
St. Elizabeth's Medical Center
Tufts University School of Medicine
Boston, MA

JAN J. PIEK
Department of Cardiology
Academic Medical Center
Amsterdam, The Netherlands

MARK POST, M.D., PH.D.
Cardiovascular Division
Beth Israel Deaconess Medical Center
Boston, MA

ROBERT D. ROSENBERG, M.D.
Department of Biology
Massachusetts Institute of Technology
Cambridge, MA

ROBERT SCHAINFELD, D.O.
Department of Medicine (Cardiology)
St. Elizabeth's Medical Center
Tufts University School of Medicine
Boston, MA

WOLFGANG SCHAPER, M.D., PH.D.
Department of Experimental Cardiology
Max-Planck-Institute
Bad Nauheim, Germany

FRANK W. SELLKE, M.D.
Division of Cardiothoracic Surgery
Department of Surgery
Beth Israel Deaconess Medical Center
Boston, MA

NICHOLAS SHWORAK, PH.D.
Angiogenesis Research Center
Beth Israel Deaconess Medical Center
Boston, MA

MICHAEL SIMONS, M.D.
Angiogenesis Research Center
Beth Israel Deaconess Medical Center
Boston, MA

ROBERT J. TOMANEK, PH.D.
Department of Anatomy
University of Iowa
Iowa City, IA

J. ANTHONY WARE, M.D.
Cardiovascular Division, Department of Medicine
Department of Molecular Pharmacology
Albert Einstein College of Medicine
Montefiore Medical Center
Bronx, NY

CLAUDIA WOLF
Department of Experimental Cardiology
Max-Planck-Institute
Bad Nauheim, Germany

CHUN YU, PH.D.
Harvard-MIT Division of Health Sciences and Technology
Massachusetts Institute of Technology
Cambridge, MA

I

DEVELOPMENTAL AND NORMAL BIOLOGY OF THE VASCULATURE

1

Embryonic Development of the Vascular System

ANTONIS K. HATZOPOULOS AND ROBERT D. ROSENBERG

The vascular system supplies nutrients, hormones, and growth factors to all tissues and organs and removes waste products. The main component of the vascular system is the endothelial cells that line the walls of all blood vessels. Endothelial cells are involved in numerous interactions with perivascular cells, adjacent tissues, and blood cells. They play major roles in clotting, thrombosis, and diseases such as atherosclerosis. Under normal conditions the adult vasculature is a stable structure. Mature endothelial cells do not divide and have a half-life of many years. However, in pathological situations such as tumor-induced angiogenesis, tissue remodeling following injury, cardiac infarction, diabetic retinopathy, psoriasis, etc., endothelial cells quickly respond and grow, vascularizing affected tissues de novo (Folkman, 1995). In these cases, a resting endothelium is quickly activated in response to angiogenic signals to break cell–cell connections, divide, migrate through connective tissue, and form new blood vessels. Many of these phenomena involve reactivation of embryonic pathways of vasculogenesis and angiogenesis. Therefore, an in-depth analysis of embryonic vascular development will help us to understand the molecular and cellular bases of adult vascular diseases and design therapeutic approaches to treat them. In this chapter we provide a description of embryonic vascular development and discuss new molecules identified over the last few years that regulate particular aspects of vascular growth and differentiation.

INITIAL STAGES IN VASCULAR DEVELOPMENT

At day 11 in mouse development, or at about the midgestation period, an extensive system of blood vessels exists that supplies nutrients to the developing embryo and simultaneously removes waste products (Plate 1). By day 10 of development all major organ primordia are in place. From this point on tissues will differentiate and grow at phenomenal rates until birth. This growth is dependent on a functional vascular network, and for this reason the cardiovascular system begins to form very early during embryogenesis (Risau and Flamme, 1995; Baldwin, 1996).

The vascular system develops from cells of mesodermal origin shortly after the end of gastrulation. During gastrulation, cells from the primitive ectoderm (or epiblast) begin to delaminate, divide, invaginate through the primitive streak, and migrate to colonize most areas between the layers of ectoderm and endoderm (Fig. 1.1). The position and time the cells invaginate determine the location they will occupy within the embryo, and this in turn determines the structures and organs they will form (Lawson et al., 1991). Cell lineage tracing experiments reveal that the heart and endothelial progenitors are derived from mesodermal cells migrating throughout the primitive streak except the most anterior area of the streak next to Hensen's node (Garcia-Martinez and Schoenwolf, 1993).

The first manifestation of vascular formation takes place in the extraembryonic yolk sac membrane where mesoderm cells form clusters called *blood islands* (Sabin, 1920) (Plate 2). Shortly thereafter, blood islands differentiate into an external layer of flat cells that will give rise to endothelium and an inner core of round cells that will form blood. The blood islands first assemble at an area of extraembryonic tissue furthest away from the embryo, called *area vasculosa* in the chicken, where they appear at the fringes of the epiblast. In rodent embryos, this area lies just below the chorion, where blood islands form as a zone surrounding the exocoelomic cavity (Jolly, 1940). Very quickly thereafter a progressive wave of blood island cell clusters forms, moving from the extraembryonic areas toward inside the embryo. The appearance of the clusters becomes more solid where they are farthest away from the area vasculosa, and the number of loose cells inside the clusters gradually diminishes. Neighboring blood islands seek each other and begin to anastomose to long channels that fill with blood cells. Most of these blood cells already express hemoglobins, which accounts for the red color of the blood islands.

In parallel, vascular formation commences inside the embryo (Plate 2). Cells of the proximal lateral mesoderm start assembling symmetrically around the body axis into structures called *preendocardial tubes* (Sabin, 1917). These tubes fuse at the area of the anterior intestinal portal. The area of the fusion will develop to the heart endocardium, which within a day will be surrounded by adjacent premyocardial cells (DeRuiter et al., 1992). The two layers of endocardium and myocardium will then proceed to a complex series of morphological changes and movements that will give rise to the embryonic heart (Fishman and Chien, 1997). The fused tube elongates anteriorly and splits into two ventral aortae that, after a loop, extend further posteriorly as the two symmetrically paired dorsal

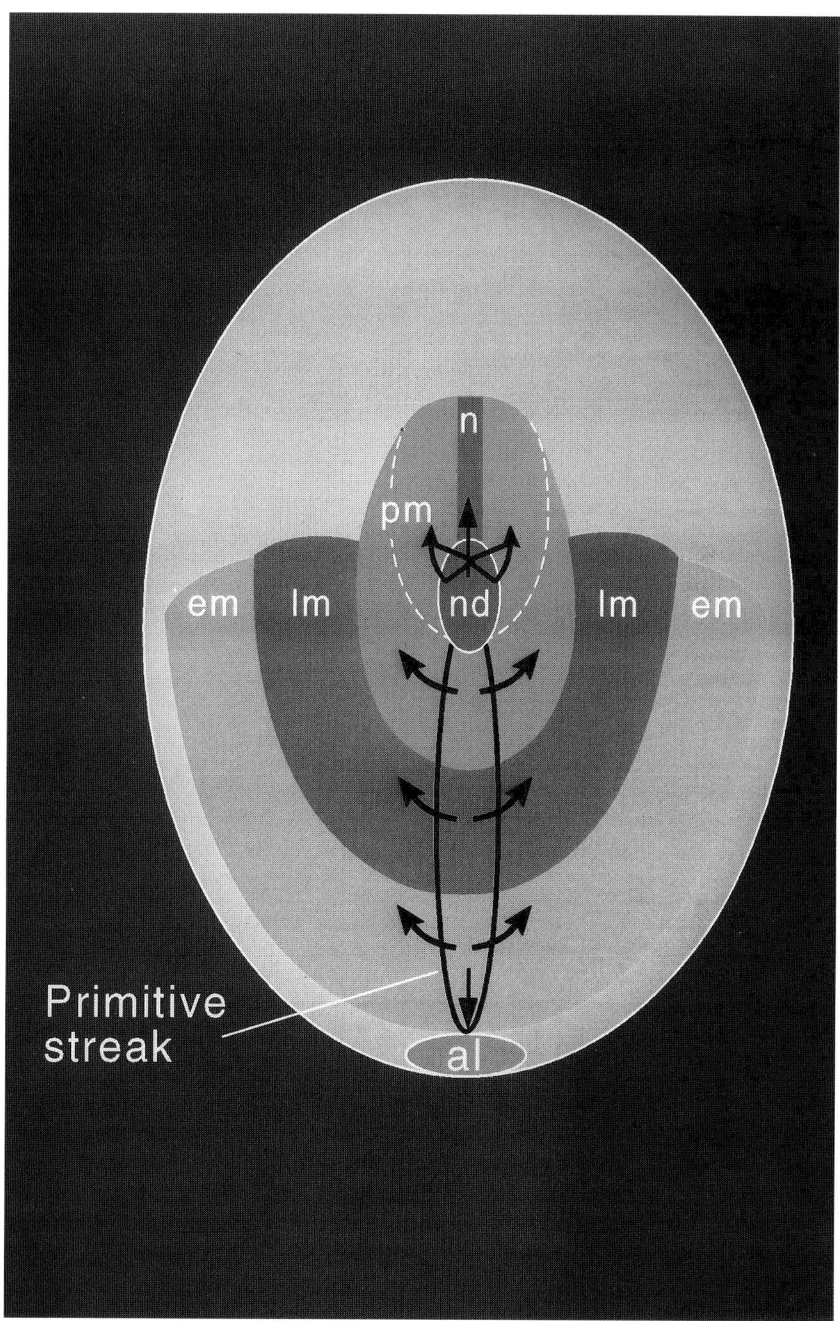

Figure 1.1. Diagram of mesodermal cell movements during gastrulation in mouse (Smith et al., 1994); nd: anterior boundary of the primitive streak (Hensen's node); n: notochord; pm: paraxial mesoderm; lm: lateral mesoderm; em: extraembryonic mesoderm; al: allantois.

aortae. The two dorsal aortae will merge later in development into a single tube that will assume a place below the notochord.

At the same time, the posterior end of the forming heart splits at the sinus venosus area into two vessels, the vitelline, or omphalomesenteric, veins, which will connect with major vessels forming in the yolk sac (Sabin, 1917). The two vitelline or omphalomesenteric arteries develop as extensions of the dorsal aortae and complete the yolk sac circulatory loop (Evans, 1909). Simultaneously, mesodermal cells in the allantois form vascular cords that will build the umbilical arteries and veins. In rodent embryos, the allantois rapidly expands inside the exocoelomic cavity and fuses with the mesoderm of the chorion at the roof of the cavity. This fusion triggers endothelial cell differentiation in this area that will produce the embryonic part of the placental circulation, which will in turn connect indirectly with the maternal circulatory system. The heart begins to contract at around the ten-somite stage, and initially, blood cells start moving back and forth inside the major blood vessels. When the circulatory loops are complete, embryonic circulation begins around the 16-somite stage.

These initial stages of vascular formation are best described by the term *vasculogenesis* to signify de novo formation of blood vessels by mesodermal precursors, also called *angioblasts* (Risau, 1991). The endocardium and the major arteries and veins develop in situ in this manner. Later in embryogenesis, the vascular tree grows by sprouting, cell division, migration, and assembly of endothelial cells derived from preexisting vessels through a process termed *angiogenesis* (Risau, 1991). Organs of mesodermal and endodermal origins, e.g., heart, lung, kidneys, and liver, vascularize by a combination of in situ assembly of angioblasts (vasculogenesis) and attraction of endothelial cells from neighboring vessels (angiogenesis) while organs of ectodermal origin such as brain are mainly vascularized by angiogenic processes (Bär, 1980; Pardanaud et al., 1989).

Classical embryological investigations have sought to ascertain the relationship between the different sites of origin of embryonic blood vessels. (For a thorough review of early literature see Wilting and Christ, 1996.) According to the in-growth theory of His (His, 1868), both intraembryonic and extraembryonic vessels are derived from the yolk sac vasculature, whereas Rabl suggested that all intraembryonic vessels sprout from the endocardium (Rabl, 1889). Subsequently Hahn, Reagan, and Sabin postulated that both somatic and splachnic mesoderm possess angiogenic potential (Hahn, 1909; Reagan, 1915; Sabin, 1917). In the previous decade, further insight in the assembly of vasculature was gained mainly due to the availability and application of antibodies against endothelial antigens such as von Willebrand factor (vWF) and lectins such as GSL IB_4 that specifically stain endothelial cells and early endothelial precursors (Coffin et al., 1991). Moreover, the development of the quail/chicken chimera system (Le Douarin, 1969) and the use of quail-specific antibodies such as QH1 and MB1 that recognize endothelial precursors expanded our understanding of how the endothelial cell lineage emerges in early embryogenesis (Pardanaud et al., 1987; Coffin and Poole, 1988; Péault et al., 1988). These studies substantiated the differentiation of endothelial cells from mesodermal progenitors and confirmed that most areas of early mesoderm contain endothelial cell precursors or angioblasts with the exception of the amnion, the sinus romboidalis, and the primitive streak. These experiments demonstrated that the major vascular channels assemble in situ as a homogeneous plexus of endothelial cells. Furthermore, they established that later in development the vascular tree expands by sprouting of preexisting vessels but also by concurrent incorporation of angioblasts that appear to be able to migrate extensively within the developing embryo (Noden, 1989).

It has been postulated that the yolk sac visceral endoderm plays a role in the induction and differentiation of blood islands (Augustine, 1981). Studies in *Xenopus* embryos have shown that members of the fibroblast growth factor (FGF) and transforming growth factor β (TGFβ) families emanating from the endoderm induce ventral specification of the mesoderm and blood island formation (Slack, 1994). In addition, it has been proposed that the endoderm in the area of the anterior intestinal portal (AIP) influences the early differentiation of the heart. (For a recent review see Nascone and Mercola, 1996.) In vitro explants of the AIP endoderm can induce the expression of both myocyte-and endothelial-cell-specific early markers when cocultured with mesoderm (Schultheiss et al., 1995; Sugi and Markwald, 1996).

One still unresolved paradox is that while formation of certain structures of mesodermal origin, e.g., skeletal muscle, depends on gastrulation, blood islands can form in isolated explants that do not undergo gastrulation (Azar and Eyal-Giladi, 1979; Mitrani and Shimoni, 1990). It is possible that posterior and extraembryonic mesoderm might be derived by direct delamination from the epiblast or primitive ectoderm, thus bypassing the need for invagination and migration through the primitive streak. At present it is unclear how the endothelial progenitor cells differentiate from mesoderm at early embryonic stages.

REMODELING OF THE VASCULAR NETWORK

An important feature of the developing vascular network is its constant remodeling during embryogenesis. The adult vasculature has little resemblance to the original vascular plan in the embryo. In the initial phase of vasculogenesis it appears that in most instances a homogeneous plexus of equal-size vessels forms. Subsequently, from this plexus, larger and smaller vessels emerge by a mechanism described by the term *intussusceptive microvascular growth* (Evans, 1909; Caduff et al., 1986) (Fig. 1.2). This process is probably driven by blood flow pressure or hemodynamics. Remodeling involves fusion of smaller vessels to larger ones and the splitting of large

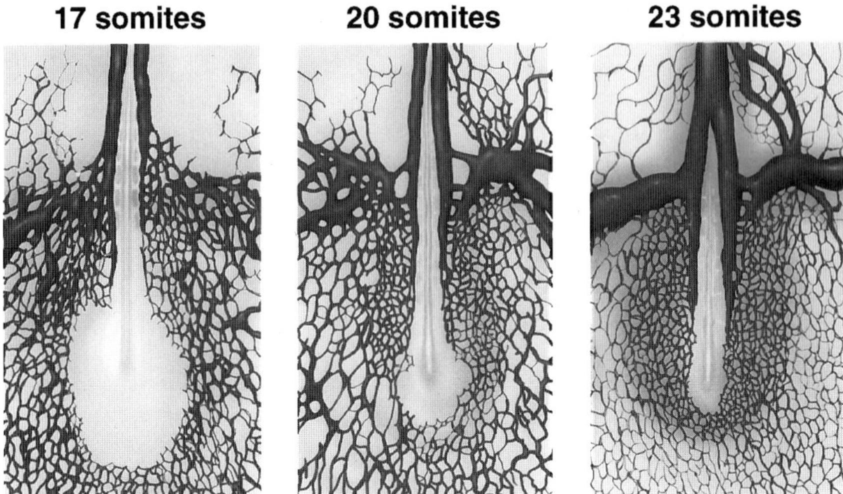

Figure 1.2. Remodeling of the primary vascular network of the vitelline arteries in chicken embryos. From a homogeneous plexus of endothelial cells at the 17-somite stage, small and large vessels emerge toward the 23-somite stage.

vessels into smaller ones (Baldwin, 1996; Wilting and Christ, 1996). Often vessels dissociate and freed endothelial cells incorporate into neighboring endothelium. In other instances, it appears that new vessels form from sprouting of preexisting vascular channels and concurrent incorporation of neighboring angioblasts (Noden, 1989). At this point it is not clear when the original pool of angioblasts is exhausted and the vascular tree simply grows by sprouting of existing blood vessels. Embryonic development of the endothelium also includes extensive cell death, triggered probably by low blood flow and lack of nutrients or other environmental factors rather than a specific genetically controlled program (Hallmann et al., 1987). Moreover, the direction of blood flow within vessels might change during development. In other instances, certain vessels initially have a transitory "mixed" function wherein they simultaneously supply and drain a developing tissue (Sabin, 1917).

One example of vascular remodeling extensively described in the literature is the formation of the aortic arches (Rosenquist, 1970). Early in development they develop as outgrowths of the ventral aorta, only to dissociate at later embryonic stages. Another example is the development and reorganization of the posterior venous system (Plate 9). Originally two symmetrical vitelline veins form at the posterior part of sinus venosus. Subsequently, the right vitelline vein regresses whereas the left vein persists. The developing liver grows around the left vitelline vein, which breaks down into numerous channels surrounding the hepatocytes. The initial layout of the postcardinal veins changes as well. Their reorganization in association with the development of nephrogenic mesoderm is depicted in Plate 9.

DIVERSITY OF VASCULAR DEVELOPMENT

The first manifestation of diversity in vascular development is apparent from the very early embryonic stages (Pardanaud et al., 1989). For example, vasculogenesis in the yolk sac is tied to hematopoiesis, and it appears that a common cell precursor, the hemangioblast, exists that can give rise to both endothelial cells and blood cell precursors (Murray, 1932). On the other hand, endothelial progenitors, or pure angioblasts, assemble to form the central part of the intraembryonic vasculature—namely, the endocardium and the dorsal aortae—and they do not appear to give rise to blood cells, except in a small paraaortic area (Cormier and Dieterlen-Lièvre, 1988). So it is likely that angioblasts and hemangioblasts might be two different cell types. Consistent with this idea, transplantation experiments in chicken/quail chimeras support the existence of two distinct populations of endothelial cell progenitors—one that contributes to formation of the dorsal aorta and dorsal vessels and another that contributes to ventral vessels and gives rise to hematopoietic precursors (Pardanaud et al., 1996).

There is also a distinction between sinusoidal and capillary circulation (Minot, 1900). Sinusoidal endothelial cells develop in direct contact with the underlying tissue as is the case of the sinusoids in the liver and the hepatocytes. Another example is the endocardium, which grows and differentiates in close association with the myocardial cells. Kidneys originally develop in similar fashion as endothelial cells from the area of the postcardinal veins form sinusoids around the pronephric tubules. Other examples of organs whose circulation is of sinusoidal origin are the parathyroid and parotid glands.

The direct contact of the sinusoidal endothelial cells with cells of the corresponding tissues is in contrast to the structure of capillaries that are surrounded by smooth muscle cells, pericytes, macrophages, fibroblasts, as well as an extensive array of extracellular matrix. The sinusoidal system is phylogenetically a more ancient form of vasculature while the appearance of capillary microcirculation is a later evolutionary event. This idea is better illustrated when one considers the development and evolution of an organ such as the heart (Fishman and Chien, 1997). The endocardium is the original vasculature of the heart that interacts with the myocardium to form an extensive system of trabeculae. Later on, the coronary circulation is established from angiogenic precursor cells that sprout and migrate out from the epicardium (Poelmann et al., 1993). Retroviral tagging of cell lineages in the heart at this stage demonstrated that the coronary vessels are derived from the epicardial region and not by sprouting from the endocardium (Mikawa and Gourdie, 1996). These experiments further showed that other cell types such as connective tissue and smooth muscle originate in the epicardium. From there they migrate to colonize the developing heart (Mikawa and Gourdie, 1996). Transplantation experiments provided evidence that the endothelial precursors for the coronary vessels originally migrate to the epicardium from the liver (Poelmann et al., 1993). It appears that the two systems, the endocardial lining of the trabeculae and the coronary vessels, are independent and do not connect except at two points, the arteries next to the outflow tract and the veins close to sinus venosus.

Lower vertebrates, such as certain species of fish, do not develop a coronary microcirculation and rely only on the sinusoidal system for the blood supply of the cardiac tissue; the contraction of the cardiac myocytes resembles a sponge, whose squeezing motions drive the blood in and out from the heart. This structure apparently is not adequate in higher vertebrates, where the greater need for blood pressure leads to a more compact cardiac tissue that requires an efficient system for adequate blood supply, an objective achieved with the evolution of the coronary circulation. Consequently, at later embryonic stages in birds and mammals, the extensive trabeculation of the early heart gradually diminishes, and the endocardium is only present in the walls lining the ventricles, while the coronary vessels carry in and out most of the blood supply to the heart tissue. Certain organisms, like frogs, have a "mixed" system of cardiac circulation—that is, a coronary circulation develops, but the heart remains extensively trabeculated, and thus both systems provide the myocytes with oxygen and nutrients.

As a result of the close interaction between myocardium and endocardium, mutations in either cell type lead to abnormal heart development. Because of this intrinsic relationship and the near proximity of the two cell lineages, it has been postulated that they might share a common precursor. Recent experiments using retroviral tagging of early mesodermal cells have shown, though, that two distinct lineages already exist by the time myocardium and endocardium precursor cells reach their location shortly after gastrulation (Cohen-Gould and Mikawa, 1996). In addition, whole mount in situs of early myocardial-specific markers, such as the homeobox-containing gene *Nkx-2.5*, show no expression in endocardium and only mark the myocardium lineage very early in development (Lints et al., 1993).

An interesting aspect of heart development is the formation of the endocardial cushions that will eventually give rise to the valves between the ventricles and the atria. The cushions are derived from specific areas of the endocardium, and this is the only known example of *trans*-differentiation of endothelium to mesenchyme (Eisenberg and Markwald, 1995).

Another example of functional diversity within the vascular tree is the lymphatic system that is derived from the veins and has certain distinct functions compared to the rest of the vasculature mainly in respect to its interaction with lymphocytes.

REGULATION OF VASCULOGENESIS

Despite the extensive description of early events in vasculogenesis, and the subsequent steps in the angiogenic phase, until 5 years ago very little was known about the molecules that regulate embryonic vascular development. Up to that point, by using either isolated endothelial cells or angiogenic assays in the chick chorioallantoic membrane and the rabbit cornea, a large number of small molecules and proteins had been shown to have angiogenic properties or to influence growth of endothelial cells (Folkman and Klagsbrun, 1987). However, their function in development, or their precise role in angiogenesis in adult pathological situations, remained obscure. In recent years two major developments have allowed considerable progress in our understanding of vasculogenesis and angiogenic responses. The first was the identification, cloning, and characterization of two groups of endothelial-specific tyrosine kinase receptors and their corresponding ligands (Mustonen and Alitalo, 1995). The second was the wide application of transgenic and germ-line inactivation techniques in mice that revealed the role of these genes during embryogenesis.

Flk-1, Flt-1, and Their Ligand, VEGF

The first group of endothelial-specific receptors—namely, flk-1 and flt-1—were cloned by polymerase chain reaction (PCR) during search for novel tyrosine kinase molecules using as template cDNAs prepared from diverse sources such as liver, adult endothelial cell lines, or differentiated embryonic stem cells (Shibuya et al., 1990; Matthews et al., 1991; Millauer et al., 1993; Yamaguchi et al., 1993). Subsequently, whole mount and tissue section in situs during embryogenesis determined that the two receptors were expressed specifically in endothelial cells (Millauer et al., 1993; Yamaguchi et al., 1993; Breier et al., 1995). Both flk-1 and flt-1 were shown to be receptors for vascular endothelial growth factor (VEGF), a potent endothelial cell mitogen and an angiogenic factor (De Vries et al., 1992; Terman et al., 1992; Millauer et al., 1993). The flk-1 molecule is one of the earliest markers of endothelial cells and their presumptive progenitors (Yamaguchi et al., 1993). It is first detected during mouse development in the extraembryonic mesoderm of the yolk sac where the blood islands form shortly after gastrulation around day 7 postcoitum. Flk-1 (or VEGFR-2) expression was also observed in the area of early endocardium and in the allantois. At day 8.0, flk-1 expression in the endocardium declines but reappears again at the 4–5-somite stage. At the 8–10 somite level, flk-1 is highly expressed in the head mesenchyme; at later stages its expression in the dorsal aorta is confined in patches at the areas of sprouting of the intersomitic arteries. Similarly, in avian embryos flk-1 is expressed early in the whole mesoderm, and later its expression is confined to endothelial cells (Eichman et al., 1993; Flamme et al., 1995a).

The expression pattern of flk-1 during development and its activity as a VEGF receptor strongly suggested that it might have an important role in both vasculogenesis and angiogenesis. The function of flk-1 was assessed in mouse development by inactivation of the *flk-1* gene following homologous recombination in embryonic stem cells. (Shalaby et al., 1995). The study of the resulting mouse lines revealed that homozygous *flk-1* −/− mouse embryos die early during gestation (between days 8.5 and 9.5) due to a complete lack of vasculature. Staining of mutant embryos showed that mesodermal progenitors did not differentiate into mature endothelial cells and thus failed to assemble in vascular channels. This defect was obvious in both extra- and intraembryonic vascular structures. In addition, a dramatic reduction in early hematopoietic precursors was observed, but at present it is unclear if flk-1 is independently involved in blood cell differentiation or whether, rather, the reduction resulted from the endothelial cell failure.

The flk-1 ligand VEGF is also expressed early in postgastrulation embryos. In situ hybridization studies in mouse and avian embryos show abundant expression in all three germ layers, albeit at higher levels in the endoderm (Breier et al., 1992; Flamme et al., 1995a). The early expression suggests that VEGF is involved in the initial stages of vasculogenesis. Moreover, overexpression of VEGF in development leads to abnormal overvascularization of the surrounding areas (Drake and Little, 1995; Flamme et al., 1995b). Later in development VEGF is expressed in tissues that secrete angiogenic signals, e.g., developing kidney or brain, while flk-1 is expressed in the responding surrounding endothelial cells, indicating that VEGF/flk-1 act in a paracrine fashion.

The inactivation of the *VEGF* gene supports the importance of this ligand/receptor system in both vasculogenesis and angiogenesis (Carmeliet et al., 1996a; Ferrara et al., 1996). Interestingly, heterozygous *VEGF* +/− embryos die between days 11 and 12 of development and display severe abnormalities in the vasculature, demonstrating that dosage levels and ligand gradients are crucial for vascular development. Careful analysis revealed that endothelial cell development was delayed but not aborted. The dorsal aorta was abnormal, and most vascular beds displayed an irregular plexus. Extensive necrosis was seen in most tissues and angiogenesis was severely impaired. The homozygous *VEGF* −/− embryos had even more severe defects and the dorsal aorta was completely missing. The fact that the *VEGF* −/− die latter than the *flk-1* −/− embryos indicates that other ligands might partially replace VEGF.

The results of the flk-1 and VEGF inactivation were particularly rewarding because they displayed the expected phenotypes based on the in vitro action of this receptor/ligand system and the expression patterns of the two molecules during embryonic development. Analysis of pathological situations such as tumor-induced angiogenesis showed that VEGF is expressed by many tumors while the flk-1 receptor is induced in the surrounding endothelial cells (Plate et al., 1992, 1993). Neutralizing antibodies against VEGF can block tumor vascularization and thus tumor growth (Kim et al., 1993). In parallel fashion, overexpression of flk-1 dominant negative forms in endothelial cells close to the angiogenic site inhibits angiogenesis (Millauer et al., 1994). These data clearly demonstrate that the dormant VEGF/flk-1 mechanism that operates during normal embryogenesis is reactivated in tumor-induced angiogenesis.

The second VEGF receptor flt-1 (or VEGFR-1) is expressed early during development in mesodermal cells, similarly to flk-1 (Breier et al., 1995; Dumont et al., 1995). Later, flt-1 is expressed in embryonic endothelial cells. One organ in which expression of flk-1 and flt-1 differs widely is the developing placenta, where flk-1 is found in the embryonic vasculature of the labyrinth area and flt-1 is present in the spongiotrophoblasts that reside between the maternal and embryonic parts of the placenta (Dumont et al., 1995). Despite the similar expression patterns in early embryos, the inactivation of the *flt-1* gene by homologous recombination showed a distinct phenotype from *flk-1* (Fong et al., 1995). *Flt-1* −/− mice also died at midsomatogenesis around day 8.5 but endothelial cells and vascular structures formed. Nevertheless, blood vessels were disorganized, enlarged, and abnormal, with endothelial cell clusters present within the vascular lumen. All major vascular structures inside the embryo (including the endocardium) and in the yolk sac were affected. These results indicate that the flt-1/VEGF system plays a significant role in the maintenance of the vasculature and might be important for proper cell–cell or cell–extracellular matrix interactions. The fact that the *flk-1* −/− and *flt-1* −/− phenotypes vary suggests that the two receptors use distinct signal transduction pathways, a notion that is also supported by their action in isolated cells in vitro.

Tie Tyrosine Kinase Receptors and Angiopoietins

A second class of endothelial-specific tyrosine kinases and their receptors has been characterized. These are the tie-1 and tie-2 (also known as tek) receptors (Dumont et al., 1992; Partanen et al., 1992; Sato et al., 1993; Schnürch and Risau, 1993). They are homologous to each other, but unlike the VEGF receptors, they contain matrix association motifs in their extracellular domains. Both are expressed very early in development. tie-2 follows flk-1 by 12 hours and tie-1 follows flk-1 by 24 hours (Dumont et al., 1995). tie-2 is expressed in the blood islands and in intraembryonic angioblasts, where it appears earlier than von Willebrand factor; it is also highly expressed in the mesoderm layer of the amnion. Contrary to flk-1 that is present in angiogenic clusters in the dorsal aorta, tie-2 is uniformly expressed in the entire length of this vessel. After day 12, the expression patterns of tie-2, flk-1, and tie-1 are almost indistinguishable in embryonic endothelial cells, but the levels of all three decline in yolk sac vasculature.

The *tie-2* gene inactivation is embryonic lethal but embryos die later, around day 10.5 (Dumont et al., 1994; Sato et al., 1995). Vascular structures are present but do not develop properly. Both angiogenesis and vascular remodeling are abolished. The original homogeneous plexus of endothelium forms but fails to differentiate into smaller and larger vessels. *tie-2* −/− embryos have grossly abnormal hearts that are hypotrabeculated.

A ligand of tie-2 named *angiopoietin-1 (Ang1)* has been isolated and characterized (Davis et al., 1996). Ang1 is expressed during embryogenesis in the proximity of blood vessel formation, mainly in smooth muscle and surrounding mesenchymal cells. Ang1 levels are particularly high in the myocardium. Inactivation of *Ang1* in mice leads to severe vascular defects that closely resemble the ones in the *tie-2* −/− mice (Suri et al., 1996). Recruitment of pericytes is minimal and the collagen-like fibers around blood vessels are sparse. As in *tie-2* null embryos, trabeculation in the heart is aborted, and the endocardium attaches loosely to the myocardium.

Human congenital venous malformations are common errors in vascular morphogenesis that result in dilated, serpiginous channels. It was recently shown that, in two families of patients with venous malformations, there was a point mutation of arginine to tryptophan in the kinase domain of the tie-2 receptor (Vikkula et al., 1996). This mutation alters a function of the tie-2 signaling pathway that is critical for the interaction between endothelial cells and smooth muscle cells; as a result, this modification leads to a disproportionate number of endothelial and smooth muscle cells through a negative feedback mechanism involving the tie-2 receptor. Taken together, the phenotypes in mice and the human mutations strongly support a role of the Ang1/tie-2 system in proper interaction of endothelial cells with extracellular matrix and underlying tissues.

A second ligand of tie-2, called *angiopoietin-2 (Ang2)*, has been recently cloned (Maisonpierre et al., 1997). Although both Ang1 and Ang2 can bind to the tie-2 receptor, only Ang1 can induce receptor autophosphorylation and thus lead to intracellular signal activation. Ang2 expression overlaps with Ang1 during development in perivascular cells but Ang2 is absent in the myocardium.

The expression pattern and in vitro action of Ang2 raised the possibility that Ang2 might inhibit the binding and consequently the stimulatory function of Ang1. Recent experiments support this notion. Overexpression of Ang2 in transgenic mice results in a heart phenotype similar to that in the *Ang1* −/− and *tie-2* −/− embryos and leads to embryonic lethality at day 10.5 (Maisonpierre et al., 1997). Moreover, there was extensive vascular discontinuity within the embryos and certain major vessels such as the cardinal veins were completely missing. These results substantiate the role of Ang2 as an angiogenic inhibitor and natural antagonist of Ang1. Probably, a fine balance exists between Ang1 and Ang2 at and around angiogenic sites. Analysis of Ang1 and Ang2 expression patterns in the rat ovary during neovascularization of this tissue in adult animals suggests that Ang2 works together with VEGF in early stages of angiogenesis to maintain the migrating endothelial cells in a plastic stage while Ang1 is required later for proper association of the newly laid out vasculature with the extracellular matrix and also for recruitment of pericytes (Maisonpierre et al., 1997).

The tie-1 receptor has been also analyzed by gene targeting in mice (Puri et al., 1995; Sato et al., 1995). The mutation is lethal and *tie-1* −/− animals die at late embryonic stages (after day 13.5) or shortly after birth. *tie-1* −/− embryos suffer from edema and localized hemorrhage. Thus, it appears that the tie-1 receptor is important for the survival and integrity of mature endothelial cells. The ligands of the tie-1 receptor are currently unknown.

The endothelial-specific tyrosine kinase receptors are expressed in early hematopoietic cells as well; their role in the development of the hematopoietic system is unclear (Batard et al., 1996; Kabrun et al., 1997). Their function in hematopoiesis will probably be revealed when conditional inactivation of these genes bypasses the endothelial-specific defects.

Taken together, the data from the inactivation of the endothelial-specific receptors indicate that diverse signaling pathways are activated in endothelial cells after the binding of the corresponding ligands. However, it is not well understood how embryonic endothelial cells transduce and sort out the various signals. The Ras GTPase-activating protein and the Ras pathway are involved, since inactivation of the GTPase-activating protein by homologous recombination causes severe defects in vascular organization and remodeling (Henkemeyer et al., 1995).

Additional Genes that Regulate Vascular Development

It is noteworthy that tissue factor (TF) knockout mice display defects similar to those in *Ang1* −/− mice in pericyte recruitment in the yolk sac vasculature (Carmeliet et al., 1996b). The embryonic lethality in TF-deficient animals also resembles the phenotype noticed in half of the thrombin receptor null embryos (Connolly et al., 1966). These observations raise the exciting possibility that coagulation mechanisms may have a significant role in embryonic blood vessel formation and development. The inactivation of thrombomodulin (TM) also leads to early embryonic lethality at day 8.5 of mouse development, indicating that the thromboresistance function of the vascular system might be crucial for early development (Healy et al., 1995). However, the exact reason for the embryonic lethality remains obscure and it can be also attributed to the expression of TM in trophoblast cells that surround the developing embryo (Weiler-Guettler et al., 1996).

A large number of proteins have been implicated in angiogenic events in investigations of vascular responses during pathological situations. These molecules include members of the FGF, TGFβ, and platelet derived growth factor (PDGF) families of growth factors and their corresponding receptors (Battegay, 1995). In most instances, inactivation of these molecules showed that they also regulate embryonic vascular formation. Mutations in this group of genes do not exclusively affect endothelial cells but instead reveal pleiotropic effects during development. Although none of the phenotypes is as dramatic as the ones in the flk-1-and tie-2-deficient mice, certain aspects of embryonic angiogenesis are impaired. *TGFβ1* −/− embryos display defects in endothelial differentiation, mainly in the yolk sac vasculature, and in hematopoiesis (Dickson et al., 1995). Inactivation of PDGFA or PDGFB results in hypertrabeculated hearts (Levéen et al., 1994; Schatteman et al., 1996). PDGFRα mutants show vascular ruptures and diminished numbers of smooth muscle cells (Schatteman et al., 1992), while the PDGFRβ knockout mice show abnormalities in capillary organization and shape within skeletal structures (Soriano, 1994). In addition, many engineered mutations in extracellular matrix proteins, such as fibronectin, or in certain cellular integrin receptors, result in abnormal vascular formation, thus demonstrating the importance of endothelial cell interactions with extracellular matrix for proper vascular development (Hynes and Bader, 1997). A summary of genes whose inactivation affects normal vascular development and their expression profile during embryogenesis is shown in Table 1.1.

A ligand/receptor system that is important for heart development is neuregulin (or heregulin) and its receptors erbB2 and erbB4. Neuregulin is expressed in the endocardium while erbB2 and erbB4 are found in the adjacent myocardium (Corfas et al., 1995; Gassmann et al., 1995; Lee et al., 1995). This pattern is opposite to the expression of Ang1 and tie-2 in the myocardium and endocardium, respectively. Inactivation of neuregulin and either erbB2 or erbB4 results in embryonic lethality at day 10.5 (Meyer and Birchmeier, 1995; Gassmann et al., 1995; Lee et al., 1995). In all three cases, null embryos have hypotrabeculated hearts and the sparse myocardium apparently fails to provide enough blood supply to the developing organism. The heart phenotypes are starkly similar to the cardiac abnormalities in *tie-2* −/− and *Ang1* −/− mice indicating that the two systems collaborate for proper interaction between endocardium and myocardium. This phenotype is in contrast to the hypertrabeculation observed in PDGF mutants. At the moment it is unclear how the various networks interact and cooperate for proper heart differentiation. It is evident, though, that endocardium and myocardium interact as coordinate partners for proper heart development.

The results of the mutations in heart development described above illustrate a distinct—and often not recognized—function of endothelia. The developing endothelium in close association with tissue parenchyma has a crucial role in the differentiation of certain organ primordia. The intimate relationship of sinusoidal endothelium with the differentiating cells of tissues such as heart, liver, and pronephros is probably instrumental at the initial stages of organogenesis. The molecular pathways involved

Table 1.1 Genes (and Their Expression Profiles) Whose Inactivation Affects Normal Vascular Development[a]

Gene	*Expression Profile*	*Phenotype*
flk-1	Early mesoderm, blood islands, endothelial precursors, embryonic endothelial cells	Failure of endothelial precursors to differentiate; no vasculature; death at embryonic days 8.5–9.5
flt-1	Similar to *flk-1*	Abnormal vasculature; large vessels; death at day 8.5–9.5
VEGF	Early germ layers, endoderm, multiple sites within the embryo	Heterozygous lethal: irregular vasculature; impaired angiogenesis; death at day 11–12
tie-2	12 hours later than *flk-1,* blood islands, endothelial precursors, embryonic endothelial cells	Vascular remodeling and angiogenesis impaired; failure of heart trabeculation; recruitment of periendothelial cells diminished; death at day 10.5
tie-1	12 hours later than *tie-2,* then similar expression	Edemas, hemorrhage; integrity and endothelial cell survival compromised; death after day 13.5 or immediately after birth
Ang1	Smooth muscle and periendothelial cells, myocardium	Vascular defects similar to *tie-2;* death at day 10.5
Ang2	Smooth muscle and periendothelial cells; patchy	Overexpression leads to similar defects as *Ang1* −/−; vessels discontinuous or missing
Neuregulin	Endocardium	Failure of heart trabeculation; death at day 10.5
erbB2	Myocardium	Failure of heart trabeculation; death at day 10.5
erbB4	Myocardium	Failure of heart trabeculation; death at day 10.5
Tissue factor	Widespread, endoderm	Abnormal yolk sac circulation; fragile vessels from lack of pericytes; death around or after day 9.5
TGFβ1	Widespread	Abnormal yolk sac endothelial cells; lack of pericytes; hematopoiesis fails; death at day 10.5
PDGFA	Widespread	Injection of anti-PDGFA antibodies between days 8.5–10.5 results in thickened myocardium, hypertrabeculation
PDGFB	Widespread	Dilated heart; hypertrabeculation; hemorrhage; pericyte loss; late embryonic lethality

(continued)

Table 1.1 Genes (and Their Expression Profiles) Whose Inactivation Affects Normal Vascular Development[a]—Continued

Gene	*Expression Profile*	*Phenotype*
PDGFRα	Widespread	Ventricular thinning; late embryonic lethality
PDGFRβ	Widespread	Hemorrhage; irregular venules; death around birth
p120-ras-GAP	Widespread	Disorganized vascular networks; death at day 10.5
Fibronectin	Widespread	Vascular defects; death at day 9–10
Collagen α1(I)	Widespread	Blood vessel rupture; death day 13
Integrin α5	Widespread	Vascular and cardiac defects; death at day 10–11
Integrin αv	Widespread	Cerebral vascular defects; embryonic/perinatal lethality
Integrin α4	Widespread	Placental and cardiac defects; death at day 10.5–14

[a] Summary of genes whose inactivation produces vascular defects in mice; all inactivation phenotypes are by gene inactivation using homologous recombination in embryonic stem cells, except: *Ang2,* overexpression in transgenic mice; *PDGFA,* injection of blocking antibodies; *PDGFRα,* natural mutation (*patch* mouse). A brief description of embryonic expression of the corresponding genes is found in the second column.

in this particular function of endothelial cells might be overlapping, yet fundamentally distinct from the angiogenic mechanisms of blood vessel formation.

TRANSCRIPTIONAL REGULATION OF VASCULAR FORMATION

The distinct temporal and spatial patterns of endothelial-specific gene expression at early embryonic stages indicate a complex sequence of transcriptional regulation. Certain endothelial-specific genes such as *TM* are first expressed very early in development in the intraembryonic proximal lateral mesoderm where the preendocardial tubes assemble (Weiler-Guettler et al., 1996). A day later *TM* is expressed in the whole vasculature similar to other endothelial markers. Other genes that appear similarly in the preendocardial tubes include the transcriptional factors GATA-4 and GATA-6 (Arceci et al., 1993; Kelley et al., 1993; Heikinheimo et al., 1994; Laverriere et al., 1994; Jiang and Evans, 1996; Morrisey et al., 1996). Unlike TM, their later expression is confined to the endocardium and not in other endothelial cells. Recent evidence implicates the GATA factors in heart development (Narita et al., 1997). In contrast to TM, flk-1 and flt-1 appear first at day 7 in the extraembryonic mesoderm in the yolk sac followed within a few hours by tie-2 and tie-1 (Breier et al., 1995; Dumont et al., 1995).

At this point little is known about the transcriptional regulation of endothelial-specific genes, especially in early development. The endothelial-specific promoter elements of genes such as *TM* have been difficult to analyze. Large promoter pieces from the *TM* gene were proven insufficient to promote endothelial-specific expression. The complete in vivo pattern of the endogenous *TM* expression could be recapitulated in transgenic animals only when the *TM* gene was replaced with *β-galactosidase* by homologous recombination (Weiler-Guettler et al., 1996).

The *flk-1* gene promoter has also been analyzed and the first results indicate the presence of a variety of tissue-specific and ubiquitous elements, either negatively or positively acting, that contribute to tissue-specific expression (Patterson et al., 1995; Rönicke et al., 1996). These elements have not yet been analyzed in transgenic animals. The transcriptional regulation of the *tie-2* gene has been studied in endothelial cells in culture as well as in transgenic mice. These studies showed that 2.0 kb of promoter sequence can drive expression in subpopulations of endothelial cells early in development (Schlaeger et al., 1995). The entire endogenous pattern, as well as high expression in adult endothelial cells, could be achieved only when a 10-kb fragment from the first intron of the *tie-2* gene was included in the promoter constructs (Schlaeger et al., 1997). Most of the enhancer activity is found within a 300-bp sequence that contains many crucial elements. Among them a binding site for the ets-1 transcription factor stands out as particularly important. Interestingly, the ets-1 is expressed in early endothelial cells during development (Pardanaud and Dieterlen-Lièvre, 1993). At around day 11, ets-1 appears to be confined in endothelial cells around angiogenic sites (Maroulakou et al., 1994). Recently a hypoxia-induced endothelial-cell-specific transcriptional factor called EPAS1 was shown to regulate the *tie-2* promoter/enhancer, thus providing a molecular mechanism to link hypoxia to angiogenesis (Tian et al., 1997).

An example of how endothelial cell specific expression is regulated in vivo comes from the analysis of the *vWF* gene promoter in transgenic mice. It has been shown that distinct parts of the promoter direct expression to different vascular beds, which provides a molecular basis to explain how heterogeneity is established and maintained in the vasculature (Aird et al., 1995). Most excitingly, the results show that vWF expression in the heart endothelium can be regulated by myocardial cells (Aird et al., 1997). It is therefore evident that endothelial-specific gene expression is established by a unique combination of endothelial-specific transcriptional elements and environmental signals.

IN VITRO MODELS OF VASCULOGENESIS

Certain in vitro models of vasculogenesis have been developed recently. Embryonic stem cells can differentiate in vitro to embryoid bodies that in many instances contain blood islands which further differentiate to vascular channels and blood cells (Doetschman et al., 1985; Wang et al., 1992). Moreover, cells were isolated from yolk sac quail epiblasts that have properties of early endothelial cells (Flamme and Risau, 1992). They depend on FGF for growth and differentiation to acetylated low density lipoprotein (AcLDL)-uptake-positive cells that form cords in vitro resembling endothelial vascular channels. A second distinct endothelial progenitor cell population with interesting properties was isolated from day-7.5 mouse egg cylinders (Hatzopoulos et al., 1998). These cells express early endothelial markers that are associated with the proximal-lateral mesoderm where the preendocardial tubes develop such as TM, GATA-4, GATA-6, and tie-2. They have an unlimited stem-cell like growth in vitro and can be differentiated to mature endothelial cells under defined conditions. In addition, they can contribute to the embryonic vasculature when injected in chicken embryos.

Recently, the isolation of putative human endothelial cell progenitors was reported from adult human blood (Asahara et al., 1997). At present, the relationship between the different progenitor cell types is unclear. Differences exist in morphology and patterns of gene expression. The isolated adult endothelial cell progenitors are spindle shaped, express both flk-1 and tie-2, have a finite life span in vitro, and appear to differentiate to AcLDL-uptake-positive cells. Thus, these progenitors resemble the cells dissociated from quail blastodiscs. The adult progenitor cells also integrate into sites of active angiogenesis after venous injection. In similar fashion, it has been previously shown that human umbilical vein endothelial cells can incorporate around angiogenic sites after injection (Ojeifo et al., 1995). It will be of great interest to compare the behavior of the embryonic endothelial cell progenitors in response to angiogenic signals in adult pathological situations. These new in vitro systems provide a novel and powerful tool with which to study transcriptional regulation and signal transduction pathways of vasculogenesis.

ZEBRAFISH, A VERTEBRATE GENETIC SYSTEM FOR CARDIOVASCULAR DEVELOPMENT

In the last few years the zebrafish has emerged as a powerful new developmental and genetic model in which to study early development in general and early vasculogenesis and heart formation specifically; it offers many advantages over other approaches (Eisen, 1996). The embryos are transparent and early development can be observed under the dissecting microscope. It is relatively inexpensive to grow a large number of progeny from a single mating pair in a short period of time. The smaller genome size (1,700 Megabases) of the zebrafish permits modern genetic analyses (Postlethwait et al., 1994; Knapik et al., 1996). Large scale mutagenesis screens induced by N-ethyl-N-nitrosourea (ENU) recently uncovered more than 600 genes that are important for early development and organogenesis (Eisen, 1996). Among them, many mutations have been characterized that alter vascular development and heart formation (Chen et al., 1996; Stainier et al., 1996). Initial analysis of individual mutants has revealed that mutations that interfere with notochord formation also impair the proper development of the dorsal aorta whereas the axial vein that lies more ventrally was less affected (Fouquet et al., 1997). These results correlate with the chicken/quail transplantation experiments that established two populations of endothelial progenitors, one for dorsal vasculature and one for ventral vessels that is also tied to blood cell differentiation. They also correspond well with the isolation of two distinct embryonic endothelial progenitors in vitro, one of which is a precursor of yolk sac hemangioblasts and one that shows early markers of preendocardial tubes. These results might also explain the observation that expression of early endothelial-specific genes between endocardial tubes and blood islands is quite diverse. Intense efforts to positionally clone the mutated genes are now underway. Identification of these genes will certainly provide new insights in the regulation of vascular development.

SUMMARY AND PERSPECTIVES

The development of the cardiovascular system has received considerable attention for a long time. There is an extensive description of endothelial cell growth and differentiation during embryogenesis in many species. Recent years have provided a great deal of information about the molecular mechanisms of vasculogenesis, angiogenesis, and heart formation. Nevertheless, there are still many unanswered questions. We still do not understand how the endothelial cell lineage emerges from mesodermal precursors. Little is known about the regulation of endothelial-specific gene expression during development and in adult endothelial cells. How the great diversity of endothelial function and structure is established during embryonic development and maintained in the mature vascular system is still relatively obscure. More importantly, we do not understand how endothelial cells interpret and integrate the diverse signals that they receive from their environment through an extensive array of ligands and their corresponding receptors. Finally, we have limited information on the important function of the endothelium in organogenesis and organ regeneration. A variety of powerful molecular, cellular, and genetic systems are now available, and they are likely to provide answers to these important questions in the near future.

Acknowledgments

We are grateful to Dr. I. Drummond and Dr. E. Knapik for helpful comments and to S. Moskowitz for artwork. Plate 1 was based on a drawing from the book *The Mouse* by R. Rugh. Figure 1.1 was reproduced from a drawing in Smith et al. (1994). Figure 1.2 was based on a drawing of H. M. Evans. Plate 9 was based on a drawing in the book *An Introduction to Embryology* by B. I. Balinsky.

REFERENCES

Aird, W. C., Jahroudi, N., Weiler-Guettler, H., Rayburn, H. B., and Rosenberg, R. D. (1995). Human von Willebrand factor gene sequences target expression to a subpopulation of endothelial cells in transgenic mice. Proc. Natl. Acad. Sci. USA 92: 4567–4571.

Aird, W. C., Edelberg, J. M., Weiler-Guettler, H., Simmons, W. W., Smith, T. W., and Rosenberg, R. D. (1997). Vascular bed-specific expression of an endothelial cell gene is programmed by the tissue microenvironment. J. Cell Biol. 138: 1117–1124.

Arceci, R. J., King, A. A. J., Simon, M. C., Orkin, S. H., and Wilson, D. B. (1993). Mouse GATA-4: a retinoic acid-inducible GATA-binding transcription factor expressed in endodermally derived tissues and heart. Mol. Cell. Biol. 13: 2235–2246.

Asahara, T., Murohara, T., Sullivan, A., Silver, M., van der Zee, R., Li, T., Witzenbichler, B., Schatteman, G., and Isner, J. M. (1997). Isolation of putative progenitor endothelial cells for angiogenesis. Science 275: 964–967.

Augustine, J. M. (1981). Influence of the entoderm on mesodermal expansion in the area vasculosa of the chick. J. Embryol. Exp. Morphol. 65: 89–103.

Azar, Y. and Eyal-Giladi, H. (1979). Marginal zone cells—the primitive-streak-inducing component of the primary hypoblast in the chick. J. Embryol. Exp. Morphol. 52: 79–88.

Bär, T. (1980). The vascular system of the cerebral cortex. Adv. Anat. Embryol. Cell. Biol. 59: 1–62.

Baldwin, H. S. (1996). Early embryonic vascular development. Cardiovasc. Res. 31: E34–E45.

Batard, P., Sansilvestri, P., Scheinecker, C., Knapp, W., Debili, N., Vainchenker, W., Bühring, H.-J., Monier, M.-N., Kukk, E., Partanen, J., Matikainen, M.-T., Alitalo, R., Hatzfeld, J., and Alitalo, K. (1996). The tie receptor tyrosine kinase is expressed by human hematopoietic progenitor cells and by a subset of megakaryocytic cells. Blood 87: 2212–2220.

Battegay, E. J. (1995). Angiogenesis: mechanistic insights, neovascular diseases, and therapeutic prospects. J. Mol. Med. 73: 333–346.

Breier, G., Albrecht, U., Sterrer, S., and Risau, W. (1992). Expression of vascular endothelial growth factor during embryonic angiogenesis and endothelial cell differentiation. Development 114: 521–532.

Breier, G., Clauss, M., and Risau, W. (1995). Coordinate expression of Vascular Endothelial Growth Factor Receptor-1 (flt-1) and its ligand suggests a paracrine regulation of murine vascular development. Dev. Dyn. 204: 228–239.

Caduff, J. H., Fischer, L. C., and Burri, P. H. (1986). Scanning electron microscope study of the developing microvasculature in the postnatal rat lung. Anat. Rec. 216: 154–164.

Carmeliet, P., Ferreira, V., Breier, G., Pollefeyt, S., Kieckens, L., Gertsenstein, M., Fahrig, M., Vandenhoeck, A., Harpal, K., Eberhardt, C., Declercq, C., Pawling, J., Moons, L., Collen, D., Risau, W., and Nagy, A. (1996a). Abnormal blood vessel development and lethality in embryos lacking a single VEGF allele. Nature 380: 435–439.

Carmeliet, P., Mackman, N., Moons, L., Luther, T., Gressens, P., Van Vlaenderen, I., Demunck, H., Kasper, M., Breier, G., Evrard, P., Müller, M., Risau, W., Edgington, T., and Collen, D. (1996b). Role of tissue factor in embryonic blood vessel development. Nature 383: 73–75.

Chen, J.-N., Haffter, P., Odenthal, J., Vogelsang, E., Brand, M., van Eeden, F. J. M., Furutani-Seiki, M., Granato, M., Hammerschmidt, M., Heisenberg, C.-P., Jiang, Y.-J., Kane, D. A., Kelsh, R. N., Mullins, M. C., and Nüsslein-Volhard, C. (1996). Mutations affecting the cardiovascular system and other internal organs in zebrafish. Development 123: 293–302.

Coffin, J. D. and Poole, T. J. (1988). Embryonic vascular development: immunohistochemical identification of the origin and subsequent morphogenesis of the major vessel primordia in quail embryos. Development 102: 735–748.

Coffin, J. D., Harrison, J., Schwartz, S., and Heimark, R. (1991). Angioblast differentiation and morphogenesis of the vascular endothelium in the mouse embryo. Dev. Biol. 148: 51–62.

Cohen-Gould, L. and Mikawa, T. (1996). The fate diversity of mesodermal cells within the heart field during chicken early embryogenesis. Dev. Biol. 177: 265–273.

Connolly, A., Ishihara, H., Kahn, M. L., Farese, R. V., and Coughlin, S. R. (1996). Role of the thrombin receptor in development and evidence for a second receptor. Nature 381: 516–519.

Corfas, G., Rosen, K. M., Aratake, H., Krauss, R., and Fischbach, G. D. (1995). Differential expression of ARIA isoforms in the rat brain. Neuron 14: 103–115.

Cormier, F. and Dieterlen-Lièvre, F. (1988). The wall of the chick embryo aorta harbours M-CFC, G-CFC, GM-CFC and BFU-E. Development 102: 279–285.

Davis, S., Aldrich, T. H., Jones, P. F., Acheson, A., Compton, D. L., Jain, V., Ryan, T. E., Bruno, J., Radziejewski, C., Maisonpierre, P. C., and Yancopoulos, G. D. (1996). Isolation of Angiopoietin-1, a ligand for the TIE2 receptor, by secretion-trap expression cloning. Cell 87: 1161–1169.

DeRuiter, M. C., Poelmann, R. E., VanderPlas-de Vries, I., Mentink, M. M. T., and Gittenberger-de Groot, A. C. (1992). The development of the myocardium and endocardium in mouse embryos: fusion of two heart tubes? Anat. Embryol. 185: 461–473.

Doetschman, T. C., Eistetter, H., Katz, M., Schmidt, W., and Kemler, R. (1985). The in vitro development of blastocyst-derived embryonic stem cell lines: formation of visceral yolk sac, blood islands and myocardium. J. Embryol. Exp. Morph. 87: 27–45.

De Vries, C., Escobedo, J. A., Ueno, H., Houck, K., Ferrara, N., and Williams, L. T. (1992). The fms-like tyrosine kinase, a receptor for vascular endothelial growth factor. Science 255: 989–991.

Dickson, M. C., Martin, J. S., Cousins, F. M., Kulkarni, A. B., Karlsson, S. and Akhurst, R. J. (1995). Defective haematopoiesis and vasculogenesis in transforming growth factor-β1 knock out mice. Development 121: 1845–1854.

Drake, C. J. and Little, C. D. (1995). Exogenous vascular endothelial growth factor induces malformed and hyperfused vessels during embryonic neovascularization. Proc. Natl. Acad. Sci. USA 92: 7657–7661.

Dumont, D. J., Yamaguchi, T. P., Conlon, R. A., Rossant, J., and Breitman, M. L. (1992). *Tek,* novel tyrosine kinase gene located on mouse chromosome 4, is expressed in endothelial cells and their presumptive precursors. Oncogene 7: 1471–1480.

Dumont, D. J., Gradwohl, G., Fong, G.-H., Puri, M. C., Gertsenstein, M., Auerbach, A., and Breitman, M. L. (1994). Dominant-negative and targeted null mutations in the endothelial receptor tyrosine kinase, tek, reveal a critical role in vasculogenesis of the embryo. Gen. Dev. 8: 1897–1909.

Dumont, D. J., Fong, G.-H., Puri, M. C., Gradwohl, G., Alitalo, K., and Breitman, M. L. (1995). Vascularization of the mouse embryo: a study of flk-1, tek, tie, and Vascular Endothelial Growth Factor expression during development. Dev. Dyn. 203: 80–92.

Eichmann, A., Marcelle, C., Breant, C., and Le Douarin, N. M. (1993). Two molecules related to the VEGF receptor are expressed in early endothelial cells during avian embryonic development. Mech. Dev. 42: 33–48.

Eisen, J. S. (1996). Zebrafish make a big splash. Cell 87: 969–977.

Eisenberg, L. M. and Markwald, R. R. (1995). Molecular regulation of atrioventricular valvuloseptal morphogenesis. Circ. Res. 77: 1–6.

Evans, H. M. (1909). On the development of the aortae, cardinal and umbilical veins, and the other blood vessels of vertebrate embryos from capillaries. Anat. Rec. 3: 498–518.

Ferrara, N., Carver-Moore, K., Chen, H., Dowd, M., Lu, L., O'Shea, K. S., Powell-Braxton, L., Hillan, K. J., and Moore, M. W. (1996). Heterozygous embryonic lethality induced by targeted inactivation of the VEGF gene. Nature 380: 439–442.

Fishman, M. C. and Chien, K. R. (1997). Fashioning the vertebrate heart: earliest embryonic decisions. Development 124: 2099–2117.

Flamme, I. and Risau, W. (1992). Induction of vasculogenesis and hematopoiesis in vitro. Development 116: 435–439.

Flamme, I., Breier, G., and Risau, W. (1995a). Vascular Endothelial Growth Factor (VEGF) and VEGF receptor 2 (flk-1) are expressed during vasculogenesis and vascular differentiation in the quail embryo. Dev. Biol. 169: 699–712.

Flamme, I., von Reutern, M., Drexler, H. C. A., Syed-Ali, S., and Risau, W. (1995b). Overexpression of Vascular Endothelial Growth Factor in the avian embryo induces hypervascularization and increased vascular permeability without alterations of embryonic pattern formation. Dev. Biol. 171: 399–414.

Folkman, J. (1995). Agiogenesis in cancer, vascular, rheumatoid and other disease. Nat. Med. 1: 27–31.

Folkman, J. and Klagsbrun, M. (1987). Angiogenic factors. Science 235: 442–447.

Fong, G.-H., Rossant, J., Gertsenstein, M., and Breitman, M. L. (1995). Role of the Flt-1 receptor tyrosine kinase in regulating the assembly of vascular endothelium. Nature 376: 66–70.

Fouquet, B., Weinstein, B. M., Serluca, F. C., and Fishman, M. C. (1997). Vessel patterning in the embryo of the zebrafish: guidance by notochord. Dev. Biol. 183: 37–48.

Garcia-Martinez, V. and Schoenwolf, G. C. (1993). Primitive-streak origin of the cardiovascular system in avian embryos. Dev. Biol. 159: 706–719.

Gassmann, M., Casagranda, F., Orioli, D., Simon, H., Lai, C., Klein, R., and Lemke, G. (1995). Aberrant neural and cardiac development in mice lacking the ErbB4 neuregulin receptor. Nature 378: 390–394.

Hahn, H. (1909). Experimentelle Studien über die Entstehung des Blutes und der ersten Gefäße beim Hünchen. Arch. Ent. 27: 37–433

Hallmann, R., Feinberg, R. N., Latker, C. H., Sasse, J., and Risau, W. (1987). Regression of blood vessels precedes cartilage differentiation during chick limb development. Differentiation 34: 98–105.

Hatzopoulos, A. K., Folkman, J., Vasile, E., Eiselen, G. K., and Rosenberg, R. D.

(1998). Isolation and characterization of endothelial progenitor cells from mouse embryos. Development 125: 1457–1468.

Healy, A. M., Rayburn, H. B., Rosenberg, R. D., and Weiler, H. (1995). Absence of the blood-clotting regulator thrombomodulin causes embryonic lethality in mice before development of a functional cardiovascular system. Proc. Natl. Acad. Sci. USA 92: 850–854.

Heikinheimo, M., Scandrett, J. M., and Wilson, D. B. (1994). Localization of transcription factor GATA-4 to regions of the mouse embryo involved in cardiac development. Dev. Biol. 164: 361–373.

Henkemeyer, M., Rossi, D. J., Holmyard, D. P., Puri, M. C., Mbamalu, G., Harpal, K., Shih, T. S., Jacks, T., and Pawson, T. (1995). Vascular system defects and neuronal apoptosis in mice lacking ras GTPase-activating protein. Nature 377: 695–701.

His, W. (1868). Untersuchungen über die erste Anlage des Wirbelthierleibes. F. C. W. Vogel, Leipsig.

Hynes, R. O. and Bader, B. L. (1997). Targeted mutations in integrins and their ligands: their implications for vascular biology. Thromb. Haemost. 78: 83–87.

Jiang, Y. and Evans, T. (1996). The Xenopus GATA-4/5/6 genes are associated with cardiac specification and can regulate cardiac-specific transcription during embryogenesis. Dev. Biol. 174: 258–270.

Jolly, J. (1940). Recherches sur la formation du systéme vasculaire de l' embryon. Arch. Anat. Microsc. T. 35: 295–361.

Kabrun, N., Bühring, H.-J., Choi, K., Ullrich, A., Risau, W., and Keller, G. (1997). Flk-1 expression defines a population of early embryonic hematopoietic precursors. Development 124: 2039–2048.

Kelley, C., Blumberg, H., Zon, L. I., and Evans, T. (1993). GATA-4 is a novel transcription factor expressed in endocardium of the developing heart. Development 118: 817–827.

Kim, K. J., Li, B., Winer, J., Armanini, M., Gillett, N., Phillips, H. S., and Ferrara, N. (1993). Inhibition of vascular endothelial growth factor-induced angiogenesis suppresses tumour growth in vivo. Nature 362: 841–844.

Knapik, E. W., Goodman, A., Atkinson, O. S., Roberts, C. T., Shiozawa, M., Sim, C. U., Weksler-Zangen, S., Trolliet, M. R., Futrell, C., Innes, B. A., Koike, G., McLaughlin, M. G., Pierre, L., Simon, J. S., Vilallonga, E., Roy, M., Chiang, P.-W., Fishman, M. C., Driever, W., and Jacob, H. J. (1996). A reference cross DNA panel for zebrafish (*Danio rerio*) anchored with simple sequence length polymorphisms. Development 123: 451–460.

Laverriere, A. C., MacNeil, C., Mueller, C., Poelmann, R. E., Burch J. B. E., and Evans, T. (1994). GATA-4/5/6, a subfamily of three transcription factors transcribed in developing heart and gut. J. Biol. Chem. 269: 23177–23184.

Lawson, K. A., Meneses, J. J., and Pedersen, R. A. (1991). Clonal analysis of epiblast fate during germ layer formation in the mouse embryo. Development 113: 891–911.

Le Douarin, N. M. (1969). Particularités du noyau interphasique chez le caille japonaise (Coturnix japonica). Utilization de ces particularités comme "marquage biologique" dans les recherches sur les interactions tissulaires et les migrationes cellulaires au cours de l'ontogénèse. Bull. Biol. Fr. Belg. 103: 435–452.

Lee, K.-F., Simon, H., Chen, H., Bates, B., Hung, M.-C., and Hauser, C. (1995).

Requirement for neuregulin receptor erbB2 in neural and cardiac development. Nature 378: 394–398.

Levéen, P., Pekny, M., Gebre-Medhin, S., Swolin, B., Larsson, E., and Betsholtz, C. (1994). Mice deficient for PDGF B show renal, cardiovascular, and hematological abnormalities. Gen. Dev. 8: 1875–1887.

Lints, T. J., Parsons, L. M., Hartley, L., Lyons, I., and Harvey, R. P. (1993). Nkx-2.5: a novel murine homeobox gene expressed in early heart progenitor cells and their myogenic descendants. Development 119: 419–431.

Maisonpierre, P. C., Suri, C., Jones, P. F., Bartunkova, S., Wiegand, S. J., Radziejewski, C., Compton, D., McClain, J., Aldrich, T. H., Papadopoulos, N., Daly, T. J., Davis, S., Sato, T. N., and Yancopoulos, G. D. (1997). Angiopoietin-2, a natural antagonist for tie2 that disrupts in vivo angiogenesis. Science 277: 55–60.

Maroulakou, I. G., Papas, T. S., and Green, J. E. (1994). Differential expression of ets-1 and ets-2 proto-oncogenes during murine embryogenesis. Oncogene 9: 1551–1565.

Matthews, W., Jordan, C. T., Gavin, M., Jenkins, N. A., Copeland, N. G., and Lemischka, I. R. (1991). A receptor tyrosine kinase cDNA isolated from a population of enriched primitive hematopoietic cells and exhibiting close genetic linkage to c-kit. Proc. Natl. Acad. Sci. USA 88: 9026–9030.

Meyer, D. and Birchmeier, C. (1995). Multiple essential functions of neuregulin in development. Nature 378: 386–390.

Mikawa, T. and Gourdie, R. G. (1996). Pericardial mesoderm generates a population of coronary smooth muscle cells migrating into the heart along with ingrowth of the epicardial organ. Dev. Biol. 174: 221–232.

Millauer, B., Wizigmann-Voos, S., Schnürch, H., Martinez, R., Møller, N. P. H., Risau, W., and Ullrich, A. (1993). High affinity VEGF binding and developmental expression suggest Flk-1 as a major regulator of vasculogenesis and angiogenesis. Cell 72: 835–846.

Millauer, B., Shawver, L. K., Plate, K. H., Risau, W., and Ullrich, A. (1994). Glioblastoma growth inhibited in vivo by a dominant-negative Flk-1 mutant. Nature 367: 576–579.

Minot, C. S. (1900). On a hitherto unrecognized form of blood circulation without capillaries in the organs of Vertebrata. Proc. Boston Soc. Nat. History 29: 185–215.

Mitrani, E. and Shimoni, Y. (1990). Induction by soluble factors of organized axial structures in chick epiblasts. Science 247: 1092–1094.

Morrisey, E. E., Ip, H. S., Lu, M. M., and Parmacek, M. S. (1996). GATA-6: a zinc finger transcription factor that is expressed in multiple cell lineages derived from lateral mesoderm. Dev. Biol. 177: 309–322.

Murray, P. D. F. (1932). The development in vitro of the blood of the early chick embryo. Proc. R. Soc. Lond. [Biol.] 11: 497–521.

Mustonen, T. and Alitalo, K. (1995). Endothelial receptor tyrosine kinases involved in angiogenesis. J. Cell Biol. 129: 895–898.

Narita, N., Bielinska, M., and Wilson, D. B. (1997). Wild-type endoderm abrogates the ventral developmental defects associated with GATA-4 deficiency in the mouse. Dev. Biol. 189: 270–274.

Nascone, N. and Mercola, M. (1996). Endoderm and cardiogenesis. Trends Cardiovasc. Med. 6: 211–216.

Noden, D. M. (1989). Embryonic origins and assembly of blood vessels. Am. Rev. Respir. Dis. 140: 1097–1103.

Ojeifo, J. O., Forough, R., Paik, S., Maciag, T., and Zwiebel, J. A. (1995). Angiogenesis-directed implantation of genetically modified endothelial cells in mice. Cancer Res. 55: 2240–2244.

Pardanaud, L. and Dieterlen-Lièvre, F. (1993). Expression of *c-ets-1* in early chick embryo mesoderm—relationship to the hemangioblastic lineage. Cell Res. Commun. 1: 151–160.

Pardanaud, L., Altmann, C., Kitos, P., Dieterlen-Lièvre, F., and Buck, C. A. (1987). Vasculogenesis in the early quail blastodisc as studied with a monoclonal antibody recognizing endothelial cells. Development 100: 339–349.

Pardanaud, L., Yassine, F., and Dieterlen-Lièvre, F. (1989). Relationship between vasculogenesis, angiogenesis and haemopoiesis during avian ontogeny. Development 105: 473–485.

Pardanaud, L., Luton, D., Prigent, M., Bourcheix, L.-M., Catala, M., and Dieterlen-Lièvre, F. (1996). Two distinct endothelial lineages in ontogeny, one of them related to hemopoiesis. Development 122: 1363–1371.

Partanen, J., Armstrong, E., Mäkelä, T. P., Korhonen, J., Sandberg, M., Renkonen, R., Knuutila, S., Huebner, K. and Alitalo, K. (1992). A novel endothelial cell surface receptor tyrosine kinase with extracellular epidermal growth factor homology domains. Mol. Cell. Biol. 12: 1698–1707.

Patterson, C., Perrella, M. A., Hsieh, C.-M., Yoshizumi, M., Lee, M.-E., and Haber, E. (1995). Cloning and functional analysis of the promoter for KDR/flk-1, a receptor for vascular endothelial growth factor. J. Biol. Chem. 270: 23111–23118.

Péault, B., Coltey, M., and Le Douarin, N. M. (1988). Ontogenic emergence of a quail leukocyte/endothelium cell surface antigen. Cell Differ. 23: 165–174.

Plate, K. H., Breier, G., Weich, H. A., and Risau, W. (1992). Vascular endothelial growth factor is a potential tumour angiogenesis factor in human gliomas in vivo. Nature 359: 845–848.

Plate, K. H., Breier, G., Millauer, B., Ullrich, A., and Risau, W. (1993). Up-regulation of vascular endothelial growth factor and its cognate receptors in a rat glioma model of tumor angiogenesis. Cancer Res. 53: 5822–5827.

Poelmann, R. E., Gittenberger-de Groot, A. C., Mentink, M. M. T., Bökenkamp, R., and Hogers, B. (1993). Development of the cardiac coronary vascular endothelium, studied with antiendothelial antibodies, in chicken-quail chimeras. Circ. Res. 73: 559–568.

Postlethwait, J. H., Johnson, S. L., Midson, C. N., Talbot, W. S., Gates, M., Ballinger, E. W., Africa, D., Andrews, R., Carl, T., Eisen, J. S., Horne, S., Kimmel, C. B., Hutchinson, M., Johnson, M., and Rodriguez, A. (1994). A genetic linkage map for the zebrafish. Science 264: 699–703.

Puri, M. C., Rossant, J., Alitalo, K., Bernstein, A., and Partanen, J. (1995). The receptor tyrosine kinase TIE is required for integrity and survival of vascular endothelial cells. EMBO J. 14: 5884–5891.

Rabl, C. (1889). Theorie des Mesoderms. Morphol. Jahrbuch 15: 113–252.

Reagan, F. R. (1915). Vascularization phenomena in fragments of embryonic bodies completely isolated from yolk sac blastoderm. Anat. Rec. 9: 329–341.

Risau, W. (1991). Vasculogenesis, angiogenesis and endothelial cell differentiation during embryonic development. *In* "The Development of the Vascular System"

(R. N. Feinberg, G. K. Sherer, and R. Auerbach, eds.), pp. 56–68. Karger, Basel.
Risau, W. and Flamme, I. (1995). Vasculogenesis. Annu. Rev. Cell Dev. Biol. 11: 73–91.
Rönicke, V., Risau, W., and Breier, G. (1996). Characterization of the endothelium-specific murine vascular endothelial growth factor receptor-2 (flk-1) promoter. Circ. Res. 79: 277–285.
Rosenquist, G. C. (1970). Aortic arches in the chick embryo: origin of the cells as determined by radioautographic mapping. Anat. Rec. 168: 351–359.
Sabin, F. R. (1917). Origin and development of the primitive vessels of the chick and of the pig. Contrib. Embryol. Carnegie Inst. Publ. Wash. 6: 61–124.
Sabin, F. R. (1920). Studies on the origin of blood-vessels and of red blood-corpuscles as seen in the living blastoderm of chicks during the second day of incubation. Contrib. Embryol. Carnegie Inst. Publ. Wash. 9: 213–262.
Sato, T. N., Qin, Y., Kozak, C. A., and Audus, K. L. (1993). tie-1 and tie-2 define another class of putative receptor tyrosine kinase genes expressed in early embryonic vascular system. Proc. Natl. Acad. Sci. USA 90: 9355–9358.
Sato, T. N., Tozawa, Y., Deutsch, U., Wolburg-Buchholz, K., Fujiwara, Y., Gendron-Maguire, M., Gridley, T., Wolburg, H., Risau, W., and Qin, Y. (1995). Distinct roles of the receptor tyrosine kinases tie-1 and tie-2 in blood vessel formation. Nature 376: 70–74.
Schatteman, G. C., Morrison-Graham, K., van Koppen, A., Weston, J. A., and Bowen-Pope, D. F. (1992). Regulation and role of PDGF receptor α-subunit expression during embryogenesis. Development 115: 123–131.
Schatteman, G. C., Loushin, C., Li, T., and Hart, C. E. (1996). PDGF-A is required for normal murine cardiovascular development. Dev. Biol. 176: 133–142.
Schlaeger, T. M., Qin, Y., Fujiwara, Y., Magram, J., and Sato, T. N. (1995). Vascular endothelial cell lineage-specific promoter in transgenic mice. Development 121: 1089–1098.
Schlaeger, T. M., Bartunkova, S., Lawitts, J. A., Teichmann, G., Risau, W., Deutsch, U., and Sato, T. N. (1997). Uniform vascular-endothelial-cell-specific gene expression in both embryonic and adult transgenic mice. Proc. Natl. Acad. Sci. USA 94: 3058–3063.
Schnürch, H., and Risau, W. (1993). Expression of tie-2, a member of a novel family of receptor tyrosine kinases, in the endothelial cell lineage. Development 119: 957–968.
Schultheiss, T. M., Xydas, S., and Lassar, A. B. (1995). Induction of avian cardiac morphogenesis by anterior endoderm. Development 121: 4203–4214.
Shalaby, F., Rossant, J., Yamaguchi, T. P., Gertsenstein, M., Wu, X.-F., Breitman, M. L., and Schuh, A. C. (1995). Failure of blood-island formation and vasculogenesis in flk-1-deficient mice. Nature 376: 62–66.
Shibuya, M., Yamaguchi, S., Yamane, A., Ikeda, T., Tojo, A., Matsushime, H., and Sato, M. (1990). Nucleotide sequence and expression of a novel human receptor-type tyrosine kinase gene (flt) closely related to the fms family. Oncogene 5: 519–524.
Slack, J. M. (1994). Inducing factors in Xenopus early embryos. Cur. Biol. 4: 116–126.
Smith, J. L., Gesteland, K. M., and Schoenwolf, G. C. (1994). Prospective fate map of the mouse primitive streak at 7.5 days of gestation. Dev. Dyn. 201: 279–289.
Soriano, P. (1994). Abnormal kidney development and hematological disorders in PDGF beta-receptor mutant mice. Gen. Dev. 8: 1888–1896.

Stainier, D. Y. R., Fouquet, B., Chen, J.-N., Warren, K. S., Weinstein, B. M., Meiler, S. E., Mohideen, M.-A. P. K., Neuhauss, S. C. F., Solnica-Krezel, L., Schier, A. F., Zwartkruis, F., Stemple, D. L., Malicki, J., Driever, W., and Fishman, M. C. (1996). Mutations affecting the formation and function of the cardiovascular system in the zebrafish embryo. Development 123: 285–292.

Sugi, Y. and Markwald, R. R. (1996). Formation and early morphogenesis of endocardial endothelial precursor cells and the role of endoderm. Dev. Biol. 175: 66–83.

Suri, C., Jones, P. F., Patan, S., Bartunkova, S., Maisonpierre, P. C., Davis, S., Sato, T. N., and Yancopoulos, G. D. (1996). Requisite role of Angiopoietin-1, a ligand of the TIE2 receptor, during embryonic angiogenesis. Cell 87: 1171–1180.

Terman, B. I., Dougher-Vermazen, M., Carrion, M. E., Dimitrov, D., Armellino, D. C., Gospodarowicz, D., and Bohlen, P. (1992). Identification of the KDR tyrosine kinase as a receptor for vascular endothelial cell growth factor. Biochem. Biophys. Res. Commun. 187: 1579–1586.

Tian, H., McKnight, S. L., and Russell, D. W. (1997). Endothelial PAS domain protein 1 (EPAS1), a transcription factor selectively expressed in endothelial cells. Gen. Dev. 11: 72–82.

Vikkula, M., Boon, L. M., Carraway, III K. L., Calvert, J. T., Diamonti, A. J., Goumnerov, B., Pasyk, K. A., Marchuk, D. A., Warman, M. L., Cantley, L. C., Mulliken, J. B., and Olsen, B. R. (1996). Vascular dysmorphogenesis caused by an activating mutation in the receptor tyrosine kinase tie2. Cell 87: 1181–1190.

Wang, R., Clark, R., and Bautch, V. L. (1992). Embryonic stem cell-derived cystic embryoid bodies form vascular channels: an in vitro model of blood vessel development. Development 114: 303–316.

Weiler-Guettler, H., Aird, W. C., Rayburn, H., Husain, M., and Rosenberg, R. D. (1996). Developmentally regulated gene expression of thrombomodulin in postimplantation mouse embryos. Development 122: 2271–2281.

Wilting, J., and Christ, B. (1996). Embryonic angiogenesis: a review. Naturwissenschaften 83: 153–164.

Yamaguchi, T. P., Dumont, D. J., Conlon, R. A., Breitman, M. L., and Rossant, J. (1993). flk-1, an flt-related receptor tyrosine kinase is an early marker for endothelial cell precursors. Development 118: 489–498.

2

Cellular Mechanisms of Angiogenesis

J. ANTHONY WARE

Alterations in endothelial cell function occur not only as part of new vessel formation, but also wound healing. Small injuries to the endothelial cell monolayer heal by migration of adjacent endothelial cells into the wound; after they reattach to the underlying matrix, they then reenter the cell cycle and divide to replace the denuded cells. In angiogenesis, the first step under most circumstances is dissolution of the underlying matrix, brought about by release of proteases (e.g., collagenases and plasminogen activator) from the stimulated endothelial cells themselves or from cells or material admitted to the subendothelial space under conditions of heightened endothelial permeability. The cells detach from the matrix and migrate by crawling along the vascular bed, and eventually readhere. Endothelial cells adhere to the underlying matrix via a number of different receptors, which become expressed on their surface in greater numbers when the cells are growing. Once the cells reattach, they reenter the cell cycle, proliferate, and align themselves into capillary sprouts or tubules. This latter stage depends on interaction of the endothelial cell with specific components of the extracellular matrix (Grant et al., 1989). Some recent evidence suggests that endothelial cells that do not become aligned to form tubules undergo *apoptosis*, or programmed cell death. Whether endothelial cell death by this mechanism is important in maintaining the orderly formation of blood vessels is not known, but seems likely. After synthesis of a new basement membrane, capillary sprouts eventually will reestablish patency with the preexisting vasculature, which allows blood flow, and will form branches in a new vascular anastomotic network.

Major injuries to the vessel wall, as well as formation of vessels larger than capillaries, require migration and proliferation of pericytes or vascular smooth muscle cells as well. Pericytes and smooth muscle cells interact in a number of important ways with endothelial cells. For instance, endothelial cells release a number of substances that can either promote or inhibit the growth of vascular smooth muscle cells, and either cell type can stimulate the other to synthesize matrix components and release proteases that can repair and remodel the vascular wall.

Although each of the stages of angiogenesis have been studied extensively over the past few years, it is important to note that their temporal sequence is not clear; most likely, these phases coincide and recur, rather than being strictly sequential. The process of angiogenesis under normal conditions is self-limiting: when sufficient vessel formation has occurred, endothelial cells become quiescent and the vessels either remain or regress if unneeded. Modification of any of these components could, at least in theory, promote or interfere with angiogenesis.

Recently, another potential mechanism by which angiogenesis may occur has been described. Endothelial cell progenitors that are formed in the bone marrow and released into the circulation have been identified (Asahara et al., 1997). These cells can differentiate into endothelial cells in vitro and become incorporated into sites of active angiogenesis in animal models of ischemic vascular damage in vivo. Presumably these cells adhere to the exposed matrix, proliferate, and subsequently differentiate into a vascular tube, but the precise events are not yet known. Another important question that this model raises concerns the identity of the unknown substance produced by the area of vascular damage that triggers the release of these cells from the bone marrow.

AGONIST RECEPTORS AND SIGNAL TRANSDUCTION

A number of cytokines have been found to induce angiogenesis in vivo and to stimulate endothelial migration and/or proliferation in vitro (Table 2.1) (Folkman, 1995; Ware and Simons, 1997). The cytokines (also called growth factors) that interact with tyrosine kinase receptors (e.g., members of the fibroblastic growth factor [FGF] and vascular endothelial growth factor [VEGF] families) are described later in the book. An important source for some of these molecules is the endothelial cells themselves. Stimulation of endothelial cells causes release of these cytokines, of which the best studied in this regard is FGF-2, which then binds to its surface receptor(s) and stimulates migration, proliferation, and capillary tubule formation (Sato and Rifkin, 1988). Endothelial cells accumulate FGF-2 in their cytoplasm as they migrate; inhibition of this endogenous FGF-2 also prevents migration (Biro et al., 1994). Several cytokines (e.g., interleukin 6) that are highly expressed in angiogenic tissue appear to facilitate vessel growth primarily by causing transcription or release of endogenous growth factors, rather than by stimulating endothelial cell growth directly (Cohen et al., 1996). (Although this observation suggests that indirect angiogenic factors can be distinguished from direct, in practice the criteria to differentiate strictly between them are difficult to define.) Many growth factors work in a cooperative or synergistic manner to

Table 2.1 Selected Endothelial Growth Factors and Their Receptors

Growth Factors	*Endothelial Cell Receptors*	*Growth Factor Tissue Distribution*	*Target Tissues Other Than Endothelial Cells (EC)*
FGF-1 (acidic)	FGFR-1,2,3,4	Brain, bone matrix, kidney, EC, retina, heart, others	Multiple
FGF-2 (basic)	FGFR-1,2	Brain, retina, pituitary, kidney, placenta, testes, monocytes, corpus luteum, heart, many others	Multiple
FGF-4	FGFR-1,2	Embryonic tissue	Megakaryocytes, multiple others
FGF-5	Unknown	Neonatal brain, CNS	CNS, hair follicles
VEGF-A	VEGFR-1 (flt-1) (fms) VEGFR-2 kdr/flk-1	Pituitary cells, monocytes (macrophages), smooth muscle, heart, lung, skeletal muscle, prostate	Monocytes, coagulation system, hematopoeitic stem cells
VEGF-B	Unknown	Heart, skeletal muscle, pancreas, prostate, many others	Unknown
VEGF-C	flt-4 (VEGFR-3)/ VEGFR-2	Heart, placenta, ovary, small intestine, others	Unknown
HGF (scatter factor)	c-met	Lung, liver, skin, blood, many others	Multiple

PDGF-BB-AB	PDGFR-β	Platelets, malignant cells, macrophages, EC, fibroblasts, vascular smooth muscle, glial cells, astrocytes, myoblasts, kidney cells	Connective tissue, smooth muscle, neutrophils
EGF	EGFR (c-erbB)	Ectodermal cells, monocytes, kidney, duodenal glands	Epithelial cells, gastric glands
IL-8	IL-8 receptor (2)	Monocytes, lymphocytes, granulocytes, fibroblasts, EC, bronchial epithelial cells, keratinocytes, hepatocytes, mesangial cells, and chondrocytes	Neutrophils, lymphocytes, basophils, monocytes
Proliferin	MRP/PLF receptor	Placenta, fibroblasts, muscle	Uterus, muscle, numerous other tissues
Thrombin	Thrombin receptor (G-protein coupled)	Blood/cell interface	Platelets, smooth muscle, brain
TNF-α	TNFR-p55 -p75	EC, macrophages, stromal cells, T cells, tumor cells, others	Multiple
PD-ECGF	None?	Platelets, other blood-borne cells	Unknown
TGF-α	TGF-αR	Macrophages, tumor cells	Multiple

induce angiogenesis (Koolwijk et al., 1996). Various environmental factors also serve as stimulants for endothelial cell function; two of the best studied are hypoxia and shear stress. Both of these can cause elevations in expression of genes known to affect blood vessel growth, such as VEGF, and both have been associated with enhanced proliferation of cultured endothelial cells. Several soluble agonists interact with surface receptors linked to G proteins to affect endothelial growth and migration (Hamm, 1998). These include thrombin, platelet activating factor, thromboxane A2, 5-hydroxytryptamine, histamine, substance P, and several others. As is the case with the cytokines, many of the agonists for these receptors are released from other cells. The G-protein-linked receptors have a common structure in that they have, in addition to a single extracellular domain near the N-terminal, seven domains that span the surface membrane, and thus are sometimes called "serpentine" or "seven-spanner" receptors. Short cytoplasmic domains that form loops connect these seven transmembrane domains; a C-terminal tail of varying length follows the seventh. Interestingly, not all of these agonists have the same effect; for instance, although both thrombin and thromboxane A2 promote DNA synthesis in cultured endothelial cells, thrombin promotes angiogenesis in vitro (Haralabopoulos et al., 1997), while the process of vascular tube formation is inhibited by thromboxane A2 mimetics (A. W. Ashton and J. A. Ware; unpublished observations). Furthermore, not all cytokines facilitate all stages of angiogenesis. For example, platelet-derived endothelial cell growth factor (PD-ECGF) does not cause proliferation of endothelial cells but is a very powerful stimulant of migration of both endothelial and mast cells. Thus, enhancement or inhibition of a single stage of endothelial function may be sufficient to regulate angiogenesis.

In addition to the large number of growth primating cytokines, there are an increasing number of substances identified that prevent endothelial response to these cytokines. Many of the growth inhibitors are regulated by characteristics of the extracellular matrix and its modifiers. It is likely that new vessel growth results from decreases in these inhibitors, as well as increases in growth promoting cytokines.

The signal transduction processes that lead from G-protein-linked receptors vary significantly according to receptor class and to a degree even within the same receptor family. Many details are not known about these pathways for any cell, and many of those that have been established in other cell types may differ considerably from those in endothelial cells. Typically, the G-protein-linked receptor pathways begin with the replacement of GDP by GTP on a Gα (alpha) subunit, which thus causes it to dissociate from the β (beta) and γ (gamma) subunits, and then activates an effector, such as adenylate cyclase, which mediates formation of cyclic AMP, or the β isoform of phospholipase C (Fig. 2.1) (Hamm, 1998). The importance of one of these Gα subunits, Gα13, to angiogenesis is shown by the lack of an organized vascular system in mice with targeted deletion of this subunit (Offermans et al., 1997). Multiple Gα subunits are activated

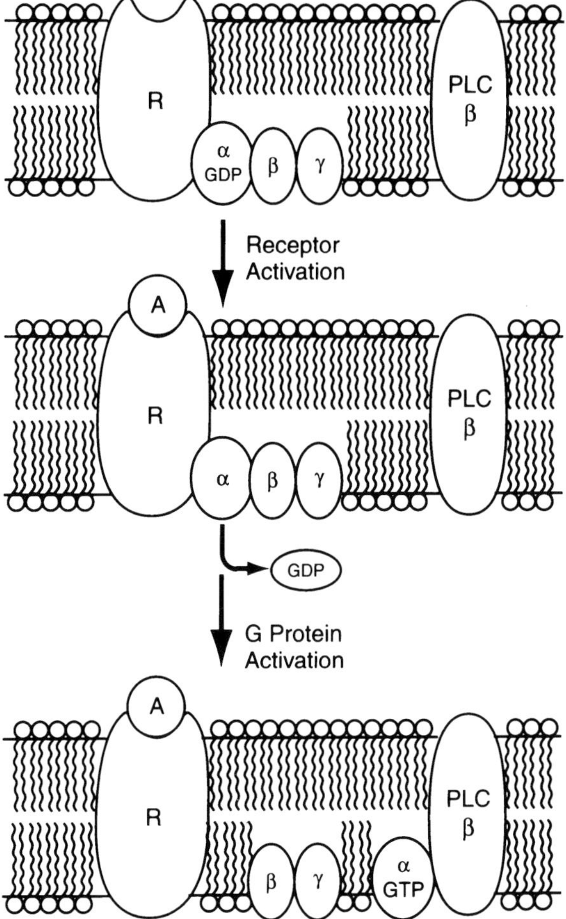

Figure 2.1. Diagram of G protein receptor-mediated signalling. Binding of an agonist causes GDP to be replaced by GTP on the Gα subunit, which dissociates from the βγ dimer and activates the effector (PLC β, in this example).

by the same agonists, and different receptors do not necessarily activate the same subunits. (Since G-protein-linked receptors for many ligands often do activate the same G proteins, however, a major unsolved question is how the specific responses of endothelial cells to various agonists that bind these receptors are controlled.) A subset of G proteins can be classified on the basis of their sensitivity to pertussis toxin, and one or more members of this subset appear to be required for endothelial cell migration and capillary tube formation in vitro, since those processes are inhibited by pertussis toxin.

Phospholipase C liberates diacylglycerol and inositol trisphosphate from the parent phosphoinositol (PI) lipids; these mediators provide at least one mechanism by which the physiological agonists can activate members of the protein kinase C (PKC) family and liberate Ca^{2+} from intracellular storage sites, respectively. Elevation of the level of cytoplasmic Ca^{2+} activates many of the enzymes (e.g., myosin light chain kinase) that are likely to be essential for cytoskeletal reorganization. Activation of PKC is also required for cytoskeletal function, and many of the proteins that bind the cytoskeleton are PKC substrates. PKC activity is necessary for advancement through certain phases of the cell cycle, and its inhibition with chemical antagonists prevents proliferation. PKC is also one of the mechanisms by which the extracellular regulated kinases (ERKs), which are also associated with mitogenesis, become activated. Both PKC and tyrosine kinases are required for autologous release of VEGF and FGF-2, which, as noted above, are amplification loops of potential importance in endothelial cell proliferation and migration.

Signal transduction downstream from the receptor tyrosine kinases involves many of these same features, since another of the isoforms of phospholipase C, PLC γ, is activated, with similar consequences of PKC activation and Ca^{2+} mobilization. Signaling associated with these receptors is more complicated, however; as a result of the binding of the growth factor (cytokine) to its specific receptor tyrosine kinase, the receptor becomes autophosphorylated on tyrosine residues in discrete sections of the cytoplasmic domain (Fig. 2.2). This event not only increases the catalytic activity of the receptor but also creates a docking site that allows the assembly of the next protein in a long sequential cascade (Malarkey et al., 1995). Some of the phosphotyrosines permit binding of adapter proteins, such as Shc or members of the Grb family. Others bind proteins that are themselves signaling proteins, such as PI3 kinase; others bind enzymes, like PLCγ that catalyze other reactions; and still others bind substrates, such as some cytoskeletal proteins, that directly mediate cellular function. Addition of VEGF to endothelial cells causes phosphorylation of several proteins on tyrosine residues, including PI3 kinase, PLCγ and Ras GTPase activating protein (Guo et al., 1995), which correlates with their activation. The features that all of these proteins have in common is the presence of certain motifs, called *src homology (SH) 2 domains,* that allow them to bind to the cytoplasmic domain of the receptor only after it becomes phosphorylated on specific tyrosine residues (Fig. 2.3). Thus, autophosphorylation of the intracellular kinase domain on many different sites leads to the initiation of several pathways of signal transduction (van der Geer et al., 1994). Studies in which receptor tyrosines that are bound by specific SH2-containing proteins are deleted reveal specific functions for the components of the signal transduction pathway. Removal of the binding tyrosine for PLCγ in the FGF receptor-1, for instance, prevents the FGF-induced PI turnover and the rise in cytoplasmic Ca^{2+}, but does not prevent mitogenesis, suggesting that PLCγ is not required for that event. On the other hand, FGF receptor internalization and downregulation are prevented by such a mutation (Mohammadi et al., 1992; Peters et al., 1992). Some sites

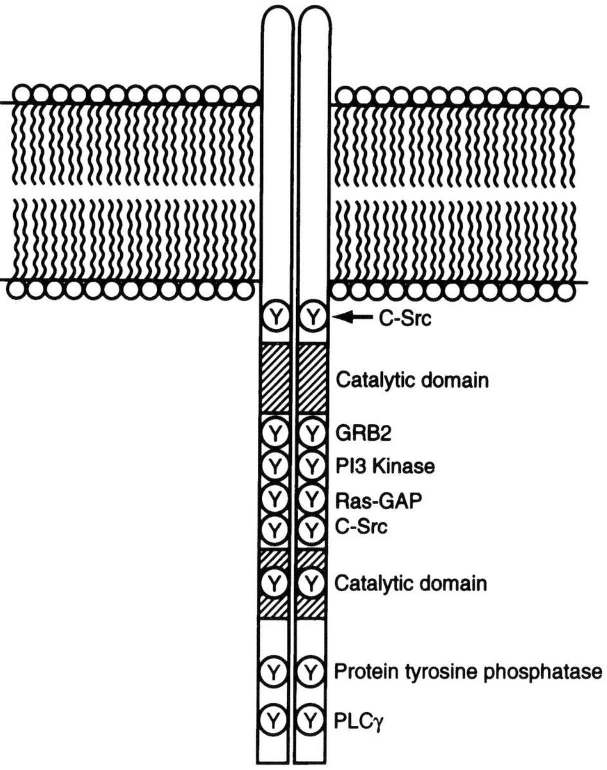

Figure 2.2. A model of a receptor tyrosine kinase dimer showing autophosphorylated tyrosine (Y) sites that are bound by SH2-binding proteins. The kinase domain of this receptor is in two parts, and is activated by phosphorylation.

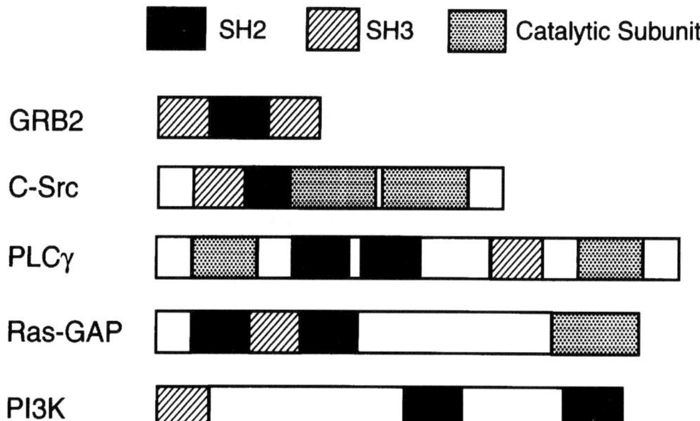

Figure 2.3. Comparison of SH2, SH3 and catalytic domains in selected proteins that bind to receptor tyrosine kinases.

on a given receptor can bind more than one type of SH2-containing protein, which, in turn, can sometimes bind to more than one receptor site.

Stimulation of the receptor tyrosine kinases, as well as receptors of other classes, activates a series of cytosolic kinases and thus creates a cascade of phosphorylation events. Regarding endothelial migration or proliferation, the ultimate targets of this cascade are either the cytoskeleton or the nucleus, where transcription factors become phosphorylated and then trigger changes in gene expression that lead to cell growth. Some of these factors (e.g., the cyclins, discussed below) directly control the cell cycle, but factors such as nf-κ b and egr-1, both of which have been associated with angiogenesis (Stoltz et al., 1996; Khachigian and Collins, 1997), probably work chiefly by promoting expression of growth factors. Still others, like the recently described Hox 3 homeobox gene, probably regulate adhesion and matrix proteolysis rather than proliferation (Boudreau et al., 1997). Although there are many aspects of signal transduction that are not yet known and many more whose relevance specifically to endothelial cell function is not yet defined, a general picture of these kinase pathways has emerged. In one pathway that has become better defined, the protooncogene Ras serves as an important mediator (Malarkey et al., 1995). In this pathway, kinases such as the ERKs that are in the mitogen-activated protein (MAP) kinase family eventually become activated, as is the case with signals that follow activation of G-protein-linked receptors, and thus the pathways converge to a certain extent (Fig. 2.4). The pathway by which

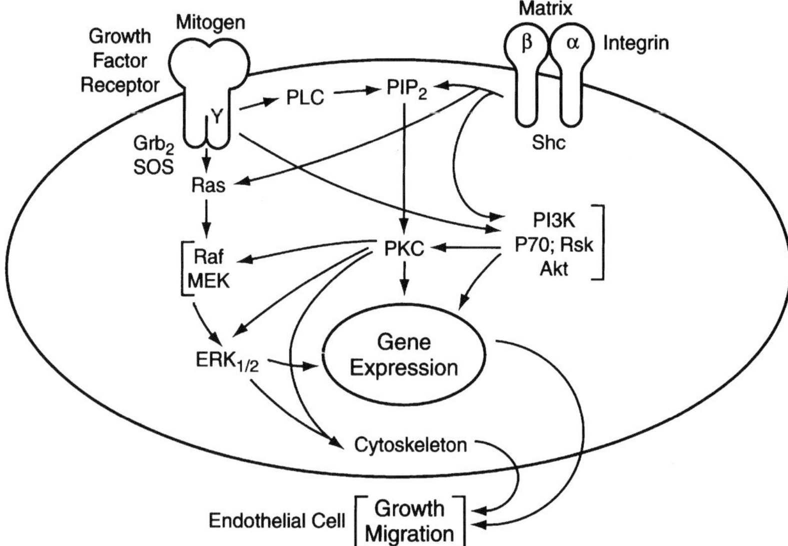

Figure 2.4. Signal transduction following stimulation of growth factor receptors or integrins. The signals generated from matrix and growth factors are coordinated and interact at several levels, eventually converging at the ERK kinases.

ERK becomes activated following receptor tyrosine kinase activation, which is sometimes called the *Ras pathway*, is much different, however, than that following G protein receptor activation. As noted above, the adapter protein Grb2 or a related Grb binds to the receptor, either directly or indirectly via another adapter protein named Shc. The Grb in turn recruits SOS to the plasma membrane, where it can then activate Ras by replacing GDP with GTP. Activated Ras binds Raf, a serine-threonine kinase, on the surface membrane, which is associated with its becoming activated. Raf then phosphorylates MEK, a kinase that is dual specific, meaning that it can phosphorylate both threonine and tyrosine on its substrate, the ERK MAP kinase. Once phosphorylated, the ERKs have many substrates that are associated with cell proliferation, such as the Rsk kinase. Use of dominant negative ERK constructs blocks DNA synthesis by several angiogenic cytokines, including FGF, suggesting that ERK activation is essential in mitogenesis (Besser et al., 1995). It is not sufficient, however; a profound reduction in endothelial cell proliferation can occur without reduction in ERK activity (Harrington et al., 1997). Thus, pathways not yet identified in addition to ERK are required for endothelial mitogenesis.

As noted above, PI3 kinase becomes activated by growth factors, including the FGFs. One of the consequences of PI3 kinase activation is the activation of p70, also known as S6 kinase, which is turn is associated with endothelial proliferation. It is clear, however, that products of PI3 kinase have other targets (see below), and that p70/S6K can become activated by means independent of PI3 kinase products (Kanda et al., 1997). PI3 kinase has been shown to mediate differentiation, mitogenesis, and migration in several cell types, but its role in angiogenesis is not yet clear.

There are mechanisms for protein–protein associations other than via SH2 domains. Other proteins that connect to the tyrosine kinase receptors have SH3 domains, which bind to polyproline motifs on a separate set of target proteins. An example of this class of proteins is cortactin, a cytoskeletal substrate for Src that binds to actin as well as the FGF receptor-1 (Zhan et al., 1994).

Although the "Ras-MAP kinase" cascade summarized above seems relatively straightforward, there are many components of signal transduction in endothelial cells that are not accounted for, and many complexities exist even with the known components. As an example of the former, key signaling molecules activated by many cytokine receptors, including TNF-α, are the JAK tyrosine kinases, whose major substrates are transcription factors known as STATs (Schindler and Darnell, 1995). How this pathway interacts with the Ras-ERK pathway outlined above in activated endothelial cells is not known. Additionally, signals generated by G-protein-linked receptors can affect distal components of this cascade. For example, elevations in cyclic AMP can activate protein kinase PKA, which inhibits ERK, probably by preventing Raf activation. "Crosstalk" between signals generated by receptors of different classes is likely to represent another mechanism for feedback control to prevent overstimulation, but many questions remain.

The complexity of a known component is emphasized when the effect of PKC on endothelial growth and migration is considered. PKC activation is required for endothelial cell proliferation following FGF-2 (Kent et al., 1995), angiogenesis following VEGF (Friedlander et al., 1995), and capillary tube formation following thrombin (Haralabopoulos, et al., 1997). Under certain experimental conditions, however, agents that activate PKC can inhibit endothelial cell cycle progression (Zhou et al., 1993) and thus proliferation. One explanation for this apparent discrepancy is the fact that PKC is not a single entity, but is a family of at least 11 gene products, some of which also have additional splicing variants. At least five of these isoenzymes are expressed in endothelial cells (Table 2.2). Different mediators can activate these isoenzymes; for example, the lipid products of PI3 kinases appear to activate selectively only a few of the PKC isoenzymes (Toker et al., 1994). Overexpression of one of these PKC isoenzymes, PKCα, in endothelial cells does not affect endothelial proliferation but does enhance their migration. On the other hand, when another isoenzyme, PKCδ (delta), is overexpressed, migration is unaffected, but endothelial cell cycle progression is blocked in S phase, and mitosis is inhibited (Harrington et al., 1997). When a third isoenzyme, PKCθ (theta), is selectively inhibited, migration, actin stress fiber formation, proliferation, cell cycle progression, and in vitro angiogenesis are all blocked (Tang et al., 1997). Thus, each of the PKC isoenzymes appears to act on selective substrates and to mediate discrete intracellular functions in endothelial cells.

It would seem logical for signaling molecules to be localized into a discrete area of the cell to promote their interaction. One such mechanism for this appears to be in the focal adhesions, discussed below. Another is perhaps in the caveolae, which are small invaginations of the

Table 2.2 Protein Kinase C Isoenzymes Expressed in Endothelial Cells[a]

Isoenzyme	*Regulation*[b]	*Function in Endothelial Cells*
α	PL, DG, Ca^{2+}	Enhances migration; thromboxane A_2 receptor downregulation
δ	PL, DG	Slows cell cycle progression
ε	PL, DG	Mediates ERK activity following shear stress
ζ	PL	Unknown
θ	PL, DG	Mediates cell cycle progression and cytoskeletal function

[a]Note: Expression of individual isoenzymes varies according to vascular source and probably species.

[b]Abbreviations: PL—phospholipids; DG—diglyceride; Ca^{2+}—calcium.

membrane of endothelial cells (Schnitzer et al., 1995), as well as some other cell types. These microdomains contain multiple signaling molecules, and also contain a distinctive protein, termed *caveolin* (Lisanti et al., 1994). Although many details are not yet known, it appears that this protein serves as a scaffold to bring several distinct signaling molecules and enzymes (e.g., one form of nitric oxide synthase) together in a small area of the cell.

Although there are questions about whether an agonist-induced Ca^{2+} rise is necessary for DNA synthesis or proliferation to occur (Kent et al., 1995; Peters et al., 1992), such a rise does occur in endothelial cells following many agonists and adherence by some integrin receptors (Leavesley et al., 1993). A Ca^{2+} rise is important in many events relevant to endothelial migration, including regulation of the cytoskeleton (see below) and activation of phospholipase A_2 with subsequent arachidonate release (Sa et al., 1995). The rise in cytoplasmic Ca^{2+} results from both influx from the extracellular space through Ca^{2+} channels and mobilization from intracellular stores. The mechanism by which Ca^{2+} influx occurs is not well understood; in endothelial cells, the voltage-dependent Ca^{2+} channels important in other cell types do not appear to be involved (Himmel et al., 1993). Intracellular triggers for Ca^{2+} influxes include an undefined tyrosine kinase (Fleming et al., 1995) and the amount of Ca^{2+}stored intracellularly (Himmel et al., 1993). A principal control of the intracellular pool of Ca^{2+} that is liberated following agonist mobilization is inositol trisphosphate (IP3), as noted above, and the sarcoplasmic reticulum Ca^{2+} pump SERCA (Cheng et al., 1996).

The role of nitric oxide (NO), whether generated by endothelial or adjacent cells, in angiogenesis is complex. Endothelial dilation mediated by NO is an early step in enhanced permeability of the endothelium, which is a prominent feature of many models by which angiogenesis is initiated, especially by VEGF. Elevation of cyclic GMP by NO, however, reduces cytoskeleton contraction and permeability induced by some agonists, both by preventing the elevation of Ca^{2+} that follows agonist stimulation and by preventing the breakdown of cyclic AMP (Draijer et al., 1995). VEGF stimulates endothelial production of NO via NO synthase (Isner, 1997). Inhibition of NO synthase prevents both angiogenesis and endothelial cell migration stimulated by VEGF, as well as TNF-α or platelet-activating factor (PAF,) but not by FGF-2 (Ziche et al., 1997; Montrucchio et al., 1997); it is not yet entirely clear whether such production is necessary for VEGF's angiogenic effect. On the other hand, NO donors have been shown to inhibit PKC-induced VEGF upregulation by preventing its transcription (Tsurumi et al., 1997). Thus, it is possible that NO is an important endogenous regulator of VEGF's effect and serves both to mediate its angiogenic effect and to limit its action after endothelial integrity and normal function are restored. It does not appear, though, that NO production is required for angiogenesis induced by all stimuli.

MATRIX PROTEASES

Quiescent endothelial cells adhere to a basement membrane, which is comprised of collagen, various proteoglycans, laminin, fibronectin, vitronectin, thrombospondin, entactin, and others. This membrane separates the endothelial cells from the interstitial matrix, which is made of many of these same components. For either angiogenesis or vascular remodeling to occur, the endothelial cells must detach and migrate, and thus limited dissolution of the matrix must occur at regions of contact with the cell surface. Activation and release of proteases from within the endothelial cells or other cells (e.g., macrophages) admitted to the subendothelial space is the principal mechanism by which proteolytic degradation of the matrix occurs. In addition to degradation of the matrix to allow endothelial migration, proteases have other potentially important roles in angiogenesis. The extracellular matrix sequesters many growth factors in a latent form, which can be released or activated by controlled proteolysis. Conversely, proteolysis of several extracellular proteins, including those of both matrix and nonmatrix origin, result in active cleavage products that inhibit angiogenesis (Sage, 1997). There are four classes of proteolytic enzymes (serine, aspartyl, cysteine, and metalloproteinases) that are potentially involved in vascular remodeling. Of these, the serine proteases and matrix metalloproteinases have been most closely associated with angiogenesis (Sage, 1997).

The serine protease plasmin/plasminogen activator system has received the most attention in this regard. Plasminogen activators convert plasminogen to active plasmin, which can degrade some matrix components directly and can also activate other matrix degrading enzymes, including the metalloproteinases. Both tissue-type plasminogen activator and plasminogen activator inhibitor-1 mRNA levels are increased during formation of capillary networks (Ito et al., 1995). For proper control of angiogenesis, it is necessary that matrix breakdown occur only in a local pericellular environment. Many of the components of this system, including plasmin, plasminogen, and the urokinase-type plasminogen activator, bind to specific sites or receptors on the surface of the endothelial cells, and this is one mechanism by which this localization is accomplished. Expression of the urokinase type of plasminogen activator (u-PA) and its receptor have been found to increase on the surface of migrating endothelial cells (Pepper et al., 1993), as does the expression of plasminogen activator inhibitor-1, which probably provides another method to localize proteolysis to the immediate environment. This receptor, in addition to binding plasminogen activator, also binds soluble vitronectin (Kanse et al., 1996), which may represent one mechanism to coordinate proteolysis and adhesion. Activation of the u-PA receptor leads to enhanced motility; signals generated in the JAK/STAT pathway, described previously in this chapter, appear to be those responsible for those effects, at least in vascular smooth muscle cells (Dumler et al., 1998). TNF-α increases cell bound u-PA activity which is responsible for a large portion of its angiogenic effect. An increase in u-PA activity was also thought to be necessary for VEGF-and FGF-2-mediated angiogenesis (Koolwijk et al. 1996). Recently, however, mice with targeted disruption of the u-PA receptor gene have been shown to have normal reendothelialization and vascular smooth muscle migration, suggesting that alternative methods of matrix proteolysis must exist (Carmeliet et al., 1998).

Recent studies have increased awareness of the role that matrix metalloproteinases (MMPs) play in matrix degradation and vascular remodeling (Griendling and Alexander, 1996). Endothelial cells, as well as macrophages and vascular smooth muscle cells, synthesize both MMPs and their tissue inhibitors (TIMPs). There are three main groups of MMPs (interstitial collagenases, stromelysins, and type 4 collagenases, which are also called *gelatinases* (Table 2.3). MMPs are produced as zymogens and can become activated by plasmin, as noted above, and cytokines. Some of the MMPs (MMP-1 [collagenase] and MMP-2 [gelatinase]) are produced constitutively, while the expression of others (MMP-3 and MMP-9) is increased markedly by stimulation of endothelial cells with cytokines such as TNF-α and direct activators of PKC. MMP-2 is commonly found in a complex with TIMP-2, its specific inhibitor. Thus, the influence of MMPs can be increased both by enhancement of transcription and by enzymatic activation, which can occur after addition of agonists such as thrombin (Zucker et al., 1995). The TIMPs appear to be constitutively expressed; therefore, the effect of stimulation with angiogenic cytokines may be to increase the relative abundance of MMPs to TIMPs. The net balance of these MMPs and their inhibitors can influence whether matrix degradation proceeds in the local environment. Increased MMP expression is found in endothelial cells undergoing migration or angiogenesis, suggesting that such upregulation is necessary for migration to occur. The observation that MMP-2 is associated with, and becomes activated by, specific endothelial adhesion receptors (Brooks et al., 1996) has suggested

Table 2.3 Endothelial Cell Matrix Metalloproteinases and Their Inhibitors

Metalloproteinases	*Other Name*	*Comments*
MMP-1	Interstitial collagenase	Induced by cytokines and PKC activators
MMP-2	Gelatinase A or type 4	Constitutive
MMP-3	Stromelysin MMP	Induced by IL-1 and PKC activators
MMP-9	Gelatinase B or type 5	Induced by IL-1 and PKC activators
Inhibitors	*Action*	
TIMP-1	Inhibits several MMPs	Constitutive
TIMP-2	Inhibits MMP-2	Constitutive

an intriguing connection between matrix proteolysis and adhesion, both important events in endothelial cell migration.

CYTOSKELETON

The cytoskeleton is the key determinant of shape in endothelial and other cell types. There is a tonic tension even in the unstimulated endothelial cell. The natural impermeability of the endothelial layer, in particular, should not be viewed as an entirely passive state; disruption of the cytoskeleton causes formation of intercellular gaps, with a resultant increase in permeability. In addition, contraction of proteins within the endothelial cell cytoskeleton is essential for endothelial cells to migrate, and also renders the endothelial barrier permeable in pathologic states. This contraction is ATP-dependent, requires an increase in cytoplasmic Ca^{2+}, and is mediated by the interaction of actin and nonmuscle myosin. This interaction is regulated by the phosphorylation status of myosin light chain (MLC), which in turn is regulated by the action of MLC kinases. In cultured endothelial cells, MLC kinases appear to differ in molecular structure from their better-studied counterparts in vascular smooth muscle cells; in addition, it appears that Rho kinase can act as a MLC kinase as well (van Hinsbergh, 1997). Rho kinase is activated by the small GTP-binding protein Rho and tyrosine phosphorylation, rather than by the Ca^{2+} calmodulin pathway used by other MLC kinases. In addition, MLC activity is controlled by one or more MLC phosphatases, which reverse the action of the kinases to provide temporal control of contraction of the endothelial cell.

Many contractile proteins comprise the endothelial cell cytoskeleton (Gallagher and Sumpio, 1997). The major protein component is actin, which is present in both filamentous (F-actin) and nonfilamentous, globular (G-actin) forms. Actin exists in equilibrium between these two forms; a number of mediators and accessory proteins control this process. When actin polymerizes (reversibly) into the F-actin form and becomes cross-linked with other actin filaments, formation of several prominent structures within the endothelial cells is possible (Fig. 2.5). These structures include tiny microspikes and asymmetric cell "ruffles" or lamellipodia at the cell periphery that are part of the so-called *migratory phenotype* and are formed by a diffuse network of short bundles. In addition, F-actin also forms much larger bundles such as stress fibers, seen in migrating cells and those exposed to high shear stress, and the dense peripheral band seen in quiescent cells. This dense peripheral band is lost upon stimulation with agonists that induce migration (Gottlieb et al., 1991). Stress fibers also contain other contractile proteins, including myosin, and, as noted above, exert tension to change the cell's shape. These stress fibers become reoriented within the cell when it is subjected to shear stress, and change the shape of the cultured endothelial cell. Microtubules surround-

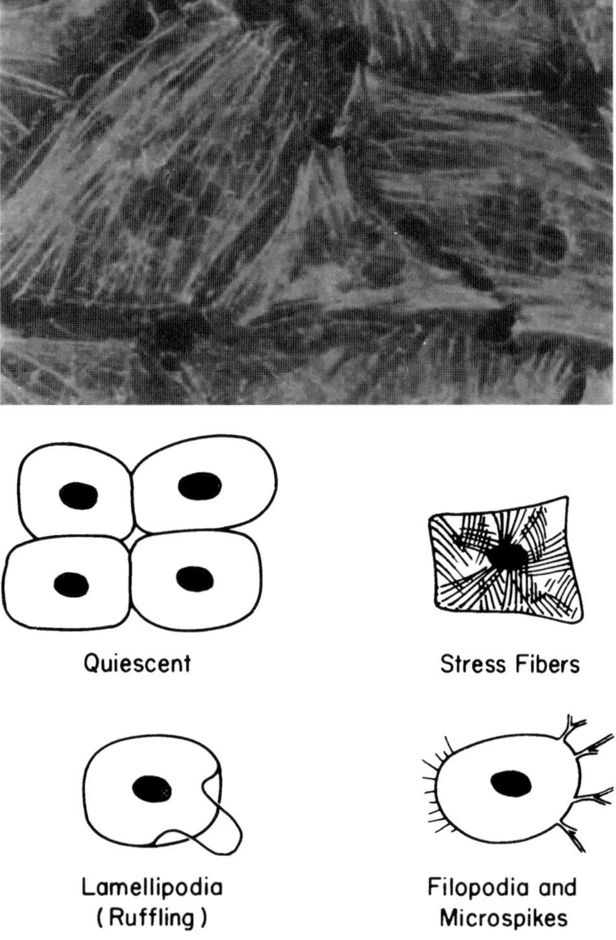

Figure 2.5 (Top) Fluorescent micrograph of endothelial cells with the F-actin stained with rhodamine phalloidin, demonstrating prominent stress fibers. (Bottom) F-actin structures are shown diagrammatically.

ing the perinuclear area also appear to be important in endothelial cell migration; with wounding of an endothelial cell monolayer, the microtubular centrosomes redistribute themselves between the leading lamellipod and the nucleus. As is the case with stress fibers, the microtubules align themselves in the direction of the applied stresses (Balboa et al., 1994), suggesting that they participate in the endothelial cell response to altered hemodynamics.

Only some of the signal transduction elements that control the formation of these cytoskeletal structures are known. Decreased levels of PIP_2 and increased levels of cytoplasmic Ca^{2+}, both results of PLC activation, favor disassembly of actin filaments by inducing capping of the ends of the actin filaments and sequestering of actin monomers. Such disassembly is necessary for filopodial extension and migration toward a stimulus. Protein kinase C activity is required for some forms of cytoskeletal contraction; an opposite effect is seen with the elevation of cyclic AMP, which reduces phosphorylation of MLC in endothelial cells without reducing cytoplasmic calcium (van Hinsberg, 1997). Cyclic AMP also leads to redistribution of F-actin and prevents the interaction between it and non-muscle myosin. Small GTP-binding proteins are required for formation of some actin structures (Amano et al., 1997). One of these proteins, Rho, mediates formation of actin stress fibers, at least in part by activating Rho kinase, while another, Rac, mediates formation of lamellipodia in fibroblasts (Machesky and Hall, 1997). Migrating endothelial cells demonstrate actin microspikes, lamellipodia and stress fibers, as well as focal adhesion complexes. Inhibition of Rho prevents the formation of the stress fibers, but not the other actin structures. Endothelial cell migration, however, is markedly delayed by Rho inhibition (Aepfelbacher et al., 1997).

There is a close relation between these F-actin structures and focal adhesion complexes, which are concentrated collections of proteins that mediate adhesion, control the cytoskeleton, and coordinate signaling between these entities and the cell interior (Fig. 2.6). Formation of these focal adhesion contacts also requires Rho activity, and is another function of Rho kinases (Burridge et al., 1997). Like stress fibers, focal adhesions also become reoriented along the direction of shear stress. Components

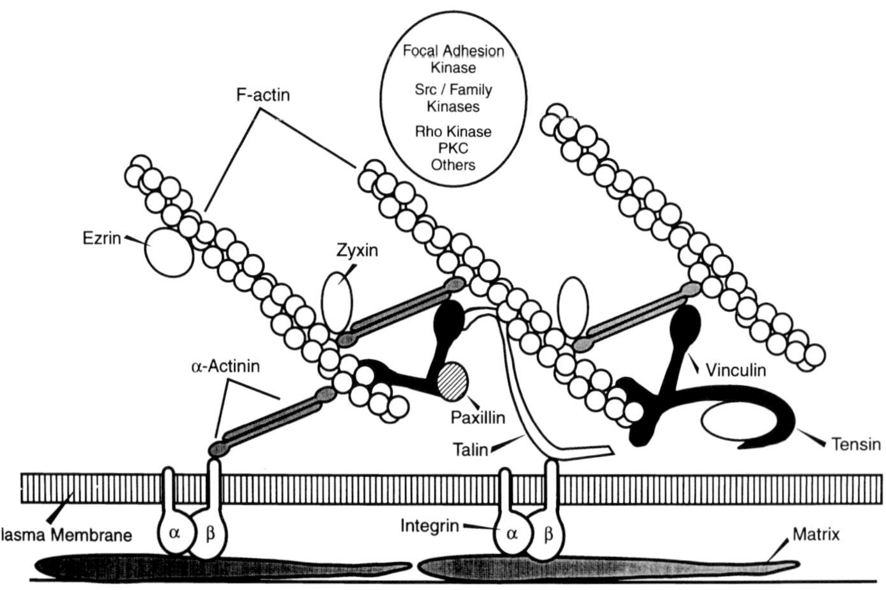

Figure 2.6 Protein-to-protein interactions in a focal adhesion. Several integrin tail-binding proteins and other components are omitted.

of the focal adhesions include the β1 and β3 integrins (90–110 kDa), vinculin (116 kDa), tensin (215 kDa), talin (220 kDa), zyxin (82 kDa), α-actinin (90 kDa), focal adhesion kinase (FAK—125 kDa), and paxillin (68 kDa) (Gallagher and Sumpio, 1997). The precise role of most of these proteins is not known. FAK becomes phosphorylated on tyrosine residues following cell attachment to certain matrix components and stimulation with either G-protein-coupled receptor agonists or tyrosine receptor agonists. Such phosphorylation in response to at least some agonists depends upon Rho activity, PKC activity, and the presence of an intact cytoskeleton. FAK does not appear to be essential for the formation of focal adhesions, but instead probably regulates the turnover of these adhesions in the migrating cell (Burridge et al., 1997). Many components of the cytoskeleton can also interact with proteins and other enzymes that participate in signal transduction. As one example, profilin, which is an actin-binding protein, associates with specific phosphoinositols and prevents the ability of phospholipase C to generate the lipid mediators described previously. Adenylate cyclase is inhibited by the formation of a complex between the stimulatory G protein and tubulin, another actin-associated protein. In addition to these specific examples, the cytoskeleton is a necessary component of many so-called "outside-in" signaling events initiated by the integrin receptors' binding to the extracellular matrix, as described in the next section. The exact contribution of the cytoskeleton to endothelial cell adhesion is not completely defined, but its disruption reduces their ability to adhere to an underlying matrix. Interestingly, many of the antiangiogenic cleavage products generated by proteolysis, such as SPARC, thrombospondin 1 and tenascin C diminish endothelial cell focal adhesions and contain counteradhesive domains (Sage, 1997).

ADHESION AND MIGRATION

Adhesion of the endothelial cells to the matrix is accomplished by several adhesive proteins, of which the most important appear to be the integrins. The integrins are critical mediators of several adhesive functions in diverse cell types. This family consists of heterodimeric transmembrane proteins with an extracellular domain that binds to one or more components of the extracellular matrix and an intracellular domain that is linked to the cytoskeleton (Shattil and Ginsberg, 1997). Integrins are comprised of two subunits, termed α and β, which are linked noncovalently. Both α, and especially β, subunits can associate with multiple subunits of the other subtype. The principal integrins expressed in endothelial cells are five members in the β1 series, plus the two vitronectin receptors αvβ3 and αvβ5 (Table 2.4). The matrix proteins bound by endothelial cell integrins include vitronectin, laminin, fibrinogen, collagen, thrombospondin, von Willebrand factor, and fibronectin. The cytoplasmic domain of integrins binds to many proteins, both cytoskeletal and signaling, only some of

Table 2.4 Endothelial Integrin Receptors

Integrin	*CD*	*Common Name*	*Ligands*
Beta 1			
α1β1	49a/29	Collagen receptor	Laminin, collagen
α2β1	49b/29	Collagen receptor	Laminin, collagen
α3β1	49c/29	Collagen receptor	Fibronectin, laminin
α5β1	49e/29	Fibronectin receptor	Fibronectin
α6β1	49f/29	Laminin receptor	Laminin
Beta3			
αvβ3	51/61	Vitronectin receptor	Vitronectin, fibrinogen, von Willebrand factor, fibronectin
Beta5			
αvβ5	51/	Vitronectin receptor	Vitronectin, fibronectin

which have been identified. The β subunits have intrinsic signals for localization to focal adhesions; such localization is blocked by the α subunit, but binding of a ligand relieves this inhibition and allows the β subunit's signal to direct the integrin heterodimer into the focal adhesion. Linkage of proteins such as talin and α-actinin to integrins also occurs at the focal adhesions (Clark and Brugge, 1995).

Integrins can act as signaling receptors as well; several cytosolic proteins become phosphorylated on tyrosine only with binding of integrins to matrix, including certain proteins (e.g., FAK, pp60src, and pp72syk) that are associated with focal adhesions. Activation of PI3 kinase and the ERKs also occurs subsequent to integrin binding, similar to the case with activation of cytokine receptors. In fact, a striking feature of recent intense investigation into integrin-mediated signaling is that the "outside-in" pathways regulated by integrins are the same as those regulated by growth factor receptors (Fig. 2.4) (Schwartz, 1997). In general, the effects appear to be synergistic between the growth factors and adhesion; for instance, activation of PKC, MAP kinase, and PI3 kinase by cytokines is enhanced markedly by adhesion. Although the details of the mechanism by which this occurs are not yet known, there is at least one pathway dependent upon Ras that employs the membrane-associated docking protein Shc, which binds to integrin subunits in fibroblasts. Ras activation is required for integrin-mediated ERK activation, but not its effects on adhesion, or formation of stress fibers or focal adhesions (Clark and Hynes, 1996). Whether the Ras dependent pathway is also required in endothelial cells is not known. Binding to the matrix via integrin receptors is essential for endothelial cell survival and angiogenesis, as apoptosis results when the cells are prevented from such binding (Meredith and Schwartz, 1997). Exactly how the extracellular matrix affects endothelial cell adhesion, cytoskeletal function, and proliferation, however, is not entirely known and is a central question in vascular biology research.

Both αvβ3 and -β5, as well as α2β1, integrin receptors are upregulated in angiogenic blood vessels (Senger et al., 1997) and participate in formation of capillary tubules in models of angiogenesis in vitro (Gamble et al., 1993). The β1 integrins do not appear to be required for endothelial cell survival but may be associated with branching of the vasculature (Brooks et al., 1994a). Cultured endothelial cells are dependent on αvβ3 for survival; if αvβ3's binding to matrix is blocked with RGD peptides, such cells in vitro, and angiogenic endothelial cells in vivo, will undergo apoptosis (Brooks et al., 1994b). The ligand that αvβ3 requires to support angiogenesis is not clear, but it is unlikely to be vitronectin; one possibility is osteopontin, an RGD-containing protein expressed at high levels in injured blood vessels (Liaw et al., 1995). Osteopontin is a natural substrate for thrombin, which appears to expose a recognition sequence for αvβ3 in osteopontin. Recent experiments have shown that αvβ3 integrin also binds the adhesion molecule PECAM (Newman, 1997) and is linked to the metalloproteinase MMP-2 that plays a prime role in matrix dissolution (Brooks et al., 1996). Additionally, proteolysis of basal membrane collagen exposes adhesion sequences that interact with αvβ3. The apparent dependence of angiogenic endothelium on αvβ3 contrasts with observations made in certain individuals who are born without β3 integrins (one of the variants of Glanzmann's thrombasthenia) (Newman et al., 1991). Although such individuals have platelet defects, they develop and give birth normally, have normal wound healing and a full life span. One possibility is that αvβ5 can, under some circumstances, support angiogenesis; this pathway appears to be used for angiogenesis resulting from exogenous VEGF or TGF-α and depends upon activation of PKC (Friedlander et al., 1995). Such activation is required for αvβ5-dependent localization of focal adhesions and FAK phosphorylation (Lewis et al., 1996). In contrast, angiogenesis mediated by TNF-α or FGF-2 depends upon αvβ3 and is not blocked by chemical PKC inhibitors (Friedlander et al., 1995). Antibody- or peptide-mediated blockade of both classes of αv integrin receptors prevents endothelial growth and angiogenesis without disturbing nonproliferating endothelial cells. In addition to causing apoptosis, disruption of the requisite adhesion events for endothelial cells in a sprouting vessel may result in their inability to align properly and thus assemble into a new capillary blood vessel.

Several other classes of adhesion receptors have been identified in endothelial cells, including members of the immunoglobulin superfamily (e.g., ICAM, VCAM, and PECAM), the selectin family (E- and P-selectin), and cadherins (Bischoff, 1997). Many of these receptors are important components of the mechanism by which neutrophils, monocytes, or lymphocytes bind to the inflamed endothelium, but their relationship to endothelial growth and migration is not known, with a few exceptions. E-selectin is one of the few adhesion receptors whose expression is restricted to endothelium. Its function appears to be required for angiogenesis, at least under some circumstances; blockade of the protein itself or of its glycoprotein ligands prevents tube formation by capillary cells. In models of wound healing in vitro, the endothelial cells in the wound front express high amounts of E-selectin (Bischoff, 1997). Furthermore, expression of E-selectin correlates with new vessel formation and addition of soluble E-selectin induces angiogenesis in some animal models. Soluble VCAM induces enhanced migration of endothelial cells and in vivo angiogenesis in animal models, suggesting that the native cell-bound molecule may have a physiologic role in those events. Those studies delivered soluble E-selectin and VCAM as recombinant proteins, but some have proposed that proteases released from macrophages cleave the cell-bound adhesion molecules to produce soluble forms in vivo.

Some adhesion proteins are clustered at the site of endothelial cell-to-cell contacts, and thus have been postulated to participate in angiogenesis. Cadherins exhibit functional adhesion activity when they form complexes with catenins, which are components of focal adhesions (Gumbiner, 1996), and the actin cytoskeleton. The principal cadherin in endothelial cells, VE-cadherin or cadherin-5, is known to inhibit cell migration, and becomes tyrosine phosphorylated (which probably inactivates it) upon stimulation with angiogenic agents. It is expressed weakly in vascular tumors but strongly at the junction points of quiescent endothelial cells (Dejana, 1997). PECAM-1 promotes homotypic endothelial cell adhesion and thus might contribute to the assembly of vascular structures. Anti-PECAM-1 antibodies prevent the formation of tight endothelial monolayers, thus suggesting that PECAM-1 stabilizes initial endothelial cell–cell contact (Newman, 1997). PECAM-1 is a particularly attractive candidate for a role in endothelial growth because of recent findings that it transmits signals into and receives signals from the cell interior. The molecule becomes tyrosine phosphorylated after either its engagement or integrin-mediated cellular adhesion (Jackson et al., 1997). Although PECAM-1 doesn't have the cytoplasmic kinase domain characteristic of receptor tyrosine kinases, its phosphorylation permits the assembly of a signaling complex that includes the tyrosine phosphatase SHP-2 and leads to activation of the Ras pathway described previously. In addition, PECAM-1 interacts in a number of ways with other adhesion molecules, and thus might facilitate endothelial migration (Newman, 1997). For instance, expression of E-selectin is enhanced by the inhibition of PECAM-1, and integrin engagement can change the phosphorylation state of, and presumably the resultant signaling pathways used by, PECAM-1.

Migrating endothelial cells develop a specific phenotype, which includes upregulation of several cell surface glycoproteins associated specifically with migration (Augustin-Voss and Pauli, 1992). As an endothelial cell migrates, the components involved in regulating adhesion and the cytoskeleton interact closely. Integrins become engaged at the leading edge of the cytoskeletal-mediated extensions (lamellipodia and filopodia) and thus interact with the matrix (Gumbiner, 1996). Focal complexes are detected at these leading edges; myosin is excluded from these regions, thus suggesting that formation of the focal adhesion complexes utilizes actin filaments alone. These focal adhesion complexes dissemble as well, both at the trailing edge of the migrating cell at the sites of cytoskeletal retraction and near the leading edge. The mechanism behind such disassembly is not fully characterized but may be partially regulated by FAK.

CELL CYCLE

Endothelial cells must proliferate for new capillaries to be formed, and to undergo mitosis, they must progress through the cell cycle. Endothelial cells in unstimulated blood vessels neither synthesize DNA nor undergo mitosis; these quiescent endothelial cells are in a resting phase of the cell cycle called G0, which is actually outside of the cycle (Fig. 2.7). After injury or stimulation with an angiogenic agent, endothelial cells reenter the cell cycle, which leads to a series of reactions that eventually results in DNA synthesis and cell division. The first change is an increase in the number

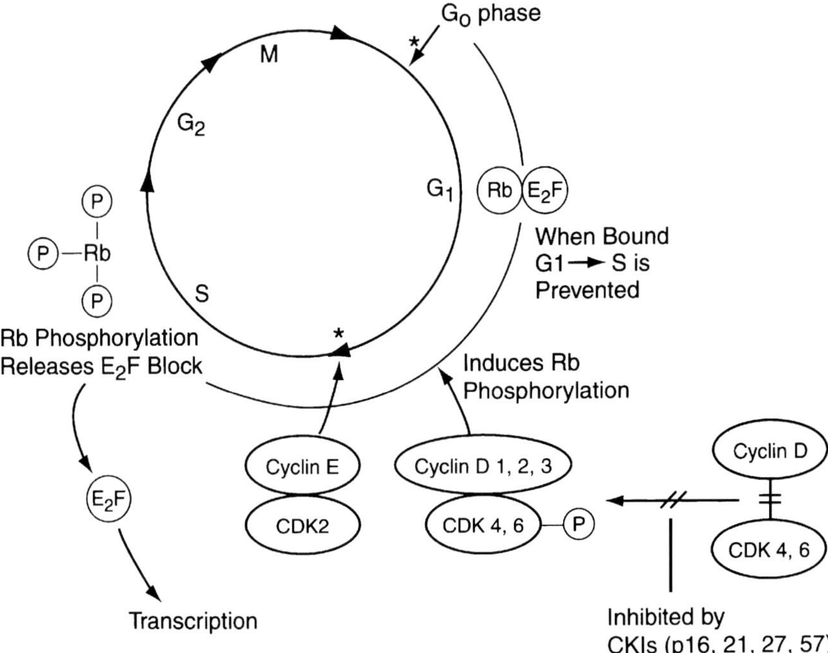

Figure 2.7 Schematic diagram of cell cycle regulation in mammalian cells. At least two checkpoints (marked *) require the presence of growth factors and signals from adhesion receptors before progression.

of endothelial cells that enter from G0 into a first so-called *gap phase* (G1). The cells then pass into S phase, during which DNA synthesis and chromosome replication occur, which is then followed by a second gap phase coupled with mitosis (G2/M). Entry from G1 into the S phase requires adherence to matrix throughout most of G1. After that, it is dispensable (Ingber et al., 1995).

The precise controls over the endothelial cell cycle are not known, for the most part. Most cytokines that promote angiogenesis are thought to promote cell cycle progression by acting on one or more of the controls that allow entry into G1 or exit from this phase to S phase so that DNA synthesis can begin.

One of the critical factors that regulates transcription of genes that control cell cycle progression is the retinoblastoma protein (Rb) (Weinberg, 1995). The function of Rb is controlled by reversible phosphorylation by cyclin-dependent kinases active in G1. When it is unphosphorylated (usually in G0 or G1), it binds to several transcription factors, of which the E2F family is the best characterized. When so bound, E2F-mediated transcription of its target genes, several of which are involved in cell cycle progression, does not occur. Phosphorylation of Rb allows for the release of E2F, which subsequently promotes transcription of its regulated genes. Rb phosphorylation and mRNA expression of E2F and other transcription factors are increased in endothelial cells as they pass through G1, as is the case in other cells in which these elements have been found to be of importance in control of the cell cycle.

Other cell cycle controls include the cyclins and the cyclin-dependent kinases (cdks). The cdks are expressed constitutively, but they remain inactive unless they combine with specific cyclin partners. Those cdks that phosphorylate Rb are cdk4, in combination with the cyclin Ds, and cdk2, which interacts with cyclin E. The expression of cyclin D is strongly induced during G1 phase in endothelial cells, and the activity of cdks 2 and 4 increase as well. Expression of cyclin D appears to be required for Rb phosphorylation and entry into S phase of the cell cycle (Assoian and Marcantonio, 1997). The presence of cytokines and contact with extracellular matrix, probably via integrin receptors, are both needed before cyclin D can become expressed. Cyclin E expression and its formation of complexes with cdk2 occur in late G1 phase, which appears to be a consequence of the ability of matrix–receptor interaction and cytokines to control inhibitors of the cdks. The most-studied group of these inhibitors is p21 and its relatives p16, p27, and p57. Intracellular signals generated separately by matrix and cytokines regulate the levels of both p21 and p27 and thus ensure timely activation of cyclin E and cdk2 late in G1 (Bottazi and Assoian, 1997). The signal transduction pathways that lead to p21 or p27 activation are not completely worked out but appear to involve the ras/ERK pathway for p21 and p70/S6K for p27. Tyrosine phosphatases also regulate p21, whose expression is reduced in endothelial cells that undergo differentiation but not in those that undergo apoptosis (Yang et al., 1996a). The last cyclin to be transcribed before DNA synthesis is cyclin A; this induction also requires both cytokines and attachment to the extracellular matrix (Bottazi and Assoian, 1997).

Another important regulator of cell cycle arrest is p53, a ubiquitous DNA-binding protein that works in late G1 phase by upregulating p21. Apoptosis can also be induced by p53, which suggests that this regulator can participate in both growth arrest and programmed cell death, depending on cellular context. During angiogenesis, p53 activity and p21 expression are suppressed; these actions appear to depend on the $\alpha v\beta 3$ integrin (Stromblad et al., 1996). P21 is induced in injured arteries, and overexpression of p21 can prevent the growth of both vascular smooth muscle and endothelial cells, as well as neointimal formation (Yang et al., 1996b).

Two of the small GTP-binding proteins whose role in controlling the cytoskeleton was discussed previously are also required for progression through certain discrete points of the cell cycle. Inhibition of Rho causes arrest in G1, before DNA synthesis (Yamamoto et al., 1993) and Rac inhibition causes arrest at G2/M in fibroblasts (Moore et al., 1997). Whether these effects are secondary to their effects on the cytoskeleton or instead are separate functions is not known.

THERAPEUTIC IMPLICATIONS

As noted in Chapter 13, therapy with currently identified growth factors, while promising, has been associated with side effects in animal models, including systemic hypotension, and renal damage, and the possibility for untoward angiogenesis or other mitogenesis is likely to cause concerns when their clinical use becomes more widespread. As possible alternatives to the use of systemic or exogenous factors, changes in matrix composition and adhesion receptors that occur in angiogenic endothelium might be exploited so that only activated endothelial cells would be affected. Another approach focuses on intracellular mediators. A number of compounds targeted at defined intracellular components of the signal transduction cascade are under development. These include inhibitors of individual PKC isoenzymes, MAP kinase antagonists, compounds that interfere with SH2 or SH3 docking domains, and Ras and Raf kinase inhibitors. These approaches, while possibly not specific for an individual cell type, are nonetheless feasible if localized or cell type-specific delivery methods become available. There are two potentially attractive aspects of such therapy. First, a blocker might be identified that interfered with a final common pathway for a critical endothelial process, and thus could be quite potent. Second, this approach raises the possibility that individual endothelial functions (e.g., expression of leukocyte-binding receptors) could be blocked while preserving others (e.g., endothelial cell migration). Thus, stimulation or inhibition of intracellular targets with agents based on intracellular mediators may prove to be an important alternative to the use of mitogens to manipulate the function of the endothelial cell, and thus subsequent blood vessel formation.

REFERENCES

Aepfelbacher, M., Essler, M., Huber, E., Sugai, M., and Weber, P. C. (1997). Bacterial toxins block endothelial wound repair. Arterioscler. Thromb. Vasc. Biol. 17: 1623–1629.

Amano, M., Chihara, K., Kimura, K., Fukata, Y., Nakamura, N., Matsuura, Y., and Kaibuchi, K. (1997). Formation of actin stress fibers and focal adhesions enhanced by Rho-kinase. Science 275: 1308–1311.

Asahara, T., Murohara, T., Sullivan, A., Silver, M., van der Zee, R., Li, T., Witzenbichler, B., Schatteman, G., and Isner, J. M. (1997). Isolation of putative progenitor endothelial cells for angiogenesis. Science 275: 964–967.

Assoian, R. K., and Marcantonio, E. E. (1997). The extracellular matrix as a cell cycle control element in atherosclerosis and restenosis. J. Clin. Invest. 100: S15–S17.

Augustin-Voss, H. G. and Pauli, B. U. (1992). Migrating endothelial cells are distinctly hyperglycosylated and express specific migration-associated cell surface glycoproteins. J. Cell Biol. 119: 483–491.

Balboa, M. A., Firestein, B. L., Godson, C., Bell, K. S., and Insel, P. A. (1994). Protein kinase C mediates phospholipase D activation by nucleotides and phorbol ester in Madin-Darby canine kidney cells. J. Biol. Chem. 269: 10511–10516.

Besser, D., Presta, M. and Nagamine, Y. (1995). Elucidation of a signaling pathway induced by FGF-2 leading to uPA gene expression in NIH 3T3 fibroblasts. Cell Growth Differ. 6: 1009–1017.

Biro, S., Yu, Z. X., Fu, Y. M., Smale, G., Sasse, J., Sanchez, J., Ferrans, V. J., and Casscells, W. (1994). Expression and subcellular distribution of basic fibroblast growth factor are regulated during migration of endothelial cells. Circ. Res. 74: 485–494.

Bischoff, J. (1997). Cell adhesion and angiogenesis. J. Clin. Invest. 100: S37–S39.

Bottazzi, M. E. and Assoian, R. K. (1997). The extracellular matrix and mitogenic growth factors control G1 phase cyclins and cyclin-dependent kinase inhibitors. Trends Cell Biol. 7: 348–352.

Boudreau, N., Andrews, C., Srebrow, A., Ravanpay, A. and Cheresh, D. A. (1997). Induction of the angiogenic phenotype by Hox D3. J. Cell Biol. 139: 257–264.

Brooks, P. C., Clark, R. A. F., and Cheresh, D. A. (1994a). Requirement of integrin $\alpha v\beta 3$ for angiogenesis. Science 264: 569–571.

Brooks, P. C., Montgomery, A. M. P., Rosenfeld, M., Reisfeld, R. A., Hu, T., Klier, G., and Cheresh, D. A. (1994b). Integrin $\alpha v\beta 3$ antagonists promote tumor regression by inducing apoptosis of angiogenic blood vessels. Cell 70: 1157–1164.

Brooks, P. C., Strömblad, S., Sanders, L. C., von Schalscha, T. L., Aimes, R. T., Stetler-Stevenson, W. G., Quigley, J. P., and Cheresh, D. A. (1996). Localization of matrix metalloproteinase MMP-2 to the surface of invasive cells by interaction with integrin $\alpha v\beta 3$. Cell 85: 683–693.

Burridge, K., Chrzanowska-Wodnicka, M., and Zhong, C. (1997). Focal adhesion assembly. Trends Cell Biol. 7: 342–347.

Carmeliet, P., Moons, L., Dewerchin, M., Rosenberg, S., Herbert, J-M., Lupu, F., and Collen, D. (1998). Receptor-independent role of urokinase-type plasminogen activator in pericellular plasmin and matrix metalloproteinase proteolysis during vascular wound healing in mice. J. Cell Biol. 140: 233–245.

Cheng, G., Lui, B. F., Yu, Y., Diglio, C., and Kuo, T. H. (1996). The exit from G(0) into the cell cycle requires and is controlled by sarco (endo) plasmic reticulum Ca^{2+} pump. Biochem. Biophys. Res. Commun. 329: 65–72.

Clark, E. A. and Brugge, J. S. (1995). Integrins and signal transduction pathways. The road taken. Science 268: 233–239.

Clark, E. A. and Hynes, R. O. (1996). Ras activation is necessary for integrin-mediated activation of extracellular signal-regulated kinase 2 and cytosolic phospholipase A2 but not for cytoskeletal organization. J. Biol. Chem. 271: 14814–14818.

Cohen, T., Nahari, D., Cerem, L. W., Neufeld, G., and Levi, B. Z. (1996). Interleukin 6 induces the expression of vascular endothelial growth factor. J. Biol. Chem. 271: 736–741.

Dejana, E. (1997). Endothelial adherens junctions: implications in the control of vascular permeability and angiogenesis. J. Clin. Invest. 100: S7–S10.

Draijer, R., Atsma, D. E., van der Laarse, A., and van Hinsbergh, V. W. M. (1995). CGMP and nitric oxide modulate thrombin-induced endothelial permeability. Circ. Res. 76: 199–208.

Dumler, I., Weis, A., Mayboroda, O. A., Maasch, C., Jerke, U., Haller, H., and Gulba, D. C. (1998). The jak/stat pathway and urokinase receptor signaling in human aortic vascular smooth muscle cells. J. Biol. Chem. 273: 315–321.

Fleming, I., Fisslthaler, B., and Busse, R. (1995). Calcium signaling in endothelial cells involves activation of tyrosine kinases and leads to activation of mitogen-activated protein kinases. Circ. Res. 76: 522–529.

Folkman, J. (1995). Clinical applications of research on angiogenesis. N. Engl. J. Med. 333: 1757–1763.

Friedlander, M., Brooks, P. C., Shaffer, R. W., Kincaid, C. M., Varner, J. A., and Cheresh, D. A. (1995). Definition of two angiogenic pathways by distinct αv integrins. Science 270: 1500–1502.

Gallagher, G. L. and Sumpio, B. E. (1997). Endothelial Cells. In "The Basic Science of Vascular Disease." Chapter 6; pp. 151–186. eds: Sidawy A. N., Sumpio B. E., De Palma R. G. Futura Publishing, Armonk.

Gamble, J. R., Matthias, L. J., Meyer, G., Kaur, P., Russ, G., Faull, R., Berndt, M. C., and Vadas, M. A. (1993). Regulation of in vitro capillary tube formation by anti-integrin antibodies. J. Cell Biol. 121: 931–943.

Gottlieb A. I., Langille, B. L., Wong, M. K., and Kim, D. W. (1991). Structure and function of the endothelial cytoskeleton. Lab. Invest. Rev. 65: 123–137.

Grant, D. S., Tashiro, K-I, Segui-Real, B., Yamada, Y., Martin, G. R., and Kleinman, H. K. (1989). Two different laminin domains mediate the differentiation of human endothelial cells into capillary like structures. Cell 58: 933–943.

Griendling, K. K. and Alexander, R. W. (1996). Endothelial control of the cardiovascular system: recent advances. FASEB J. 10: 283–292.

Gumbiner, B. M. (1996). Cell adhesion: the molecular basis of tissue architecture and morphogenesis. Cell 84: 345–357.

Guo, D., Jia, Q., Song, H. Y., Warren, R. S., and Donner, D. B. (1995). Vascular endothelial cell growth factor promotes tyrosine phosphorylation of mediators of signal transduction that contain SH2 domains. Association with endothelial cell proliferation. J. Biol. Chem. 270: 6729–6733.

Hamm, H. E. (1998). The many faces of G protein signaling. J. Cell Biol. 273: 669–672.

Haralabopoulos, G. C., Grant D. S., Kleinman H. K., and Maragoudakis M. E. (1997). Thrombin promotes endothelial cell alignment in Matrigel in vitro and angiogenesis in vivo. Am. J. Physiol. 273: C239–245.

Harrington, E. O., Loffler, J., Nelson, P. R., Kent, K. C., Simons, M., and Ware, J. A. (1997). Enhancement of migration by PKC alpha and inhibition of proliferation and cell cycle progression by PKC delta in capillary endothelial cells. J. Biol. Chem. 272: 7390–7397.

Himmel, H. M., Whorton, A. R., and Strauss, H. C. (1993). Intracellular calcium, currents, and stimulus-response coupling in endothelial cells. Review. Hypertension 21: 112–127.

Ingber, D. E., Prusty, D., Sun, Z., Betensky, H., and Wang, N. (1995). Cell shape, cytoskeletal mechanics, and cell cycle control in angiogenesis. J. Biomech. 28: 1471–1484.

Isner J. M. (1997). Oligonucleotide therapeutics—novel cardiovascular targets. Nat. Med. 3: 834–835.

Ito, K., Ryuto, M., Ushiro, S., Ono, M., Sugenoya, A., Kuraoka, A., Shibata, Y., and Kuwano, M. (1995). Expression of tissue-type plasminogen activator and its inhibitor couples with development of capillary network by human microvascular endothelial cells on Matrigel. J. Cell. Physiol. 162: 213–224.

Jackson, D. E., Kupcho, K. R., and Newman, P. J. (1997). Characterization of phosphotyrosine binding motifs in the cytoplasmic domain of platelet/endothelial cell adhesion molecule-1 (PECAM-1) that are required for the cellular association and activation of the protein-tyrosine phosphatase, SHP-2. Biol. Chem. 272: 24868–24875.

Kanda, S., Hodgkin, M. N., Woodfield, R. J., Wakelam, M. J., Thomas, G., and Claesson-Welsh, L. (1997). Phosphatidylinositol 3'-kinase-independent p70 S6 kinase activation by fibroblast growth factor receptor-1 is important for proliferation but not differentiation of endothelial cells. J. Biol. Chem. 272: 23347–23353.

Kanse, S. M., Kost, C., Wilhelm, O. G., Andreasen, P. A., and Preissner, K. T. (1996). The urokinase receptor is a major vitronectin-binding protein on endothelial cells. Exp. Cell Res. 224: 344–353.

Kent, K. C., Mii, S., Harrington, E. O., Chang, J. D., Mallette, S., and Ware, J. A. (1995). Requirement for protein kinase C activation in bFGF-induced endothelial cell proliferation. Circ. Res. 77: 231–238.

Khachigan, L. M. and Collins, T. (1997). Inducible expression of Egr-1-dependent genes. Circ. Res. 81: 457–461.

Koolwijk, P., van Erck, M. G., de Vree, W. J., Vermeer, M. A., and Weich, H. A. (1996). Cooperative effect of TNF α, bFGF, and VEGF on the formation of tubular structures of human microvascular endothelial cells in a fibrin matrix. Role of urokinase activity. J. Cell Biol. 132: 1177–1188.

Leavesley, D. I., Schwartz, M. A., Rosenfeld, M., and Cheresh, D. A. (1993). Integrin β1-and β3-mediated endothelial cell migration is triggered through distinct signaling mechanisms. J. Cell Biol. 121: 163–170.

Lewis, J. M., Cheresh, D. A., and Schwartz, M. A. (1996). Protein kinase C regulates αvβ5-dependent cytoskeletal associations and focal adhesion kinase phosphorylation. J. Cell Biol. 134: 1323–1332.

Liaw, L., Lindner, V., Schwartz, S. M., Chambers, A. F., and Giachelli, C. M. (1995).

Osteopontin and B_3 integrin are coordinately expressed in regenerating endothelium in vivo and stimulate Arg-Gly-Asp-dependent endothelial migration in vitro. Circ. Res. 77: 665–672.

Lisanti, M. P., Scherer, P. E., Vidugiriene, J., Tang, Z., Hermanowski-Vosatka, A., Tu, Y. H., Cook, R. F., and Sargiacomo, M. (1994). Characterization of caveolin-rich membrane domains isolated from an endothelial-rich source: implications for human disease. J. Cell Biol. 126: 111–126.

Machesky, L. M., and Hall, A. (1997). Role of actin polymerization and adhesion to extracellular matrix in Rac- and Rho-induced cytoskeletal reorganization. J. Cell Biol. 138: 913–926.

Malarkey, K., Belham, C. M., Paul, A., Graham, A., McLees, A., Scott, P. H., and Plevin, R. (1995). The regulation of tyrosine kinase signaling pathways by growth factor and G-protein-coupled receptors. Biochem. J. 309: 361–375.

Meredith, J. E. Jr., and Schwartz, M. A. (1997). Integrins, adhesion and apoptosis. Trends Cell Biol. 7: 146–147.

Mohammadi, M., Dionne, C. A., Li, W., Li, T., Spivak, T., Honegger, A. M., Jaye, M., and Schlessinger, J. (1992). Point mutation in FGF receptor eliminates phosphatidylinositol hydrolysis without affecting mitogenesis. Nature 358: 681–684.

Montrucchio, G., Lupia, E., de Martino, A., Battaglia, E., Arese, M., Tizzani, A., Bussolino, F., and Camussi, G. (1997). Nitric oxide mediates angiogenesis induced in vivo by platelet-activating factor and tumor necrosis factor-α. Am. J. Pathol. 151: 557–563.

Moore, K. A., Sethi, R., Doanes, A. M., Johnson, T. M., Pracyk, J. B., Kirby, M., Irani, K., Goldschmidt-Clermont, P. J., and Finkel, T. (1997). Rac1 is required for cell proliferation and G2/M progression. Biochem. J. 326: 17–20.

Newman, P. J. (1997). The biology of PECAM-1. J. Clin. Invest. 100: S25–29.

Newman, P. J., Seligsohn, U., Lyman, S., and Coller, B. S. (1991). The molecular genetic basis of Glanzmann thrombasthenia in the Iraqi-Jewish and Arab populations in Israel. Proc. Natl. Acad. Sci. USA 88: 3160–3164.

Offermanns, S., Mancino, V., Revel, J-P, and Simon, M. I. (1997). Vascular system defects and impaired cell chemokinesis as a result of $G\alpha_{13}$ deficiency. Science 275: 533–535.

Pepper, M. S., Sappino, A.-P., Stöcklin, R., Montesano, R., Orci, L., and Vassalli, J.-D. (1993). Upregulation of urokinase receptor expression on migrating endothelial cells. J. Cell Biol. 122: 673–684.

Peters, K. G., Marie, J., Wilson, E., Ives, H. E., Escobedo, J., Del Rosario, M., Mirda, D., and Williams, L. T. (1992). Point mutation of an FGF receptor abolishes phosphatidylinositol turnover and Ca^{2+} flux but not mitogenesis. Nature 358: 678–681.

Sa, G., Murugesan, G., Jaye, M., Ivashchenko, Y., and Fox, P. L. (1995). Activation of cytosolic phospholipase A2 by basic fibroblast growth factor via a p42 mitogen-activated protein kinase-dependent phosphorylation pathway in endothelial cells. J. Biol. Chem. 270: 2360–2366.

Sage, E. H. (1997). Pieces of eight: bioactive fragments of extracellular proteins as regulators of angiogenesis. Trends Cell Biol. 7: 182–186.

Sato, Y., and Rifkin, D. B., (1988). Autocrine activities of basic fibroblast growth factor: regulation of endothelial cell movement, plasminogen activator synthesis, and DNA synthesis. J. Cell Biol. 107: 1199–1205.

Schindler, C. and Darnell, J. E. (1995). Transcriptional responses to polypeptide ligands: the JAK-STAT pathway. Annu. Rev. Biochem. 64: 621–651.

Schnitzer, J. E., McIntosh, D. P., Dvorak, A. M., Liu, J., and Oh, P. (1995). Organized endothelial cell surface signal transduction in caveolae distinct from glycosylphosphatidylinositol-anchored protein microdomains. Science 269: 1435–1439.

Schwartz, M. A. (1997). Integrins, oncogenes, and anchorage independence. J. Cell Biol.139: 575–578.

Senger, D. R., Claffey, K. P., Benes, J. E., Perruzzi, C. A., Sergiou, A. P., and Detmar, M. (1997). Angiogenesis promoted by vascular endothelial growth factor: regulation through $\alpha_1\beta_1$ and $\alpha_2\beta_1$ integrins. Proc. Natl. Acad. Sci. USA 94: 13612–13617.

Shattil, S. J. and Ginsberg, M. H. (1997). Integrin signaling in vascular biology. J. Clin. Invest. 100:S91–S95.

Stoltz, R. A., Abraham, N. G., and Schwartzman, M. L. (1996). The role of NF-κB in the angiogenic response of coronary microvessel endothelial cells. Proc. Natl. Acad. Sci. USA 93: 2832–2837.

Stromblad, S., Becker, J. C., Yebra, M., Brooks, P. C., and Cheresh, D. A. (1996). Suppression of p53 activity and p21WAF1/CIP1 expression by vascular cell integrin $\alpha v\beta 3$ during angiogenesis. J. Clin. Invest. 98: 426–433.

Tang S., Morgan K. G., Parker C., and Ware J. A. (1997). Requirement for protein kinase C theta for cell cycle progression and formation of actin stress fibers and filopodia in vascular endothelial cells. J. Biol. Chem. 272: 28704–28711.

Toker, A., Meyer, M., Reddy, K. K., Falk, J. R., Aneja, R., Aneja, S., Parra, A., Burns, D. J., Ballas, L. M., and Cantley, L. C. (1994). Activation of protein kinase C family members by the novel polyphosphoinositides PtdIns-3,4-P2 and PtdIns-3,4,5-P3. J. Biol. Chem. 269: 32358–32367.

Tsurumi, Y., Murohara, T., Krasinski, K., Chen, D., Witzenbichler, B., Kearney, M., Couffinihal, T. and Isner, J. M. (1997). Reciprocal relation between VEGF and NO in the regulation of endothelial integrity. Nat. Med. 3: 879–885.

van der Geer, P., Hunter, T., and Lindberg, R. A. (1994). Receptor protein-tyrosine kinases and their signal transduction pathways. Ann. Rev. Cell Biol. 10: 251–337.

van Hinsberg, V. W. M. (1997). Endothelial permeability for macromolecules. Arterioscler. Thromb. Vasc. Biol. 17: 1018–1023.

Ware, J. A., and Simons, M. (1997). Angiogenesis in ischemic heart disease. Nat. Med. 3: 158–164

Weinberg, R. A. (1995). The retinoblastoma protein and cell cycle control. Cell. 81: 323–330.

Yamamoto, M., Marui, N., Sakai, T., Morui, N., Kozaki, S., Ikai, K., Imamura, S., and Narumiya, S. (1993). ADP-ribosylation of the rhoA gene product by botulinum C3 exoenzyme causes Swiss 3T3 cells to accumulate in the G1 phase of the cell cycle. Oncogene 8: 1449–1455.

Yang, C., Chang, J., Gorospe, M., and Passaniti, A. (1996a). Protein tyrosine phosphatase regulation of endothelial cell apoptosis and differentiation. Cell Growth Differ. 7: 161–171.

Yang, Z. Y., Simari, R. D., Perkins, N. D., San, H., Gordon, D., Nabel, G. J., and Nabel, E. G. (1996b). Role of the p21 cyclin-dependent kinase inhibitor in limiting intimal cell proliferation in response to arterial injury. Proc. Natl. Acad. Sci. USA 93: 7905–7910.

Zhan, X., Plourde, C., Hut, X., Friesel, R., and Maciag, T. (1994). Association of fibroblast growth factor receptor-1 with c-Src correlates with association between c-Src and cortactin. J. Biol. Chem. 269: 20221–20224.

Zhou, W., Takuwa, N., Kumadu, M., and Takuwa, Y. (1993). Protein kinase C-mediated bidirectional regulation of DNA synthesis, RB protein phosphorylation, and cyclin-dependent kinases in human vascular endothelial cells. J. Biol. Chem. 268: 23041–23048.

Ziche, M., Morbidelli, L., Choudhuri, R., Zhang, H. T., Donnini, S., Granger, H. J., and Bicknell, R. (1997). Nitric oxide synthase lies downstream from vascular endothelial growth factor-induced but not basic fibroblast growth factor-induced angiogenesis. J. Clin. Invest. 99: 2625–2634.

Zucker, S., Conner, C., DiMassmo, B. I., Ende, H., Drews, M., Seiki, M., and Bahou, W. F. (1995). Thrombin induces the activation of progelatinase A in vascular endothelial cells. Physiologic regulation of angiogenesis. J. Biol. Chem. 270: 23730–23738.

3

Heparan Sulfate Proteoglycans

NICHOLAS W. SHWORAK AND ROBERT D. ROSENBERG

Heparan sulfate proteoglycans (HSPGs)[1] are highly charged macromolecules consisting of different core proteins with covalently linked heparan sulfate chains (HS) of varying monosaccharide sequence. These molecules are involved in a multitude of biologic processes including regulation of mesoderm induction, extension of neurites, positioning of the heart, interactions of cells with adhesive proteins, proliferation of smooth muscle cells during atherogenesis, metabolism of lipoproteins, inhibition of thrombosis on the endothelial surface, and induction of angiogenesis (Rosenberg et al., 1997; Yanagishita and Hascall, 1992). Heparan sulfate proteoglycans are produced by virtually all cell types while a related molecule, heparin, an extremely modified form of heparan sulfate, is exclusively generated by mast cells.

Angiogenesis involves several events that are regulated by interactions between HSPGs and various effector proteins that occur at cell surfaces or within the interstitial extracellular matrix. In particular, the HS component (and heparin) binds tightly to both numerous angiogenic growth factors, including basic fibroblast growth factors and vascular endothelial growth factor, as well as angiogenic inhibitors such as platelet factor 4 and

[1]Abbreviations used in this chapter: CS, chondroitin sulfate; FGFs, fibroblast growth factors; GAG, glycosaminoglycan; GlcA, glucuronic acid; GlcA 2S, 2-*O*-sulfated glucuronic acid; GlcN, glucosamine; GlcNAc, *N*-acetylglucosamine; GlcN(Ac/S), *N*-acetyl or *N*-sulfated glucosamine; GlcNAc 6S, 6-*O*-sulfated *N*-acetylglucosamine; GlcNS 3S, 3S-*O*-sulfated *N*-sulfated glucosamine; GPI, glycosyl phosphatidylinositol; HexA, unspecified uronic acid, either GlcA or IdoA; HS, heparan sulfate chains; HSPG, heparan sulfate proteoglycan; IdoA, iduronic acid; IdoA 2S, 2-*O*-sulfated iduronic acid; NST, *N*-deacetylase/*N*-sulfotransferase; PAPS, 3'-phosphoadenosine 5'-phosphosulfate; PECAM, platelet-endothelial cell adhesion molecule; PG, proteoglycan; 2-OST, 2-*O*-sulfotransferase; 3-OST, 3-*O*-sulfotransferase; 6-OST, 6-*O*-sulfotransferase. For all sequences given, the linkages and configurations are →4-D-GlcApβ1→, →4-D-GlcNp(Ac/S)α1→, and →4-L-IdoApα1→.

thrombospondins. These interactions can affect growth factor stability, bioavailability, oligomerization, receptor activation, and internalization. In addition, there are high affinity interactions between HSPGs and proteases, protease inhibitors, extracellular matrix components including collagens and fibronectin, and cell adhesion molecules such as PECAM (DeLisser et al., 1997; Folkman and Shing, 1992; Norrby, 1997). Detailed investigations over the past decade have revealed that the HS component is a complex mixture of numerous individual fine structures. Thus, selective interactions with discrete protein ligands occur by distinct motifs, each comprised of a defined monosaccharide sequence.

In this chapter, we review structural features of the protein and carbohydrate components that define HSPGs, determine their unique functional properties, and distinguish this diverse group of molecules from other protein glycoconjugates. We also examine the biosynthetic machinary that generates HS, with particular emphasis on the mechanisms by which specific HS structures are formed. These observations provide a conceptual framework for elucidating the roles of HSPGs, bearing defined monosaccharide sequences, in multiple facets of angiogenesis, as well as other biologic processes.

NOMENCLATURE AND GENERAL STRUCTURAL FEATURES OF PROTEIN GLYCOCONJUGATES

Proteoglycans and Glycoproteins Have Distinctive Features

The unique characteristics of HSPGs are best illuminated by comparing key structural features of protein glycoconjugates. Proteoglycans (PGs) and glycoproteins are the two major categories of hybrid molecules that contain both protein and carbohydrate. PGs are comprised of a core protein to which is attached one or more (up to >100) very long, unbranched polysaccharide chains of the glycosaminoglycan (GAG) variety. In contrast, glycoproteins typically contain small, frequently branched, polysaccharide structures. Due to the difference in the size of the glycan moieties, most of the mass of a typical PG is predominantly carbohydrate, whereas protein is the major component of glycoproteins. For most PGs, the GAG moieties are attached through *O*-linkages at specific serine residues within a consensus sequence containing Ser-(Gly or Ala)-XXX-(Gly or Ala); however, *N*-glycosylation of asparagine positions can also occur. Although glycanation is usually complete, certain proteins (e.g., receptors for transferrin and "homing lymphocytes") can be synthesized either with or without GAG substituents and are designated as "part-time PGs." Both *N*- and *O*-linkages are common for glycoproteins, with the former occurring within the context Asn-XXX-(Ser or Thr) and the latter present on serine or threonine residues that occur in protein regions exhibiting surface accessibility and favorable primary and secondary structural features. Both types of glycoconjugates can be highly modified by addition of polysaccharides. The most extreme PG example is the mast cell glycoconjugate serglycin, which contains up to 24 consecutive Ser-Gly repeats that are heavily GAG-substituted. Mucins are glycoproteins having >50 % of their mass as *O*-linked saccharides, and glycoprotein regions that contain tightly packed *O*-glycosylation are referred to as mucin domains. Despite the above differences, PGs can also exhibit the small glycoprotein type glycans and can even contain mucin-type domains. Thus, PGs can also be glycoproteins; however, the GAG component conveys unique functional properties to the hybrid molecule (reviewed in Kjellén and Lindahl, 1991; Montreuil et al., 1986). This component is the common denominator that is used to classify PGs.

Comparison of Glycosaminoglycans: Heparan Sulfate Is the Most Structural Diverse GAG

The five major varieties of GAGs are the three glucosaminoglycans (heparan sulfate (HS)/heparin, keratan sulfate, and hyaluronan [hyaluronic acid]), the galactosaminoglycans chondroitin 4-sulfate/chondroitin 6-sulfate (collectively referred to as chondroitin sulfate or CS), and dermatan sulfate (Table 3.1). Each GAG is a copolymer of a repeated disaccharide comprised of an amino sugar linked to either a uronic acid or a galactose. The amino sugar is *N*-acetylglucosamine (GlcNAc) in the glucosaminoglycans and is *N*-acetylgalactosamine in the galactosaminoglycans. The second sugar of the copolymer is galactose for keratan sulfate and a uronic acid (HexA, either glucuronic or iduronic acid) for the remaining GAGs. Specifically, hyaluronan, chondroitin 4-sulfate, and chondroitin 6-sulfate only contain glucuronic acid (GlcA), whereas HS, heparin, and dermatan sulfate contain both GlcA and iduronic acid (IdoA). All of these GAGs are produced as proteoglycans, except for hyaluronan, which occurs only as a pure polysaccharide. Heparin is exclusively found in granules of mast cells, whereas the remaining GAGs occur in the extracellular matrix and are highly abundant in connective tissues. HS is the most ubiquitous form in that most cell types synthesize this GAG, including vascular endothelial and smooth muscle cells (reviewed in Ruoslahti, 1988).

Hyaluronan is the simplest of the GAG species, being comprised only of an unmodified copolymer. Interestingly, degradation of extracellular matrix creates short hyaluronan fragments that are very angiogenic. In contrast to hyaluronan, the copolymers of the remaining GAGs undergo modifications (epimerization and sulfations) that enhance structural diversity (Table 3.1). Both types of modifications occur to a variable extent and consequently generate complex mixtures containing multiple structures. Chondroitin 4-sulfate and chondroitin 6-sulfate contain only a single type of sulfation (on either the 4-*O*- or 6-*O*-position of *N*-

Table 3.1 Comparison of the Structural Features of Different Glycosaminoglycans

		Copolymer Composition						
		Amino Sugars			*Acid or Neutral Sugars*			
GAG Form[a]	*Typical Chain Length (Saccharides)*	*Saccharide*	*Sulfation Position*	*Linkage*	*Saccharide*	*Sulfation Position*	*Linkage*[b]	*Linkage to Core Protein*
Hyaluronan	5,000–15,000	*N*-acetylglucosamine		β-(1→4)	Glucuronic acid		β-(1→3)	No core protein
Chondroitin 4-sulfate	100–200	*N*-acetylgalactosamine	4-*O*-	β-(1→4)	Glucuronic acid		β-(1→3)	Serine
Chondroitin 6-sulfate	100–200	*N*-acetylgalactosamine	6-*O*-	β-(1→4)	Glucuronic acid		β-(1→3)	Serine
Dermatan sulfate	100–200	*N*-acetylgalactosamine	4-*O*-	β-(1→4)	Glucuromic acid or iduronic acid		β-(1→3) or α-(1→3)	Serine
Keratan sulfate	25–100	*N*-acetylglucosamine	6-*O*-	β-(1→3)	Galactose	6-*O*-	β-(1→4)	Asparagine
Heparin	30–100	*N*-acetylglucosamine or glucosamine	*N*-, 6-*O*-, 3-*O*-	α-(1→4)	Glucuronic acid or iduronic acid	2-*O*-	β-(1→4) or α-(1→4)	Serine
Heparan sulfate	100–200	*N*-acetylglucosamine or glucosamine	*N*-, 6-*O*-, 3-*O*-	α-(1→4)	Glucuronic acid or iduronic acid	2-*O*-	β-(1→4) or α-(1→4)	Serine

[a] Alternative names of various GAGs include heparitin sulfate (heparan sulfate), chondroitin sulfate A (chondroitin 4-sulfate), chondroitin sulfate B (dermatan sulfate), chondroitin sulfate C (chondroitin 6-sulfate), and hyaluronic acid (hyaluronan).

[b] The linkages generated from C1 of D-glucuronic acid and L-iduronic acid are physically identical but are differentially designated as β or α, respectively, on the basis of the D or L configurations.

acetylgalactosamine, respectively) and so are the most homogeneous of the modified GAGs.

Keratan is slightly more complex as two positions can be sulfated. For example, along the length of the keratan copolymer one can find four distinct disaccharide structures: unmodified, monosulfated on either the GlcNAc or the galactose, or substituted on both residues. Dermatan sulfate is sulfated in only one position but is comparably heterogeneous, as it contains two types of uronosyl residues (GlcA and IdoA) (reviewed in Ruoslahti, 1988).

HS is the most complex species and contains at least 21 distinct disaccharides. Thus the complexity of HS is comparable to that of proteins. HS and heparin exhibit extremely similar structures. The predominant distinguishing feature is that HS is less extensively modified than heparin. It now appears that a common biosynthetic machinery, described below, generates both forms and so heparin can be considered to be a biosynthetic variant of heparan. Both HS and heparin contain sulfates in five distinct positions—three potential sites on glucosaminyl residues and one site each on glucuronosyl and iduronosyl residues (Table 3.1, Fig. 3.1). Complexity is further enhanced by two factors. First, the amino group of glucosaminyl residues can have three forms: (1) acetylated, (2) *N*-sulfated

R_1 = H or SO_3^-
R_2 = H or SO_3^- or Ac

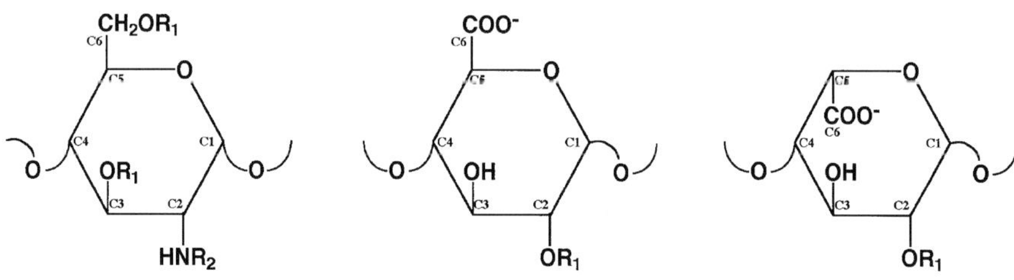

R_2 = H: Glucosamine (GlcN) Glucuronic acid (GlcA) Iduronic acid (IdoA)

R_2 = Ac: *N*-acetylglucosamine (GlcNAc)

R_2 = SO_3^-: *N*-sulfated glucosamine (GlcNS)

Figure 3.1. Monosaccharides found in heparan sulfate and heparin. Displayed are the hexosamines and hexuronic acids found in heparin and heparan. In general, glucosaminyl residues (GlcN, GlcNAc, and GlcNS) may be sulfated on the C1 amine (amino sulfation, *N*-sulfation) or on C3 or C6 hydroxyls (ester sulfation, *O*-sulfation). In amino sulfation the acetyl group of GlcNAc is replaced with a sulfate moiety. The uronosyl residues (GlcA and IdoA) may contain ester sulfates on the C2 hydroxyls. Ac is an acetyl group ($COCH_3$). The linkages and configurations are →4-D-GlcNp(Ac/S)α1→, →4-D-GlcApβ1→, and →4-L-IdoApα1→.

or (3) unmodified. The degree to which glucosamine residues are *N*-sulfated is idiosyncratic, with ~40% modification occurring in HS but >80% in heparin. The unmodified amino group does not occur in heparin but is enriched in HS from specific basement membranes and basal laminae, especially those surrounding capillaries and vascular smooth muscle cells of the kidney (van den Born et al., 1995). Second, HS and heparin also contain both GlcA and IdoA. The IdoA residues are generated by C-5 epimerization of GlcA moieties already present in the GAG copolymer. The resulting IdoA is less sterically constrained than GlcA; consequently HS, heparin and dermatan are the most flexible GAGs (reviewed in Casu, 1989; Lindahl et al., 1994). Such flexibility and the structural complexity of HS facilitate specific interactions of this GAG with a broad array of protein effector molecules.

Structure and Glycanation of Heparan Sulfate Proteoglycans

With the exception of hyaluronan, GAGs are synthesized in situ upon a protein core. The protein core defines the potential sites for GAG attachment as well as the types of GAGs which can be generated at each site; thus, HSPGs are generated from specific core proteins. The core proteins also exhibit structural features inherent to proteoglycan function. Within the cardiovascular system three major varieties of HSPGs are generated, which belong to the syndecan, glypican, and perlecan core protein families (Fig. 3.2).

The syndecan core protein family comprises four members in humans and mouse, but only a single homologue in *Drosophila* and *Caenorhabditis elegans.* Syndecan family core proteins exhibit cell-type specific distributions with vascular endothelial and smooth muscle cells expressing syndecans-1, -2, and -4. Syndecan-1 is specifically targeted to basolateral surfaces in polarized cuboidal epithelial cells, whereas syndecan-4 can be recruited into focal adhesions (Baciu and Goetinck, 1995; Miettinen et al., 1994) Syndecans are type I integral membrane proteins (the COOH-terminus occurs on the intracellular side of the cell membrane) that exhibit two divergent and two homologous domains. The divergent regions are an NH_2-terminal leader sequence that is absent in the mature protein, and an extracellular region containing multiple glycosaminoglycan (GAG) attachment sites as well as a dibasic protease cleavage sequence. Sequences are conserved about these structures, which suggests that this domain may function as a potentially cleavable protein scaffold onto which GAGs are attached. The distinct syndecan-4 residues 56–109 enable the extracellular domain to interact directly with cell surface molecules, which might facilitate the formation of signaling complexes (McFall and Rapraeger, 1997).

Amino acid sequences are highly conserved within the membrane spanning region, and the short cytoplasmic tail, which contains four fixed tyrosine residues and terminates with the shared sequence Glu-Phe-Tyr-Ala (reviewed in Bernfield et al., 1992; Carey, 1997) that comprises a PDZ domain-binding motif (Songyang et al., 1997). Residues flanking and

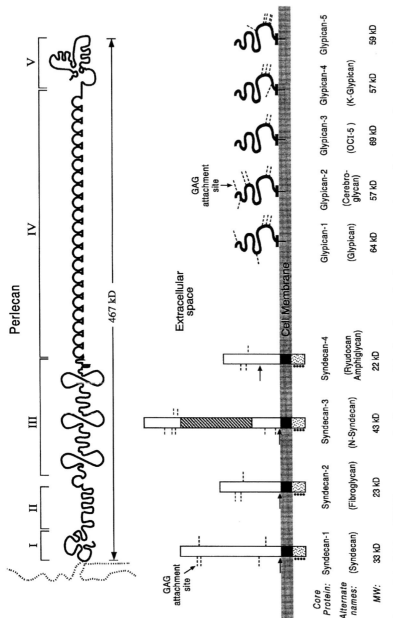

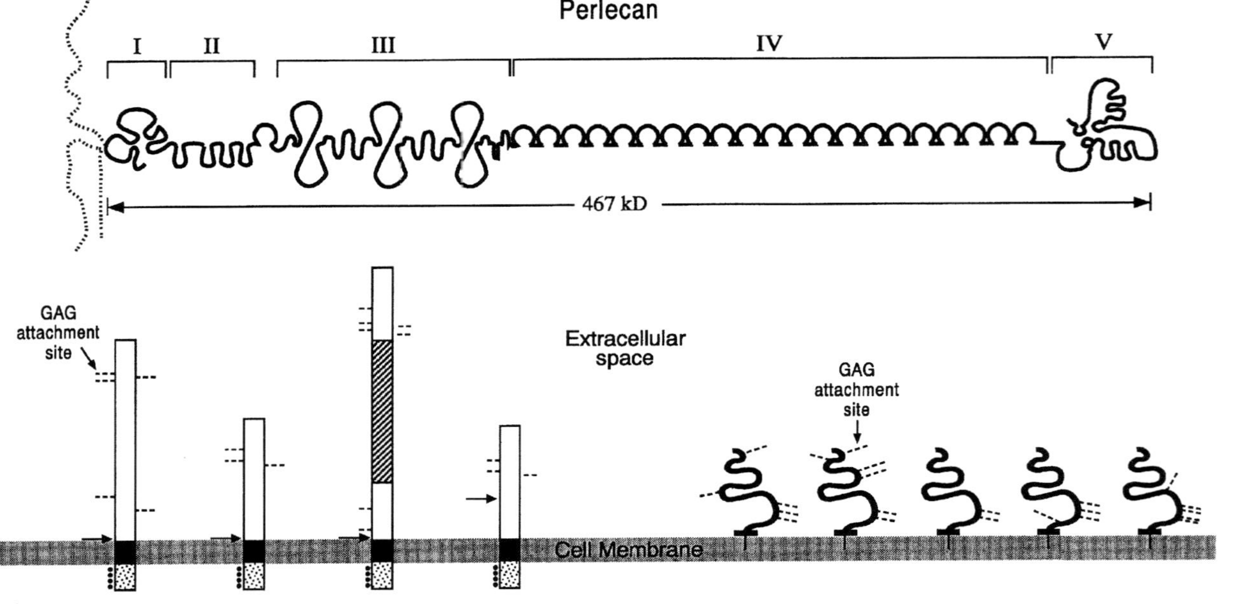

Figure 3.2. Major HSPG core protein families. Displayed are the human members of the membrane spanning syndecans, the GPI-anchored glypicans, and the matrix-localized perlecan. Potential and identified GAG attachment sites are indicated by dotted lines. For the syndecans, indicated are the homologous transmembrane domain (black) and intracellular domain (stipple) with conserved tyrosines (dots), as well as potential dibasic cleavage site (arrows) and the Thr, Ser, Pro-rich domain of syndecan-3 (crosshatch). The structure of perlecan is also displayed and includes a region for HS attachment (I), as well as domains which are homologous to the LDL receptor (II), laminin short arm (III), neural cell adhesion molecule (IV), and laminin A globular end (V).

within the transmembrane regions of syndecan family members allow for homooligomerization, which is speculated to result from extracellular HS/protein interactions that produces tight approximation of proteoglycans. Oligomerization allows the cytoplasmic tails to interact with either intracellular microfilaments or focal adhesions, depending upon the core protein (Asundi and Carey, 1995; Baciu and Goetinck, 1995). In the former instance, a specific tyrosine residue appears to be involved in regulating this association (Carey et al., 1996). The phosphorylation of intracytoplasmic serine residues and possibly tyrosine residues may play a critical role in the above process (Itano et al., 1996).

For syndecan-4, oligomerization involving unique residues Leu^{186}-Lys^{194} permits the cytoplasmic tail to interact with and activate protein kinase C (Asundi and Carey, 1995; Oh et al., 1997b). Potentially, this interaction could be modulated by phosphorylation of the nearby Ser^{183} through a calcium independent isozyme of protein kinase C (Horowitz and Simons, 1998). Phosphorylation occurs much more efficiently for syndecan dimers than monomers and does not shift the concentration dependency of dimerization (Oh et al., 1997a), which raises the possibility that serine phosphorlyation serves to regulate interactions between dimeric cytoplasmic tails and intracellular effectors. Interestingly, FGF-2 treatment counteracts this process by stimulation of a phosphatase (Horowitz and Simons, 1998).

Modulation of oligomerization and/or intracellular interactions may also involve syntenin, a putative adapter protein, which contains a tandem repeat of PDZ domains that bind the syndecan dimer by the common COOH-terminal sequence Phe-Tyr-Ala (Grootjans et al., 1997). PDZ domains, an approximately 90-amino acid motif, function as independent modules for protein–protein interaction and occur in diverse membrane-associated proteins including members of the MAGUK family of guanylate kinases, many protein phosphatases and kinases, neuronal nitric oxide synthase, several dystrophin-associated proteins, and adapter/scaffolding proteins (Ponting et al., 1997). Typically, structurally different PDZ domains selectively bind the COOH-terminal tripeptide of distinct targets, including transmembrane receptors, ion channels, and cytoskeletal components (Songyang et al., 1997). Both PDZ domains of syntenin are required for binding dimeric syndecan; however, interactions with additional components could occur through recognition sequences for SH2 and SH3 domains or could possibly involve PDZ–PDZ interactions (Brenman et al., 1996; Grootjans et al., 1997). Thus, syntenin may link oligomerized syndecan complexes to intracellular effector systems.

The glypican core protein family is comprised of five human or mouse members as well as the *Drosophila* homologue *dally*. Glypican family members possess an extracellular region with GAG attachment sites, 14 invariant cysteine residues, which stabilize a highly compact tertiary structure, and a C-terminal glycosyl phosphatidylinositol (GPI) anchor. The extracellular regions of the different family members are quite similar, which suggests that these areas may be involved in important cellular functions such as binding to ligands or interaction with Golgi components to direct glycanation. Glypican family core proteins are selectively expressed on different cell types with only glypican-1 present on vascular endothelial cells/smooth muscle cells (reviewed in Saunders et al., 1997; Weksberg et al., 1996). These core proteins are mainly targeted to apical surfaces, which is partially dependent upon the extent of glycanation (Mertens et al., 1996).

Perlecan represents the final class of core protein to be considered with only a single human or mouse family member but with multiple splice variants possible (Noonan et al., 1991). The intact core protein contains five separate regions with a variety of intriguing structural motifs decorated by posttranslational modifications such as GAG chains, *O*-linked nonsulfated oligosaccharides, as well as long chain fatty acids. Perlecan is secreted by multiple cell types including vascular endothelial cells/smooth muscle cells and interacts with collagens, laminin and other components within the basement membrane (Murdoch et al., 1992).

The biosynthetic mechanism that determines glycanation of core proteins has been extensively investigated over the past decade, but only partially defined. The glycanation of core proteins is initiated by four specific enzymes which generate a unique linkage region tetrasaccharide. The tetrasaccharide acceptor site is represented by a Ser-Gly (Ala)-XXX-Gly (Ala) sequence with subsequent attachment of HS, rather than chondroitin sulfate (CS), favored by multiple acidic amino acids at a distance of seven to nine residues, the occurrence of tryptophan residues in close proximity, and the presence of adjacent tracts of Ser-Gly repeats. However, the relative intracellular concentrations of metabolic intermediates required for HS versus CS biosynthesis and the overall structures of core proteins also play a critical role in specifying the linkage of a particular GAG. The attachment of HS to glypican family members is unusually selective, frequently approaching 100%; the linkage of HS to the *N*-terminal of perlecan is highly specific frequently approximating 80% with CS linked to the remaining sites, whereas the coupling of HS to syndecan family members is favored averaging 60% with the remaining sites decorated with CS. Under certain conditions, occasional acceptor sites in the above core proteins may be unsubstituted (Esko and Zhang, 1996).

STRUCTURE AND FUNCTION OF HS BIOSYNTHETIC ENZYMES

While alterations in expression of HS-carrying core proteins can affect HS composition on the cell surface and/or extracellular matrix, enzymatic modification of HS chains on existing protein cores may also significantly affect the HS matrix. Examination of the characteristics of HS biosynthetic enzymes reveals molecular mechanisms for the generation of specific HS sequences with distinct biologic activities. The fine structure of HS attached to core proteins is established by a complex biosynthetic pathway (Fig. 3.3). The generation of HS is initiated by HS copolymerase which

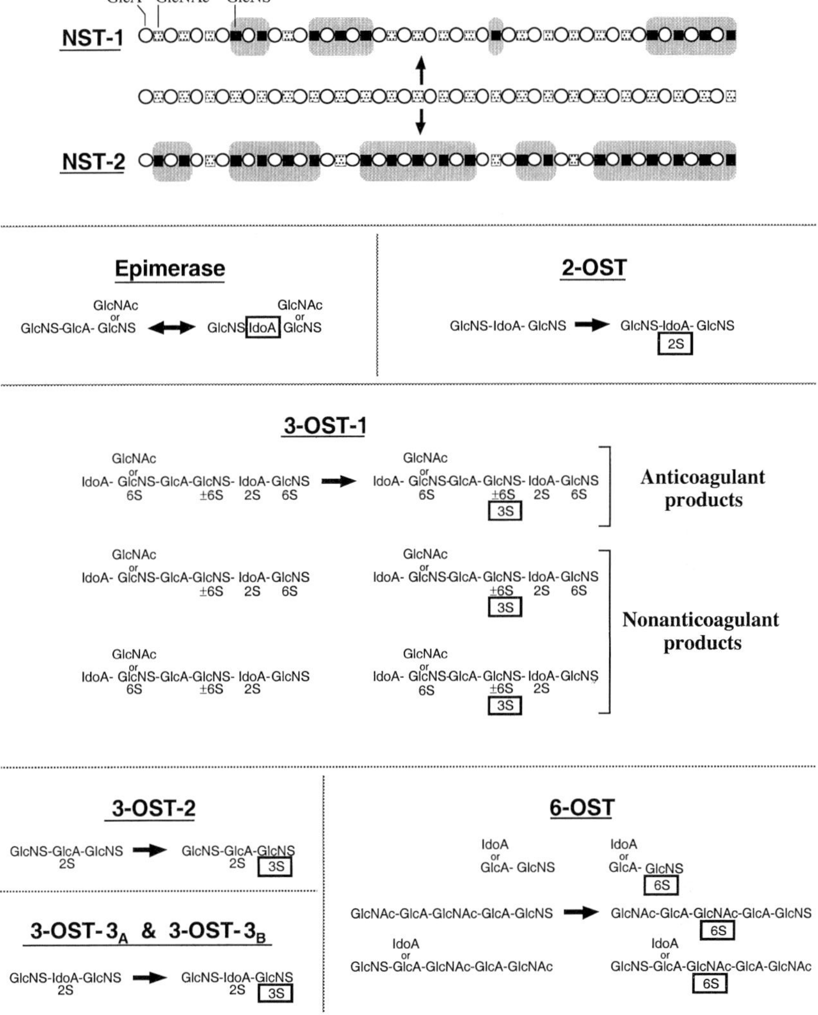

Figure 3.3. Biochemical specificities of heparan biosynthetic enzymes. Specificities are based on biochemical activities of cell extracts (epimerase, 2-OST, 6-OST) (reviewed in Lindahl, 1989) or from expression of cloned cDNAs of NST (Cheung et al., 1996; Ishihara et al., 1993a) and 3-OST isoforms (J., Liu, N. W. Shworak, J. J. Schwartz, L. M. S. Fritze, and R. D. Rosenberg; and L., Zhang, N. W. Shworak, J. Liu, and R. D. Rosenberg, manuscripts in preparation). Shading indicates blocks of GlcNS generated by NST isoforms.

sequentially transfers glucuronic acid (GlcA) and *N*-acetylglucosamine (GlcNAc) residues from their respective sugar nucleotides to the tetrasaccharide linkage region to produce GAGs with about 100 disaccharide units of →4-D-GlcApβ1→4-D-GlcNpAcα1→. The homogenous copolymer is structurally altered at rare GlcNAc residues by *N*-deacetylase/*N*-sulfotransferase (NST), which replaces *N*-acetyl groups with *N*-sulfate groups, with the process spreading in both directions to generate modified domains of about five disaccharide units separated by relatively unmodified regions of about 18 disaccharide units. The C5 glucuronosyl/iduronosyl epimerase then catalyzes transformation of occasional D-GlcA residues into L-iduronic acid (IdoA) residues if *N*-sulfate groups are present at the immediate upstream position. The equilibrium distribution of this reaction lies far in the direction of GlcA but epimerization is favored by sulfation of a IdoA. The iduronosyl 2-*O*-sulfotransferase then sulfates selected IdoA residues (creates IdoA 2S) provided that *N*-sulfated glucosamine (GlcNS) groups are located at the immediate upstream position and 6-*O*-sulfated glucosamine (GlcN(Ac/S) 6S) groups are absent from the immediate downstream position. The glucuronsyl 2-*O*-sulfotransferase also sulfates rare GlcA residues (creates GlcA 2S) which prevent subsequent epimerization to IdoA. The glucosaminyl 6-*O*-sulfotransferase (6-OST) then frequently sulfates GlcN(Ac/S) residues provided that *N*-sulfate groups are present at either the immediate upstream or downstream positions (reviewed in Lindahl, 1989). Finally, the glucosaminyl 3-*O*-sulfotransferase (3-OST-1) sulfates occasional GlcNS and GlcNS 6S residues (creates GlcNS 3S and GlcNS 3S 6S, respectively) when →IdoA→GlcN(Ac/S) ±6S→GlcA→ is present in the immediate upstream position and the downstream location is filled by an →IdoA2S→GlcNS ±6S→. Thus, the above enzymatic reactions that generate distinct HS fine structures represent, at the very minimum, a partially ordered biochemical pathway with clear-cut precursor/product relationships.

Until recently, all biosynthetic enzymes were postulated entities based upon the biochemical activities of cell lysates. During the past 5 years, virtually all of these proteins have been purified, cDNAs encoding three families of HS sulfotransferases have been molecularly cloned, and the primary structures of NST, 2-OST, and 3-OST enzymes have been determined (Eriksson et al., 1994; Habuchi et al., 1995; Hashimoto et al., 1992; Kobayashi et al., 1997; Lind et al., 1993; Liu et al., 1996; Shworak et al., 1997). To date, only a single 2-OST isoform has been cloned, whereas, two NST family members have been isolated (NST-1 and NST-2) (Eriksson et al., 1994; Hashimoto et al., 1992), and five 3-OST isoforms have been identified (3-OST-1, 3-OST-2, 3-OST-3A, 3-OST-3B, and 3-OST-4) (Fig. 3.4) (Shworak et al., 1997).

The available data on the initial and final sulfation enzymes in the biosynthetic pathway provide intriguing clues about potential mechanisms for generating HS with regions of defined monosaccharide sequence. We note that NST-1 and NST-2 were cloned from hepatic cells and mast cells, respectively, but are also expressed in other cell types (Eriksson et al., 1994; Hashimoto et al., 1992). The cellular expression of these cDNAs reveals the two enzymes exhibit alternate specificities that initially lead to a varying extent of *N*-sulfation of HS (i.e., NST-1 generates about 40% *N*-sulfation of HS whereas NST-2 produces about 80% *N*-sulfation of HS), which subsequently results in different patterns of *O*-sulfation and epimerization (Fig. 3.3) (Cheung et al., 1996; Ishihara et al., 1993a). The sulfation specificity of the 3-OSTs has been determined with recombinantly expressed enzyme. The sulfation of GlcNS residues by each isoform requires a specific upstream uronic acid; GlcA for 3-OST-1, GlcA 2S is preferred by 3-OST-2, and IdoA 2S is necessary for 3-OST-3_A and -3_B (Fig. 3.3). The specificities of these enzymes are also dependent upon additional residues in the neighborhood of the site of sulfation. We note that the forms 3-OST-2, 3-OST-3_A, and 3-OST-3_B do not appear to be present in endothelial cells, and sulfate HS structures that are distinct from the 3-OST-1 precursor sequence; hence, these isoforms produce GAGs with potential interaction sites for biologic targets other than antithrombin (i.e., only 3-OST-1 generates the antithrombin binding site). It is of interest that HS modified by the 3-OST-3 isoform has been identified in the glomerular basement membrane where it has been hypothesized to be involved in regulating permeability to proteins (Edge and Spiro, 1990). Based upon these data, we speculate that isoforms of biosynthetic enzyme exist in different cell types which sulfate HS at specific sites based upon the surrounding monosaccharide sequence and hence are capable of producing GAGs with regions of defined structure. The regulation of the concentrations of these enzymes, provided that they serve as limiting components in a biosynthetic pathway, would establish particular levels of HSPG with regions of defined monosaccharide sequence.

An examination of the deduced structures of the cloned HS sulfotransferases reveals several common as well as distinctive features and provides a foundation for exploring the molecular basis of heparan sequence diversity. All of these enzymes exhibit multiple potential *N*-glycosylation sites, constant with the analysis of the purified proteins (Brandan and Hirschberg, 1988; Eriksson et al., 1994; Liu et al., 1996; Pettersson et al., 1991); whereas potential *O*-glycosylation sites have been detected for 3-OST-2, -3_A, -3_B, -4(Fig. 3.4). Most HS sulfotransferases are type II integral membrane proteins (described in Wickner and Lodish, 1985); however, 3-OST-1 exhibits the unusual configuration of an intraluminal Golgi resident and is generated from a precursor protein by signal peptidase cleavage of a 20 amino acid, NH_2-terminal leader sequence (Shworak et al., 1997) (Fig. 3.4). Localization of 3-OST-1 to the *trans*-Golgi lumen is speculated to involve the interaction of COOH-terminal residues with integral membrane proteins, as previously established for intraluminal residents of the endoplasmic reticulum (Munro and Pelham, 1987). Cellular secretion of 3-OST-1 is high (Liu et al., 1996; Shworak et al., 1997), which testifies to a leaky retention mechanism and raises the possibility that mod-

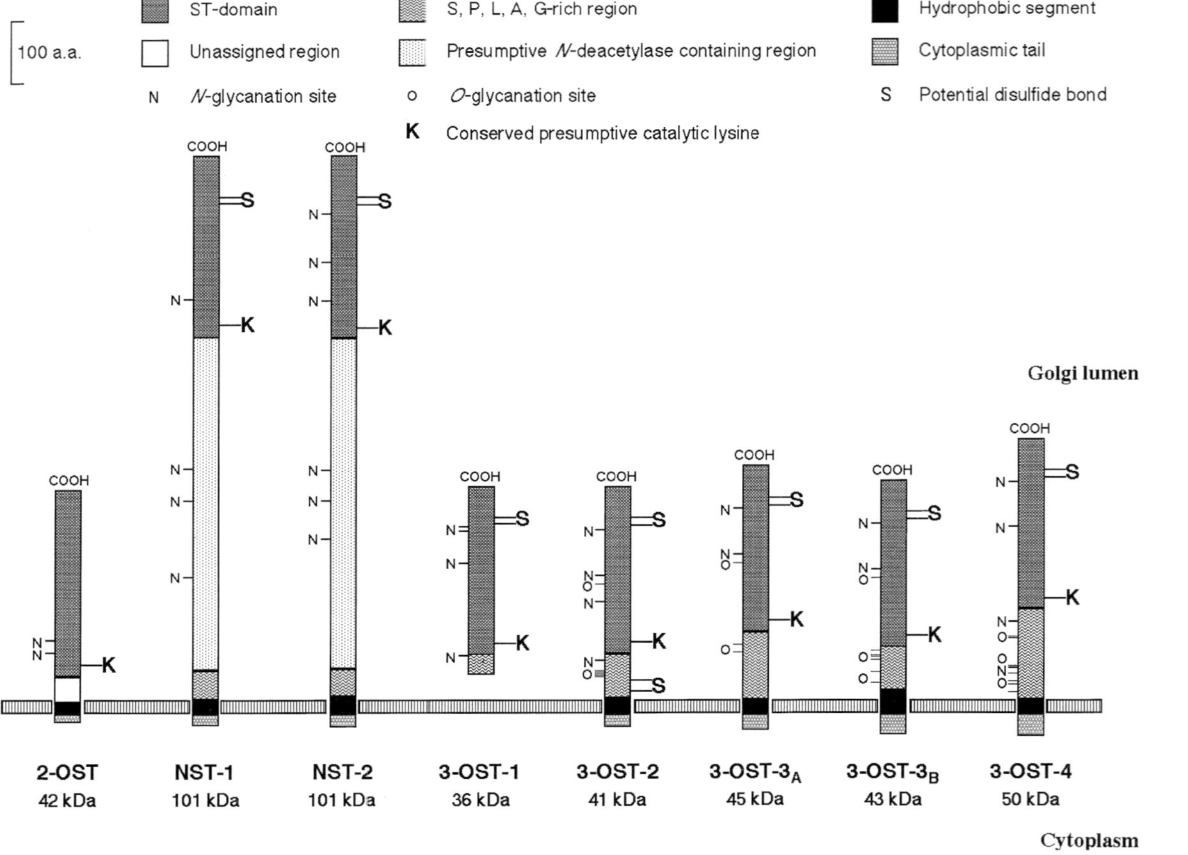

100 a.a.
ST-domain
Unassigned region
N N-glycanation site
S, P, L, A, G-rich region
Presumptive N-deacetylase containing region
o O-glycanation site
K Conserved presumptive catalytic lysine
Hydrophobic segment
Cytoplasmic tail
S Potential disulfide bond
Golgi lumen
Cytoplasm
COOH
2-OST
42 kDa
NST-1
101 kDa
NST-2
101 kDa
3-OST-1
36 kDa
3-OST-2
41 kDa
3-OST-3A
45 kDa
3-OST-3B
43 kDa
3-OST-4
50 kDa

ulation of enzyme retention could serve as a mechanism to control the cellular generation of anticoagulant HS.

The architecture of the type II HS sulfotransferases is akin to that of the glycosyltransferases (Eriksson et al., 1994). Thus, the majority of the protein is intraluminal but is anchored by a single hydrophobic membrane spanning segment, followed by a short, positively charged, NH_2-terminal, cytoplasmic tail (Fig. 3.4). Residues within and flanking the transmembrane domain are expected to define localization to Golgi subcompartments, as has been demonstrated for glycosyltransferases (Machamer, 1993). Indeed, NST-1 has been immunolocalized to the *trans*-Golgi network and the NH_2-terminal 161 residues shown to convey retention within the Golgi (Humphries et al., 1997). The glycosyltransferase structural analogy further predicts the intraluminal component to be comprised of a large COOH-terminal catalytic region that is joined to the membrane spanning domain by a short flexible stem domain (Eriksson et al., 1994). This connecting region of the NST and the type II 3-OST enzymes ranges from 39 to 104 amino acids and is extremely enriched in S, P, L, A, and G (60%–79% of all residues). Interestingly, the NH_2-terminal 32 residues of 3-OST-1 exhibit a similar enrichment (50%). This unusual composition creates a stem region that is predominantly devoid of secondary structure and so should allow for unconstrained movement of the catalytic domain. However, the stem portion of 3-OST-2 contains two cysteines that potentially could form a disulfide bond and thereby partially restrict freedom of motion (Fig. 3.4). Within each HS sulfotransferase family, the presumptive catalytic regions are highly homologous, whereas the remaining NH_2-terminal portions (comprised of the stem region, the transmembrane domain, and the cytoplasmic tail) appear unrelated. This relationship is most extreme for 3-OST-3_A and 3-OST-3_B, with the presumed catalytic regions differing by only a single amino acid.

Critical features of the catalytic region have been revealed by comparing HS sulfotransferases to more than 40 previously identified sulfotransfer-

---

Figure 3.4. Predicted domain organization and structural features of HS sulfotransferases. Schematic localization of features relative to primary sequence for Chinese hamster 2-OST, rat NST-1, mouse NST-2, and human 3-OST isoforms (Eriksson et al., 1994; Hashimoto et al., 1992; Kobayashi et al., 1997; Orellana et al., 1994; Shworak et al., 1997). The complete structures of 3-OST-2, 3-OST-3_A, and 3-OST-3_B have been elucidated from the isolation of full-length cDNAs, whereas 3-OST-4 has been identified from partial length cDNAs and genomic clones (N. W. Shworak, J. Liu, L. M. Petros, M. Kobayashi, N. G. Copeland, N. A. Jenkins and R. D. Rosenberg, manuscript in preparation). Molecular weights are given for unglycosylated enzymes and only selected potential disulfide bonds are presented. Domain patterns designate common predicted function but not necessarily homology of primary sequences. The ST-domains and the presumptive *N*-deacetylase regions exhibit high potential for secondary structure and so are likely to be globular structures.

ases (isolated from animals, plants, and bacteria), including chondroitin-, aryl-/phenol-, *N*-hydroxyarylamine-, alcohol-/hydroxysteroid-, flavonol-, and nodulation factor sulfotransferases (Shworak et al., 1997). This analysis reveals a homologous COOH-terminal region of 260–290 residues, the putative sulfotransferase domain (ST-domain), that exhibits at least ~30% similarity (Shworak et al., 1997). The conservation of sequence across this diverse class of enzymes probably reflects common structural and functional constraints imposed by the obligate cofactor PAPS, which is the sulfate donor required for all sulfotransferase reactions. In particular, the sequence $(L/I/V/f/a)_{3-4}$-X_{3-5}-(K/r)-(S/t/g)-(G/a)-(T/s)-X_2-(V/L/i/m/f) (lowercase represents infrequent variants) occurs near the amino terminus of the ST-domain (Fig. 3.4) and appears to be a critical active site component, as indicated for mammalian and plant cytosolic sulfotransferases by affinity labeling with a PAPS analog and by mutational analysis (Marsolais and Varin, 1995; Zheng et al., 1994). Within this consensus sequence, the central basic residue is typically lysine (96% of all enzymes) and is considered essential for stabilization of a transition state intermediate, as the Lys→Ala mutant of flavonol 3-sulfotransferase has a 300-fold reduction in enzymatic activity with minimal affect on PAPS binding (Marsolais and Varin, 1995). This conserved lysine occurs in all HS sulfotransferases (Fig. 3.4) and likely serves an equivalent catalytic role. The ST-domain encompasses to the entire anticipated catalytic region of 2-OST and 3-OST isoforms, but only the COOH-terminal third of NST enzymes. The remaining ~520 catalytic residues of the NST forms presumablely contain the *N*-deacetylase activity. The ST-domain is likely to contain the predominant determinants which recognize distinct precursor structures given that the COOH-terminal 286 residues of 3-OST-1 (ST-domain with additional 26 residues) maintain wild-type substrate specificity and sulfotransferase activity (Shworak et al., 1997). Furthermore, 3-OST-3_A and 3-OST-3_B, exhibit the same sulfation specificity (Fig. 3.3) and possess virtually identical ST-domains.

SUMMARY

We have summarized recent advances in our knowledge of HSGPs, which can have covalently linked HS containing regions of defined monosaccharide sequence that interact with receptors and proteins to regulate many different aspects of angiogenesis. Indeed, given the various cellular processes thought to be controlled by GAGs, one should anticipate the existence of numerous discrete HS sequences. However, it remains unclear how the biosynthetic mechanism is able to generate and specifically regulate the concentrations of each of these components. Based upon the available data, we speculate that the various classes of sulfotransferases exist as multiple isoforms, each able to recognize and modify slightly different monosaccharide sequences. Cell type specific expression of these isoforms would then dictate the synthesis of a particular array of GAGs. The actual levels of a given HS population with regions of defined monosaccharide sequence could then be regulated by controlling the concentrations/activities of key enzymes present in limiting amount. Identification of such key enzymes that control important cell signaling events should lead to the development of novel therapeutic approaches to modulate the complex process of angiogenesis.

REFERENCES

Asundi, V. K. and Carey, D. J. (1995). Self-association of N-syndecan (syndecan-3) core protein is mediated by a novel structural motif in the transmembrane domain and ectodomain flanking region. J. Biol. Chem. 270: 26404–26410.

Baciu, P. C. and Goetinck, P. F. (1995). Protein kinase C regulates the recruitment of syndecan-4 into focal contacts. Mol. Biol. Cell 6: 1503–1513.

Bernfield, M., Kokenyesi, R., Kato, M., Hinkes, M. T., Spring, J., Gallo, R. L., and Lose, E. J. (1992). Biology of the syndecans: a family of transmembrane heparan sulfate proteoglycans. Annu. Rev. Cell Biol. 8: 365–393.

Brandan, E. and Hirschberg, C. B. (1988). Purification of rat liver N-Heparan-sulfate sulfotransferase. J. Biol. Chem. 263: 2417–2422.

Brenman, J. E., Chao, D. S., Gee, S. H., McGee, A. W., Craven, S. E., Santillano, D. R., Wu, Z., Huang, F., Xia, H., Peters, M. F., Froehner, S. C., and Bredt, D. S. (1996). Interaction of nitric oxide synthase with the postsynaptic density protein PSD-95 and alpha1-syntrophin mediated by PDZ domains. Cell 84: 757–767.

Carey, D. J. (1997). Syndecans: multifunctional cell-surface co-receptors. Biochem. J. 327: 1–16.

Carey, D. J., Bendt, K. M., and Stahl, R. C. (1996). The cytoplasmic domain of syndecan-1 is required for cytoskeleton association but not detergent insolubility. Identification of essential cytoplasmic domain residues. J. Biol. Chem. 271: 15253–15260.

Casu, B. (1989). Method of structural analysis. *In* "Heparin, Chemical and Biological Properties: Clinical Applications" (D. A. Lane and U. Lindahl, eds.) pp. 25–49. Edward Arnold, London.

Cheung, W.-F., Eriksson, I., Kusche-Gullberg, M., Lindahl, U., and Kjellén, L. (1996). Expression of the mouse mastocytoma glucosaminyl *N*-deacetylase/*N*-sulfotransferase in human kidney 293 cells results in increased *N*-sulfation of heparan sulfate. Biochemistry 35: 5250–5256.

DeLisser, H. M., Christofidou-Solomidou, M., Strieter, R. M., Burdick, M. D., Robinson, C. S., Wexler, R. S., Kerr, J. S., Garlanda, C., Merwin, J. R., Madri, J. A., and Albelda, S. M. (1997). Involvement of endothelial PECAM-1/CD31 in angiogenesis. Am. J. Pathol. 151: 671–677.

Edge, A. S. and Spiro, R. G. (1990). Characterization of novel sequences containing 3-*O*-sulfated glucosamine in glomerular basement membrane heparan sulfate and localization of sulfated disaccharides to a peripheral domain. J. Biol. Chem. 265: 15874–15881.

Eriksson, I., Sandbäck, D., Ek, B., Lindahl, U., and Kjellén, L. (1994). cDNA cloning and sequencing of mouse mastocytoma glucosaminyl N-deacetylase/N-sulfotransferase, an enzyme involved in the biosynthesis of heparin. J. Biol. Chem. 269: 10438–10443.

Esko, J. D. and Zhang, L. (1996). Influence of core protein sequence on glycosaminoglycan assembly. Curr. Opin. Struct. Biol. 6: 663–670.

Folkman, J. and Shing, Y. (1992). Control of angiogenesis by heparin and other sulfated polysaccharides. Adv. Exp. Med. Biol. 313: 355–364.

Grootjans, J. J., Zimmermann, P., Reekmans, G., Smets, A., Degeest, G., Durr, J., and David, G. (1997). Syntenin, a PDZ protein that binds syndecan cytoplasmic domains. Proc. Natl. Acad. Sci. USA 94: 13683–13688.

Habuchi, H., Habuchi, O., and Kimata, K. (1995). Purification and characterization of heparan sulfate 6-sulfotransferase from the culture medium of Chinese hamster ovary cells. J. Biol. Chem. 270: 4172–4179.

Hashimoto, Y., Orellana, A., Gil, G., and Hirschberg, C. B. (1992). Molecular cloning and expression of rat liver *N*-heparan sulfate sulfotransferase. J. Biol. Chem. 267: 15744–15750.

Horowitz, A. and Simons, M. (1998). Regulation of syndecan-4 phosphorylation in vivo. J. Biol. Chem., 273: 10914–10918.

Humphries, D. E., Sullivan, B. R., Aleixo, M. D., and Snow, J. L. (1997). Localization of human heparan glucosaminyl *N*-deacetylase/*N*-sulphotransferase to the *trans*-Golgi network. Biochem. J. 325: 351–357.

Ishihara, M., Guo, Y., Wei, Z., Yang, Z., Swiedler, S. J., Orellana, A., and Hirschberg, C. B. (1993a). Regulation of biosynthesis of the basic fibroblast growth factor binding domains of heparan sulfate by heparan sulfate-N-deacetylase/N-sulfotransferase expression. J. Biol. Chem. 268: 20091–20095.

Ishihara, M., Tyrrell, D. J., Stauber, G. B., Brown, S., Cousens, L. S., and Stack, R. J. (1993b). Preparation of affinity-fractionated, heparin-derived oligosaccharides and their effects on selected biological activities mediated by basic fibroblast growth factor. J. Biol. Chem. 268: 4675–4683.

Itano, N., Oguri, K., Nagayasu, Y., Kusano, Y., Nakanishi, H., David, G., and Okayama, M. (1996). Phosphorylation of a membrane-intercalated proteoglycan, syndecan-2, expressed in a stroma-inducing clone from a mouse Lewis lung carcinoma. Biochem. J. 315: 925–930.

Kjellén, L. and Lindahl, U. (1991). Proteoglycans: structures and interactions. Annu. Rev. Biochem. 60: 443–475.

Kobayashi, M., Habuchi, H., Yoneda, M., Habuchi, O., and Kimata, K. (1997). Molecular cloning and expression of Chinese hamster ovary cell heparan-sulfate 2-sulfotransferase. J. Biol. Chem. 272: 13980–13985.

Lind, T., Lindahl, U., and Lidholt, K. (1993). Biosynthesis of heparin/heparan sulfate. Identification of a 70-kDa protein catalyzing both the D-glucuronosyl- and the *N*-acetyl-D-glucosaminyltransferase reactions. J. Biol. Chem. 268: 20706–20708.

Lindahl, U. (1989). Biosynthesis of heparin and related polysaccharides. *In* "Heparin, Chemical and Biological Properties: Clinical Applications" (D. A. Lane and U. Lindahl, eds.) pp. 159–191. Edward Arnold, London.

Lindahl, U., Lidholt, K., Spillmann, D., and Kjellén, L. (1994). More to "heparin" than anticoagulation. Thromb. Res. 75: 1–32.

Liu, J., Shworak, N. W., Fritze, L. M. S., Edelberg, J. M., and Rosenberg, R. D. (1996). Purification of heparan sulfate D-glucosaminyl 3-*O*-sulfotransferase. J. Biol. Chem. 271: 27072–27082.

Machamer, C. E. (1993). Targeting and retention of Golgi membrane proteins. Curr. Opin. Cell Biol. 5: 606–612.

Marsolais, F., and Varin, L. (1995). Identification of amino acid residues critical for catalysis and cosubstrate binding in the flavonol 3-sulfotransferase. J. Biol. Chem. 270: 30458–30463.

McFall, A. J. and Rapraeger, A. C. (1997). Identification of an adhesion site within the syndecan-4 extracellular protein domain. J. Biol. Chem. 272: 12901–12904.

Mertens, G., Van der Schueren, B., van den Berghe, H., and David, G. (1996). Heparan sulfate expression in polarized epithelial cells: the apical sorting of glypican (GPI-anchored proteoglycan) is inversely related to its heparan sulfate content. J. Cell Biol. 132: 487–497.

Miettinen, H. M., Edwards, S. N., and Jalkanen, M. (1994). Analysis of transport and targeting of syndecan-1: effect of cytoplasmic tail deletions. Mol. Biol. Cell. 5: 1325–1339.

Montreuil, J., Bouquelt, S., Debray, H., Fournet, B., Spik, G., and Strecker, G. (1986). Glycoproteins. *In* "Carbohydrate Analysis: A Practical Approach" (M. F. Chaplin and J. F. Kennedy, eds.) pp. 143–203. IRL Press, Oxford.

Munro, S. and Pelham, H. R. (1987). A C-terminal singal prevents secretion of luminal ER proteins. Cell 48: 899–907.

Murdoch, A. D., Dodge, G. R., Cohen, I., Tuan, R. S., and Iozzo, R. V. (1992). Primary structure of the human heparan sulfate proteoglycan from basement membrane (HSPG2/perlecan). A chimeric molecule with multiple domains homologous to the low density lipoprotein receptor, laminin, neural cell adhesion molecules, and epidermal growth factor. J. Biol. Chem. 267: 8544–8557.

Noonan, D. M., Fulle, A., Valente, P., Cai, S., Horigan, E., Sasaki, M., Yamada, Y., and Hassell, J. R. (1991). The complete sequence of perlecan, a basement membrane heparan sulfate proteoglycan, reveals extensive similarity with laminin A chain, low density lipoprotein-receptor, and the neural cell adhesin molecule. J. Biol. Chem. 266: 22939–22947.

Norrby, K. (1997). Angiogenesis: new aspects relating to its initiation and control. APMIS 105: 417–437.

Oh, E. S., Couchman, J. R., and Woods, A. (1997a). Serine phosphorylation of syndecan-2 proteoglycan cytoplasmic domain. Arch. Biochem. Biophys. 344: 67–74.

Oh, E. S., Woods, A., and Couchman, J. R. (1997b). Multimerization of the cytoplasmic domain of syndecan-4 is required for its ability to activate protein kinase C. J. Biol. Chem. 272: 11805–11811.

Orellana, A., Hirschberg, C. B., Wei, Z., Swiedler, S. J., and Ishihara, M. (1994). Molecular cloning and expression of a glycosaminoglycan *N*-acetylglucosaminyl *N*-deacetylase/*N*-sulfotransferase from a heparin-producing cell line. J. Biol. Chem. 269: 2270–2276.

Pettersson, I., Kusche, M., Unger, E., Wlad, H., Nylund, L., Lindahl, U., and Kjellén, L. (1991). Biosynthesis of heparin. Purification of a 110-kDa mouse mastocytoma protein required for both glucosaminyl *N*-deacetylation and *N*-sulfation. J. Biol. Chem. 266: 8044–8049.

Ponting, C. P., Phillips, C., Davies, K. E., and Blake, D. J. (1997). PDZ domains: targeting signalling molecules to sub-membranous sites. Bioessays 19: 469–479.

Rosenberg, R. D., Shworak, N. W., Liu, J., Schwartz, J. J., and Zhang, L. (1997). Heparan sulfate proteoglycans of the cardiovascular system. Specific structures emerge but how is synthesis regulated? J. Clin. Invest. 99: 2062–2070.

Ruoslahti, E. (1988). Structure and biology of proteoglycans. Annu. Rev. Cell Biol. 4: 229–255.

Saunders, S., Paine-Saunders, S., and Lander, A. D. (1997). Expression of the cell surface proteoglycan glypican-5 is developmentally regulated in kidney, limb, and brain. Dev. Biol. 190: 78–93.

Shworak, N. W., Liu, J., Fritze, L. M. S., Schwartz, J. J., Zhang, L., Logeart, D., and Rosenberg, R. D. (1997). Molecular cloning and expression of mouse and human cDNAs encoding heparan sulfate D-glucosaminyl 3-*O*-sulfotransferase. J. Biol. Chem. 272: 28008–28019.

Songyang, Z., Fanning, A. S., Fu, C., Xu, J., Marfatia, S. M., Chishti, A. H., Crompton, A., Chan, A. C., Anderson, J. M., and Cantley, L. C. (1997). Recognition of unique carboxyl-terminal motifs by distinct PDZ domains. Science 275: 73–77.

van den Born, J., Gunnarsson, K., Bakker, M. A. H., Kjellén, L., Kusche-Gullberg, M., Maccarana, M., Berden, J. H. M., and Lindahl, U. (1995). Presence of N-unsubstituted glucosamine units in native heparan sulfate revealed by a monoclonal antibody. J. Biol. Chem. 270: 31303–31309.

Weksberg, R., Squire, J. A., and Templeton, D. M. (1996). Glypicans: a growing trend. Nat. Genet. 12: 225–227.

Wickner, W. T. and Lodish, H. F. (1985). Multiple mechanisms of protein insertion into and across membranes. Science 230: 400–407.

Yanagishita, M. and Hascall, V. C. (1992). Cell surface heparan sulfate proteoglycans. J. Biol. Chem. 267: 9451–9454.

Zheng, Y., Bergold, A., and Duffel, M. W. (1994). Affinity labeling of aryl sulfotransferase IV. Identification of a peptide sequence at the binding site for 3'-phosphoadenosine-5'-phosphosulfate. J. Biol. Chem. 269: 30313–30319.

4

Molecular Mechanisms of the Fibroblast Growth Factor Family

KURT A. ENGLEKA AND THOMAS MACIAG

The "fibroblast" in fibroblast growth factor(FGF) is derived from its initial characterization as a potent mitogen for the murine 3T3 fibroblast-like cell line. However, the moniker should not be misconstrued as a restrictive one for what is now a multimembered growth factor family. FGFs regulate cellular proliferation and differentiation in a wide variety of cell types besides fibroblasts, including neuronal, epithelial and vascular cells. Therefore, FGFs function in a preponderance of cellular and tissue generative processes as well as neoplastic disorders. FGFs are produced by and display direct activity for endothelial and smooth muscle cells and induce the formation of blood vessels from preexisting vessels. In this regard, the characterization of the FGF growth factor system in cellular proliferation and tissue differentiation has illuminated much about the molecular mechanisms underlying vascular development and physiology.

CLASSIFICATION OF FGF GENES AND THEIR RECEPTORS

The FGF gene family consists of a growing number of structurally related polypeptide ligands (Coulier et al., 1997). The first two FGF proteins identified, purified and with genes subsequently isolated and sequenced were the FGF prototypes. Although earliest classification was according to target cell type or tissue of origin, the first two FGFs were distinguished by their isoelectric points and thus became known as acidic or basic FGF. These are now called FGF-1 and FGF-2, respectively. The two prototypes are mitogenic for a wide variety of cell types and were the first endothelial cell growth factors described. Their shared property of binding to the glycosaminoglycan heparin classified the FGF prototypes as heparin-binding growth factors, aided in the development of FGF purification schemes centered around immobilized heparin, and suggested an important role for heparan sulfate proteoglycans as regulators of FGF-mediated responses.

Indeed, the FGF proteins function in conjunction with cell surface heparan sulfates to bind and activate FGF-specific transmembrane receptor proteins. The isolation of the first receptor for FGF by ligand-affinity purification identified the FGF receptors as protein tyrosine kinases. These linked FGF signal transduction to intracellular tyrosine phosphorylation signaling pathways also utilized by the receptors for other mitogens including epidermal growth factor, insulin, platelet-derived growth factor, and the endothelial-specific vascular endothelial cell growth factor. The trimeric interactions of FGF ligand with heparan sulfate and tyrosine kinase receptor at the cell surface are transduced into activated cytoplasmic signaling pathways that eventually result in specific gene expression leading to cell survival, migration, growth, or differentiation.

Currently, the multicomponent FGF system consists of at least seventeen potential FGF polypeptide ligands, a heterogeneous group of heparan sulfate proteoglycan coreceptors, and a family of transmembrane tyrosine kinase receptors containing at least four members (Fig. 4.1). FGF ligands and associated FGF tyrosine kinase receptors have been isolated from vertebrate (mammalian, avian, bony fish) and invertebrate organisms (*Caenorhabditis elegans, Drosophila melanogaster,* and *Strongylocentrotus purpuratus* [sea urchin]), and they are highly conserved across species, indicating divergence from very ancient but fundamental genes that may have undergone duplication and genetic selection or drift.

FGF ligands have been identified by protein purification methods as well as nucleic acid selective procedures and are classified as FGFs on a structural basis rather than by any characteristic property such as heparin-binding or growth-promoting activity. As FGF-1 and FGF-2 were isolated initially, much of what is known concerning the FGF system involves these ligands. However, the remainder of the FGF ligands display important properties common and others distinct from FGF-1 and FGF-2.

FGF-3 through FGF-6 were isolated by their transforming ability and several of these have been identified as oncogenes in human tumors (Goldfarb, 1990). FGF-3 is the product of the *int*-2 gene which is activated via proviral insertion of mouse mammary tumor virus (MMTV). Three FGF genes (*fgf*-3, *fgf*-4, and *fgf*-8) cooperate with the *Wnt*-1 gene, another gene activated by MMTV provirus insertion (*int*-1), in induced murine mammary tumorigenesis. FGF-4 was independently isolated by its transforming ability from both human gastric tumors and Kaposi's sarcoma and is one of the most frequently isolated oncogenes in transformation assays. The genes for FGF-3 and FGF-4 are tandemly linked on chromosome 11 in humans and are coamplified in certain tumors. FGF-4 also directs, as do the FGF prototypes, FGF-8, and FGF-10, the outgrowth and patterning of the limb during development. This, in addition to the

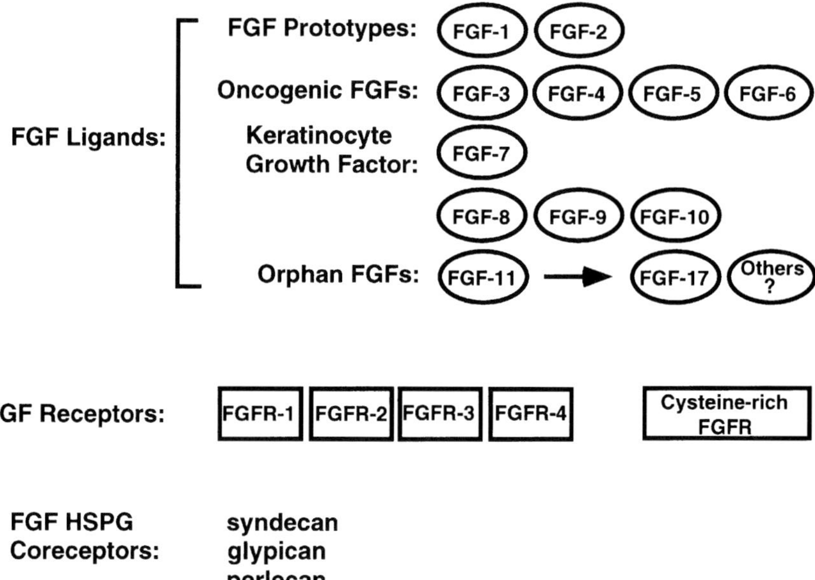

Figure 4.1. The FGF system. The FGF system is complex. It is multicomponent consisting of a variety of FGF polypeptide ligands, tyrosine kinase receptors (FGFRs), and heparan sulfate proteoglycan (HSPG) molecules. The FGF ligands and tyrosine kinase receptors are each expressed from individual genes that encode distinct structural properties. In addition, transcriptional and translational regulation produces isoforms of each ligand or receptor component that further increases the complexity of the system.

regulated expression of the various FGF genes in early embryogenesis and the ability of certain FGF proteins to induce the formation of mesoderm from embryonic precursors, indicates a prevalent role for the FGF gene family in development. FGF-5 was detected by its transformation potential in cultured cells and is allelic with *angora*, a regulator of the hair growth cycle in mice. The final oncogenic FGF gene, FGF-6, was isolated based on its homology to FGF-4.

In addition to these oncogenic FGF forms, additional FGFs have been identified and have been named numerically in approximate order of their discovery. FGF-7 was isolated by its restricted mitogenic action on keratinocytes yet retains its FGF classification based upon structural homology. FGF-8 and FGF-9 were isolated as active factors from tissue culture cell lines. FGF-10 was isolated by homology-based polymerase chain reaction and may function most similarly to FGF-7 in acting on epithelia exclusively. FGF-11 and FGF-12 are FGF-related human cDNA clones (Coulier et al., 1997) that correspond to FGF homologous factor (FHF)-3 and FHF-1, respectively. FGF-13 (FHF-2), FGF-14 (FHF-4), and FGF-15 through FGF-17 are the latest FGFs identified and are classified as FGFs based on nucleic acid homology. Because little is known about the biological functions of FGF-11 through FGF-17, caution should be exercised relative to their value as biological response mediators. FGF-11 through FGF-17 should be considered orphan members of the FGF gene family until their biologic targets are established.

Similarly, after the initial isolation of the first FGF receptor (FGF receptor-1), three other receptors (FGF receptors 2 through 4) were identified by nucleic acid amplification-based methods and were classified as FGF receptors by homology and specific affinity for FGF polypeptide ligands (Jaye et al., 1992; Johnson and Williams, 1993). Recently, however, the FGF receptors have been shown to mediate signal transduction in conjunction with members of the integrin family of extracellular matrix receptors (Miyamoto et al., 1996; Plopper et al., 1995) and certain cell adhesion molecules (Williams et al., 1994).

In addition to the protein tyrosine kinase receptors, a critical component of the FGF receptor system appears to include the heparan sulfate glycosaminoglycan chains contained in cell-associated proteoglycans. These proteoglycans include glypican (Brunner et al., 1991), members of the syndecan family (Chernousov and Carey, 1993), and the basal lamina proteoglycan perlecan (Aviezer et al., 1994). Such proteoglycans may function as coreceptors in mediating FGF-induced signaling. FGF receptor proteins independent of the protein tyrosine kinase and proteoglycan types include a cysteine-rich FGF receptor also identified both as a medial Golgi protein and an E-selectin receptor. This receptor binds FGF in a heparin-independent manner and may be involved in intracellular FGF trafficking (Zuber et al., 1997). Soluble FGF-binding proteins have also been characterized that appear to be secreted ligand-binding domains derived from FGF protein tyrosine kinase receptors. Such binding proteins may play a role in delivering FGFs via the circulation.

As might be expected for factors with potent and widespread mitogenic activity, control of FGF function is highly regulated. One mechanism is through the relative amount of each component of the FGF signaling system present at a certain time and place in vivo. This includes expression for both the FGF ligand and associated protein tyrosine kinase receptors and also, since the FGF proteins are heparan-sulfate-binding growth factors, the coincidental presence of heparan sulfate proteoglycans.

The FGF ligands and their tyrosine kinase receptors are expressed from each of their distinct genes in a tissue-and temporal-specific manner together or separately during many developmental stages and in the adult. The promoters for several FGF ligands and receptors have been analyzed and contain multiple *cis*-acting regulatory elements. Expression is therefore modulated by a variety of agents including protein kinase C activators and the tumor suppressor protein p53 for FGF-2, for example (Stachowiak et al., 1994; Ueba et al., 1994). FGF ligand and receptor gene products are further diversified by varied transcriptional termination and by RNA metabolism including alternative mRNA splicing and alternative translational initiation. The result of such transcriptional and translational control is the regulated expression of multifarious RNA species for many FGF ligands or receptor types. This RNA sequence diversity extends to untranslated regions whose role is unknown but whose expression is regulated, indicating functional importance. Although the reason for such complexity is unclear, the structural determinants encoded in the various primary sequences of different FGF ligands and receptors and their associated isoforms allow diversified function such as in mediating cellular fates, influencing interactions with heparin-like molecules, and determining receptor affinities.

Further, because of the heterogeneous nature and varied amounts of heparan sulfates that exist in vivo, their interactions with FGF gene family members may be hypothesized to provide exquisite regulation of FGF activity. For example, there are heparan sulfate proteoglycans which are differentially expressed during development that display altered specificity for FGF ligands and modify FGF action (Nurcombe et al., 1993).

STRUCTURE AND FUNCTION COMPARISONS AND INFORMATION

As previously stated, membership in the FGF gene family is based upon structural homology. Generally, FGF genes encode proteins of at least 155 amino acids and share 30%–60% amino acid identity in a common 120-amino-acid core sequence. Separately, each FGF is highly conserved across species with homologies ranging from 70% to 100% (Coulier et al., 1997). FGFs show distant homology to the three-dimensional core structures of Kunitz trypsin inhibitors and the proinflammatory cytokines interleukin-1α and interleukin-1β as analyzed by x-ray crystallography and nuclear magnetic resonance studies. In simplest terms FGF-1 and FGF-2 each consist of a β-barrel structure with a trifold pyramid-like cap sitting atop the barrel. This arrangement gives the molecules an approximate threefold symmetry.

Although the FGF proteins are structurally related, may all bind heparin, and interact specifically with FGF receptors, the FGF translation products display important differences which stem from sequence diversity. These include the status of conserved cysteine residues, the localization of heparin-and receptor-binding sites, and structural determinants of cellular localization and secretion (Fig. 4.2).

Status of FGF Cysteine Residues

The cysteines present within FGF ligands have generated interest in how they may impact FGF structure and function, especially whether they are involved in disulfide bond formation. The identified FGF family members contain from one to multiple cysteines. Only one cysteine is conserved absolutely throughout the FGF gene family while another is conserved in

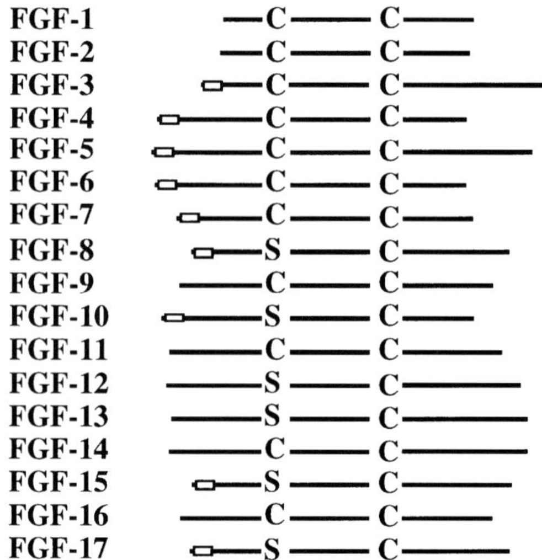

Figure 4.2. General structure of FGF ligands. The family of FGF ligands is aligned showing highly conserved cysteines present in each member. A classical signal sequence for secretion is depicted by a box at the amino terminus for those members that contain one as predicted from their primary sequence.

all but FGF-8, FGF-10, FGF-12, FGF-13, FGF-15, FGF-17, and the *C. elegans* FGF (Coulier et al., 1997). The nonconserved cysteines are located at heterologous positions among the family members and even at different sites when considering the same FGF member between species. The available FGF crystal structures indicate that the conserved cysteines are not exposed to solvent and do not appear to form intramolecular bonds. The cysteine residues are also not required for mitogenic activity for FGF-1 and FGF-2. However, it has been shown that cysteine residues may become structurally accessible after exposure to heparin, oxidants such as copper ions, or heat stress and allow the formation of disulfide-bonded FGF-1 dimers or FGF/α2-macroglobulin complexes.

Localization of Heparin- and Receptor-Binding Sites

Mutational analysis or the use of FGF peptide fragments has allowed identification of putative heparin-binding sites within FGF ligands. For example, mutagenesis studies have defined residues 65 to 81 as the domain in FGF-1 responsible for heparin-mediated potentiation of biologic activity (Imamura et al., 1995). These protein structure–function studies have localized single amino acid point mutations to contiguous binding sites responsible for heparin-binding and heparin-mediated activity. Three-dimensional structural analysis has also allowed the determination of FGF structure in the presence of heparin fragments. In these studies each FGF binds one molecule of a heparin fragment and this interaction does not induce a radical conformational change in the FGF structure. Similar to the results from protein structure–function studies, the heparin-binding sites in the three dimensional structures consist of contiguous and noncontiguous sites within the ligands. Notably, however, the heparin-binding sites isolated by the two approaches do not necessarily coincide. Physical measurements have also indicated that FGF-2 forms dimers and other higher order oligomers in the presence of heparin fragments. The ligands in FGF-2 dimers appear oriented differently depending on the nature of the heparin entity (Herr et al., 1997). The resulting orientation determines receptor competency with some dimers being inactive and others active. This may in part explain observed differential effects of heparin and heparan sulfates on FGF activity.

As might be expected, the identified heparin-binding sites contain many basic amino acids which form ionic interactions with negatively charged heparan sulfate moieties. However, acidic and neutral amino acids are also implicated, suggesting that other interactions are involved. Furthermore, the heparin-binding residues are not absolutely conserved among the FGF ligands within the FGF family or for a single FGF family member among various species. This is consistent with evidence showing that FGF ligands interact with heparin and heparin-like molecules in distinct ways as in the different affinities each FGF displays for heparin and the dependence of different FGF family members on heparin for optimal activity. For example, the heparan sulfate proteoglycan glypican inhibits FGF-7 binding to its receptor while FGF-1 binding is enhanced (Bonneh-Barkay et al., 1997).

The elucidation of the precise receptor-binding site within the FGF ligand and the stoichiometry of the FGF:heparin:FGF receptor interaction is presently unclear. Such information will aid in determining the molecular mechanism of receptor oligomerization, a molecular phenomenon thought to be necessary for subsequent activation of intracellular signaling.

Although FGF mutants or protein fragments have implicated a putative receptor-binding region, structural analysis has produced evidence for either one or two receptor-binding sites on each FGF molecule. The one-site model suggests that FGF receptors are unable to undergo the necessary dimerization required for tyrosine kinase activation in the presence of monomeric FGF. However, a mechanism for receptor dimerization and activation is suggested by receptor-competent, heparin-stabilized dimerization of FGF-2 (Herr et al., 1997). In this model, each member of the heparin-induced FGF-2 homodimer binds one receptor molecule, resulting in the obligatory receptor oligomerization. Alternatively, in the two-site model, the second receptor-binding site in the FGF ligand has lower affinity than does the primary site but may be involved in binding to a second receptor to facilitate receptor dimerization.

Structural Determinants of FGF Secretion and Localization

The presence or absence of a classical signal sequence is a distinguishing feature among the FGF ligands. FGF-1, FGF-2, FGF-9, FGF-11 through-14, and FGF-16 lack a hydrophobic signal sequence at the amino terminal domains to direct translocation into the endoplasmic reticulum and the Golgi apparatus for secretion to the extracellular space. FGF-1 and FGF-2 appear not to be secreted, consistent with a lack of a signal peptide, but are released from cells by an alternative mechanism of protein export. FGF-1 export appears to be independent of the endoplasmic reticulum, as drugs that inhibit this pathway do not inhibit FGF release (Jackson et al., 1992). FGF-1 is released from cells during heat shock in a latent form in a manner that appears to involve dimerization through a highly conserved cysteine residue. However, FGF-2 is not released under similar conditions of stress, suggesting that the FGF prototype release pathways have diverged (Shi et al., 1997). Release of FGF-2 may involve exocytosis or an ATP-dependent pathway as drugs which block exocytosis (Mignatti et al., 1992) or reduce intracellular ATP block FGF-2 release. Recent work implicates the $\alpha 1$ subunit of the Na^+, K^+-ATPase enzyme in FGF-2 export (Florkiewicz et al., 1998).

Secreted forms of the FGF gene family may also contain structural determinants that restrict their release. FGF-3 contains a structural feature for retention in the Golgi apparatus. Similarly, unlike other FGF-2 isoforms, an amino-terminal extended isoform of FGF-2 localizes to the endoplasmic reticulum. Once secreted, FGF translation products appear to remain associated with cells and extracellular matrix and do not circulate in the bloodstream, having a half-life of approximately 3 minutes (Edelman et al., 1993). Thus, there appears to be strong selection against the bioavailability of the FGF translation products that prevents ill-coordinated proliferative, angiogenic, and neurotrophic events beyond the necessary sites of activity. An overabundance of FGF-1 on synthetic sponges placed in rat peritoneum results in hyperplasia and neovascularization within the sponge, illustrating the potent effects of this growth factor in the absence of any negative controls on availability (Thompson et al., 1988).

FGF-1 is the least complicated FGF gene family member from a translation perspective since its open reading frame is flanked by termination codons. In contrast, different isoforms of FGF-2 and FGF-3 with modified amino termini are generated by the highly regulated use of alternative initiation codons for translation at upstream CUG (as compared to the traditional AUG) start codons from the same mRNA species. This regulation may occur through *cis*-acting elements in the FGF-2 mRNA. These alternative initiations result in amino-terminal additions extended from the sequence of the lower molecular weight AUG-initiated isoforms. The additional amino acid sequences contain distinct structural determinants that actively direct intracellular traffic and mediate certain cellular functions. For FGF-2, three CUG-initiated forms of 22, 22.5, and 24 kDa contain multiple functional nuclear localization sequences and are associated with the nucleus. Certain arginine residues present in the amino-terminal extended FGF-2 forms are methylated and may function in regulating cellular localization. The AUG-initiated form of FGF-2 (18 kDa) contains a single nuclear localization sequence yet is predominantly cytosolic. The 18-kDa AUG-initiated FGF-2 modulates cell motility and proliferation through the extracellular interaction with FGF tyrosine kinase surface receptors, whereas high molecular weight CUG initiated FGF-2 appears to act as a mitogen and an inducer of anchorage-independent growth through an intracellular mechanism. Similarly, high molecular weight forms of FGF-3 are CUG-initiated and contain a functional nuclear localization sequence that determines cellular fate and presumably function. In addition to these amino terminal variations, the 5' untranslated region of CUG-initiated forms of FGF-2 contains an internal ribosome entry site for cap-independent translation (Vagner et al., 1995). This feature may allow translation of extended FGF-2 mRNAs under conditions in vivo when cap-dependent translation is normally inhibited, such as during heat stress or viral infection.

Possible roles for internalized and intracellularly transported FGFs have been proposed following the identification of certain FGF translation products in the cytoplasm and nucleus. Upon binding to FGF tyrosine kinase receptors on the cell surface, exogenous FGF-1 and FGF-2 undergo receptor-mediated internalization into lysosomal compartments before conversion to degradation intermediates, some of which are stable at least up to 24 hours. A fraction of such internalized FGF-1, FGF-2, and FGF-3 is detected in the nucleus in its full-length form. FGF-1 transits from the cytosol to the nucleus during the G1 stage of cell cycle (Zhan et al., 1993) and initiation of maximal DNA synthesis by FGF-1 requires the presence of the growth factor during the entire G0 to G1 transition (Zhan et al., 1993).

Biochemical evidence that internalized FGF-1 exits the endocytic pathway and translocates across cellular membranes to the cytosol or the nucleus was demonstrated by the addition of the lipid farnesyl group to a susceptible synthetic FGF-1 protein (Wiedlocha et al., 1995), a modification known only to occur in the cytosol and possibly the nucleus but not at the cell surface or inside compartments of the endocytic pathway. Further evidence for nuclear localization as a requirement for FGF-1-mediated mitogenesis comes from studies utilizing FGF-1 in the form of FGF-1/diptheria toxin fusion proteins that are internalized by the toxin pathway. In these studies, FGF-receptor-negative cells underwent one round of DNA synthesis which correlated with the presence of nuclear FGF-1 fusion protein (Wiedlocha et al., 1996). However, the FGF-1/diptheria toxin fusion proteins stimulated a complete cellular proliferative response only in the presence of FGF receptors. This suggests FGF-1 nuclear localization is necessary but not sufficient for proliferation and also involves a FGF receptor-dependent component, such as receptor-mediated tyrosine phosphorylation. In this regard, nuclear association of structurally intact and functionally active FGF receptors in response to exogenous FGF-1 (Prudovsky et al., 1996) and FGF-2 (Maher, 1996) has also been demonstrated.

FGF nuclear localization is structure-dependent. As discussed previously, the higher molecular mass, CUG-initiated forms of FGF-2 (24, 22.5, and 22 kDa) and FGF-3 contain nuclear localization sequences and are detected in the nucleus. A FGF-1 deletion mutant lacking a putative nuclear localization sequence in its amino-terminal region displays diminished mitogenic activity which is restored by the addition of a heterologous nuclear localization sequence (Imamura et al., 1989). The FGF-1 nuclear localization sequence confers nuclear localization to a cytosolic reporter protein (Zhan et al., 1992) and, interestingly, synthetic peptides containing the FGF-1 nuclear localization sequence stimulate DNA synthesis in a receptor-independent manner (Lin et al., 1996).

Although the precise nature of FGF intracytoplasmic and intranuclear functions are unclear, FGF prototypes bind to DNA (Sosnowski et al., 1996; Zhan et al., 1992). FGF-2 appears to increase the transcription of genes encoding ribosomal RNA in the nucleolus (Bouche et al., 1987), induce transcription in a cell-free system (Nakanishi et al., 1992), and bind chromatin (Gualandris et al., 1993). Further roles for intracellular FGFs await the elucidation of receptor-dependent versus -independent effects, the distinction between the metabolic pathways of endogenously synthesized versus exogenous FGFs, and the role of intracellular receptor-like or other binding proteins in FGF metabolism.

FGF RECEPTOR STRUCTURE AND FUNCTION

The most translationally mature protein products for FGF receptors 1 through 4 contain an extracellular region and an intracellular domain separated by a single transmembrane-spanning region (Fig. 4.3). Each individual FGF tyrosine kinase receptor is more related across species than are the FGF receptors 1 through 4 within a single species (Coulier et al., 1997; Johnson and Williams, 1993). This may indicate that FGF receptors arose from evolutionary duplication(s) and subsequent divergence to retain functional overlap but also distinctive function. In general, FGF receptor-1, FGF receptor-2, and FGF receptor-3 display greater than 80% identity in the extracellular and kinase domains with FGF receptor-4 having slightly less homology (Coulier et al., 1997). The identified invertebrate receptors are significantly less related to the vertebrate FGF receptors sharing approximately 30% homology in the extracellular domain and approximately 50% to 70% in the intracellular kinase domain (Coulier et al., 1997).

The receptor ectodomain comprises FGF ligand-, metal-, and heparin-/matrix molecule-binding functions. The main structural features of the

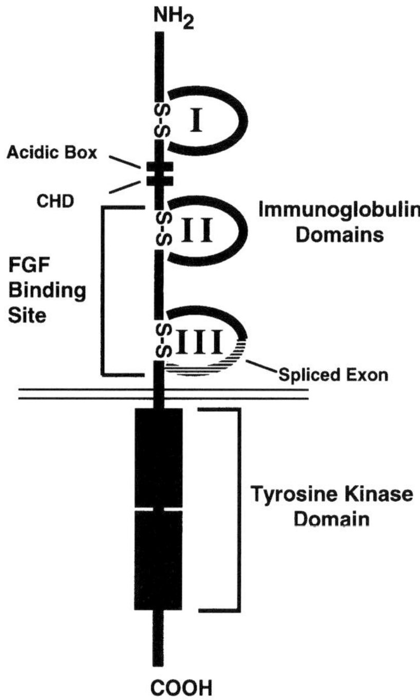

Figure 4.3. General structure of FGF tyrosine kinase receptors. A fully formed FGF tyrosine kinase receptor contains an amino-terminal (NH_2) extracellular domain consisting of three immunoglobulin domains (IgI–III) with characteristic disulfide bonds (S–S). The negatively charged acidic box is unique to FGF receptors and may mediate interactions between cell adhesion molecules (CAMs) and FGF receptors together with the neighboring CAM homology domain (CHD). The first Ig domain is dispensable for ligand binding while the second and third comprise the ligand-binding site. An alternatively spliced exon in the third Ig domain determines ligand binding specificity. The extracellular domain also contains sites susceptible to glycosylation. A single membrane-spanning region separates the ligand-binding region from the carboxy-terminal (COOH) intracellular domain. The critical tyrosine kinase region contains a short spacer region unique to FGF receptors. The intracellular domain contains a number of tyrosine residues within both the kinase domain and the carboxyl tail that become phosphorylated upon activation. These mediate the activity and substrate interactions of the receptor. Receptor isoforms generated from RNA splicing contain either deletions of various FGF receptor regions or substitutions of alternative sequence. Deletion of the first immunoglobulin domain separately or together with the acidic box results in two Ig-loop forms. Other forms lack the transmembrane domain (nonmembrane-bound) or part of the kinase domain (kinase defective). Isoforms also exist containing more than one of these variations.

extracellular region are three cysteine-linked structures called immunoglobulin (Ig)-like domains. Ligand–receptor interactions are mediated by sequences in the IgII and IgIII domains since FGF receptors lacking the first Ig loop display relatively unaltered affinity for FGF ligands. In addition, sequence conservation for IgI between species is lower than is that of IgII and IgIII and the sequence conservation between IgI compared to IgII and IgIII within a species is also lower (Coulier et al., 1997).

Domains IgI and IgII are separated by a stretch of acidic amino acids unique to vertebrate FGF receptors. This region binds metal cations including Mg^{2+}, Ca^{2+}, and Cu^{2+} (Kan et al., 1996; Patstone and Maher, 1996) and resembles metal-binding regions which mediate interactions between some cell adhesion molecules. Furthermore, the acidic region is adjacent to a highly conserved 20-amino-acid region termed the CAM homology domain (CHD) which is also homologous to sequences within some cell adhesion molecules. Consistent with these structural features, certain cell adhesion molecules can either directly or indirectly interact with FGF receptors via the CHD and, in so doing, activate the FGF receptor tyrosine phosphorylation signaling pathway (Williams et al., 1994). It is possible that just as the interactions of cell adhesion molecules are mediated by metal ions, the interactions of some cell adhesion molecules with the CHD in the FGF receptor are regulated by divalent cation binding to the adjacent acidic box.

A FGF receptor heparin-binding site is located within the CHD and is essential for heparin-mediated FGF activation (Kan et al., 1993). Thus, one function of the heparin-binding domain within the FGF receptor may be to link to the FGF ligand via mutual binding to heparan sulfates. In addition, this site may also mediate FGF receptor interactions with heparan sulfate components of the extracellular matrix. The high affinity interaction (apparent $K_d=10^{-9}$ M) of heparin with the FGF receptor requires Ca^{2+} or Mg^{2+} at physiological concentrations (Kan et al., 1996).

The extracellular region of FGF receptors is separated from the intracellular domains on the cytoplasmic face of the membrane by a single-spanning membrane segment. The intracellular region encodes the tyrosine kinase domain containing a short 14-amino-acid spacer unique to FGF receptors. The cytoplasmic region also contains conserved tyrosine residues which become phosphorylated upon activation. The kinase domain and autophosphorylation sites are critical for FGF intracellular signal transduction as evidenced by mutation analysis, although some autophosphorylation sites are not required for ultimate mitogenic activity.

Receptor variants differ from the fully formed FGF receptors in the ectodomain, intracellular juxtamembrane domain, and the intracellular kinase domain and result from RNA alternative splicing. FGF receptor isoforms exist that lack one or more Ig domains, the acidic region or the transmembrane domain. This latter configuration results in a potentially secreted FGF receptor isoform. Some receptor isoforms have a truncated carboxy terminus resulting in a partially deleted and subsequently defective tyrosine kinase domain. Others may or may not contain regions of alternative sequence encoding potential intracellular phosphorylation sites. Furthermore, receptors may contain one or more of these variations. Many tissues or cells express multiple FGF receptors and variants. The receptor isoforms are expressed in both embryonic and adult tissues resulting in cell-and tissue-specific expression and responsivity to different FGF gene family members (Fernig and Gallagher, 1994; Johnson and Williams, 1993; McKeehan and Kan, 1994).

Mutually exclusive alternative splicing of an exon in the IgIII domain determines ligand-binding specificities of the FGF receptors (Fernig and Gallagher, 1994; Jaye et al., 1992; Johnson and Williams, 1993). Therefore, different FGF ligands bind different FGF receptor isoforms dependent on the particular FGF receptor member and its IgIII splice variants. For example, FGF-1 binds to all isoforms with high affinity while FGF-7 binds to only one, a IgIII splice variant of FGF receptor-2. Ligand-binding specificity may be mediated by variable IgIII sequences binding directly to FGFs or, alternatively, through a more indirect mechanism.

FGF-MEDIATED SIGNALING

FGF gene family members mediate their biological effects via binding to both lower-affinity ($K_d=10^{-9}$ M) cell-associated heparan sulfate molecules and the higher-affinity ($K_d=10^{-10}$ to 10^{-12} M), mostly proteinaceous but also glycosylated transmembrane protein tyrosine kinase receptors (also see Chapter 2). Signaling is activated by dimerization of FGF receptors mediated by the extracellular interassociations of FGF, heparan sulfate proteoglycans, and the extracellular domains of tyrosine kinase receptors. The heparan sulfate cofactor appears necessary to facilitate optimal FGF activity, although it may not be required for absolute binding. However, the intracellular tyrosine kinase activity of FGF receptors is necessary for FGF-mediated responses since mutations in the kinase domain abrogate kinase activity and result in receptors that retain FGF-binding ability yet fail to mediate FGF-mediated responses.

FGF receptors can form either homo-or heterodimers. The FGF receptor dimerization reaction has been exploited using enzymatically inactive FGF receptor forms to eliminate the activity of endogenous FGF receptors in a dominant negative fashion. This approach has revealed much about FGF signaling in vivo. In addition, mutations in FGF receptors have been identified that give rise to defects in bone formation leading to craniofacial and skeletal abnormalities and achondroplasia, a common form of dwarfism (Shiang et al., 1994). These mutations cause an increase in FGF receptor activity by inducing FGF-independent interactions between the mutant FGF receptors and consequentially an increased level of FGF-independent autophosphorylation. Often, the identified mutations result in introduction of a free cysteine residue capable of forming an intermolecular disulfide between two mutant FGF receptors (Neilson and Friesel, 1995).

Receptor dimerization results in receptor auto/transphosphorylation of specific tyrosine residues in the cytoplasmic domains of the involved receptors. The phosphorylated tyrosines serve to both stimulate kinase activity and to bind and thus recruit specific cytoplasmic substrates to the receptor. Receptor tyrosine kinases may activate intracellular signaling directly by phosphorylating and activating enzymatic proteins which contain phosphotyrosine-binding domains or by binding nonenzymatic adaptor proteins which then interact with effector molecules (Fig. 4.4).

The FGF receptors, although related, display important differences relative to intracellular signaling pathways due to differences in FGF receptor cytoplasmic domain sequences. For example, both activated FGF receptor-1 and FGF receptor-4 bind phospholipase Cγ (PLC-γ), a common target of receptor protein tyrosine kinases. However, unlike FGF receptor-1, FGF receptor-4 binds, phosphorylates, and activates PLC-γ only weakly and does not phosphorylate the adaptor protein Shc, activate Raf-1 and mitogen-activated protein kinase (MAPK) proteins, or induce immediate-early gene expression (Vainikka et al., 1992; Wang et al., 1994). The FGF receptor-4 signaling differences appear due to the absence of three tyrosine residues common to the intracytoplasmic domains of FGF receptor-1, -2, and -3 although the site for PLC-γ binding is conserved. Such structural differences are manifested in differences in FGF-mediated responses as activation of only FGF receptor-1 leads to cell growth (Wang et al., 1994).

ROLE OF FGF'S IN VASCULAR BIOLOGY

An essential role for FGF function is illustrated by the profound phenotypes induced by abnormal FGF expression or defective FGF receptor-mediated signaling in animal models. These include hyperplasia and marked tissue-specific developmental dysmorphogenesis (Amaya et al., 1991; Coffin et al., 1995; Guo et al., 1993; Lee et al., 1995; Nguyen et al., 1996; Peters et al., 1994; Robinson et al., 1995 a, b; Simonet et al., 1995; Werner et al., 1993). In addition, identified mutations in FGF receptors are linked to skeletal disorders, some lethal, in humans (Muenke and Schell, 1995). Such drastic and varied phenotypes are the likely result of the pleiotropic nature of the FGF growth factor system in stimulating proliferation. This capability is further potentiated by the effects of FGF gene family members on vascular cells. Unlike other broad-spectrum mitogens, certain FGF ligands promote endothelial cell differentiation from embryonic precursors (Flamme and Risau, 1992) and directly induce angiogenesis (Folkman and Shing, 1992). Therefore, FGF gene family members may promote not only general cellular growth but also the critical vascularization required during tissue formation. The FGF ligands are thus doubly suited to promote a preponderance of cellular and tissue generative

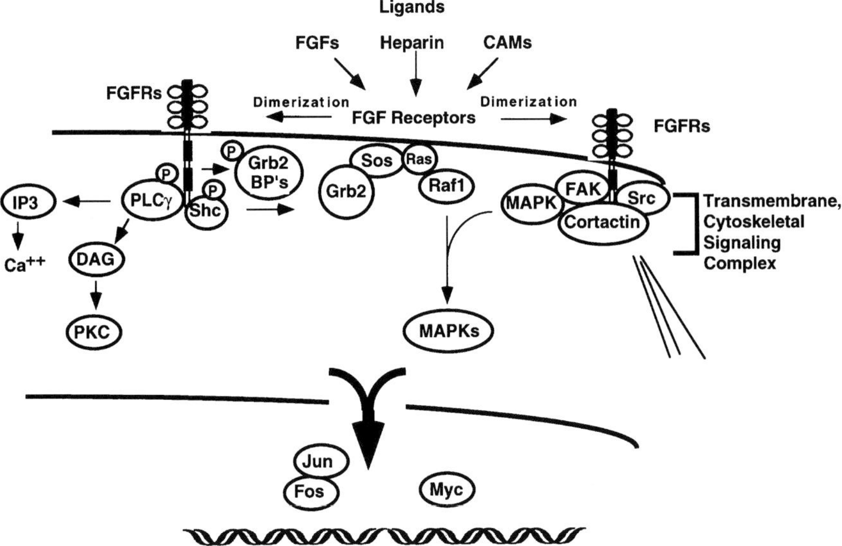

Figure 4.4. FGF signal transduction. Optimal activation of FGF tyrosine kinase receptors occurs in the presence of bound FGF ligand in conjunction with heparin or the physiological equivalent, the heparan sulfate component of proteoglycans. FGF receptor activation has also been shown to occur upon interaction with certain cell adhesion molecules (CAMs). Such interactions at the cell surface induce dimerization and activation of receptor molecules. The result is an auto-and transphosphorylation of receptor tyrosines as well as phosphorylation of identified intracellular substrates. Putative cytoplasmic substrates include phospholipase Cγ (PLC-γ), the adaptor protein Shc and Grb2-binding proteins 80K-H, SNT-like proteins, and FRS2. Transduction of FGF cytoplasmic signaling pathways has been shown to occur via the Ras/Raf1 pathway, eventually leading to the mitogen-activated protein kinase (MAPK) module of enzymes. In addition, FGF receptors along with focal adhesion kinase (FAK) and MAPK appear in focal adhesion complexes upon ligand-mediated integrin clustering. FGF receptors also associate with the Src tyrosine kinase and the Src substrate cortactin, a fibrillar actin-binding protein. The ultimate activation of nuclear transcription factors results in regulation of gene expression resulting in FGF-mediated proliferation, migration, and differentiation. Not shown is FGF-mediated activation of the STAT signaling pathway.

processes in which both proliferation and angiogenesis are necessary. These include the development of the vascular system during embryogenesis, the normal tissue repair and regeneration required for placental development, ovulation, and endometrial cycling, and after wounding and ischemia. Indeed, it is anticipated that the function of the FGF ligands will ultimately be shown to be synergistic with other potent angiogenic factors, most notably the vascular endothelial growth factor gene family.

Importantly, angiogenesis is also critical to the progression of a number of pathological processes. FGF-mediated angiogenic events are involved in cancer since solid tumor growth beyond a few millimeters in size is dependent on the induction of a blood supply to support the growing mass. Pathological vascularization is a feature of diabetic retinopathy and chronic inflammatory diseases such as rheumatoid arthritis, psoriasis, and periodontitis. Angiogenic events also play a direct role in the pathology of atherosclerosis, ischemic heart disease, and in the smooth muscle cell proliferation which occurs during restinosis following vascular intervention, transplantation, or injury. In many instances FGF-mediated responses are involved in general regulation of vessel hemostasis as well. For example, FGF-2 increases low-density lipoprotein binding, uptake, and degradation in smooth muscle cells (Hsu et al., 1994) and acts as a hypotensive agent (Cuevas et al., 1991).

FGF-related effects in the vasculature are not limited to the endothelial cell within vessels. FGF gene family members are expressed in myocardium (Casscells et al., 1990; Kardami and Fandrich, 1989; Weiner and Swain, 1989) and are upregulated, in the adult heart, by ischemia or hemodynamic stress (Padua et al., 1995; Schneider et al., 1992). FGF-2 stimulates cardiac-specific gene expression during cardiomyogenesis (Parker et al., 1992). FGF gene family members are present in vascular smooth muscle cells and cause vascular smooth muscle cell chemotaxis and proliferation (Lindner and Reidy, 1993; Winkles et al., 1987). The initial smooth muscle cell proliferation which serves as a prelude to intimal thickening observed after arterial injury in vivo correlates with the presence of FGF (Lindner and Reidy, 1993; Olson et al., 1992). Delivery of FGF-2 to sites of arterial injury increases intimal thickening and smooth muscle cell proliferation (Edelman et al., 1992) and antibodies which neutralize FGF-2 activity inhibit smooth muscle cell proliferation after injury (Lindner and Reidy, 1991). Further, the expression of an ectopic gene encoding a secreted form of FGF-1 in the arterial wall induces marked intimal hyperplasia (Nabel et al., 1993). Since FGF-2 and FGF receptor-1 are immunolocalized in the foci of human atherosclerotic plaques (Hughes and Hall, 1993), they may contribute to the proliferation and vascularization characteristic of advanced plaque growth.

FGFs regulate the migratory and proliferative aspects of angiogenesis. FGF-1 and FGF-2 are produced by and are chemotactic and mitogenic for endothelial cells. The FGF prototypes also sustain human endothelial cells in culture in a proliferative state and induce their migration along a FGF gradient. FGF-mediated endothelial cell migration and proliferation in vivo during angiogenesis is evidenced by the upregulation of immunoreactive FGF in regenerating endothelial cells after injury whereas little immunoreactivity is present in quiescent endothelium (Lindner et al., 1989). The FGF-mediated migratory and proliferative phases of early angiogenesis are coupled to FGF-induced matrix-resorbing activity. FGF-mediated signaling generates components of proteolytic systems which degrade matrix and downregulates enzymes involved in the buildup of matrix components (Feres-Filho et al., 1996).

The ability of FGF gene family members to regulate matrix metabolism is countered by the ability of heparan sulfate proteoglycans associated with the extracellular matrix and cell surface molecules to regulate both the bioavailability and activity of the FGF gene family members. Heparan sulfates may act in a passive manner to sequester FGF ligands in vivo and prevent interactions with cellular FGF tyrosine kinase receptors. In addition, since FGF ligands are sensitive to denaturation and heparin protects FGF from enzymatic and physical degradation in vitro, the heparan sulfate interaction may optimize storage of certain FGF ligands in vivo. The ability of heparan sulfates to sequester FGF in an inactive state may explain observations showing immunolocalization of matrix-associated FGF adjacent to amitotic cells. However, FGF can be specifically released from heparan sulfate sites by treatment with excess heparin, high salt concentrations, or by enzymatic digestion with heparanases and elastases. Glycolytic or proteolytic release may occur during tissue remodeling or reconstruction and allow FGF to interact with its tyrosine kinase receptors. Further, heparan sulfate may facilitate redistribution of FGF in a manner regulating its sphere of activity. Alternatively, matrix-binding and release may provide for controlled, sustained release of certain FGF ligands, which has been shown to result in maximum activity in vivo as compared to bolus administration (see Chapter 13). Further regulation of FGF activity stems from cell–matrix interactions that determine the state of the cell in its response to FGF. The angiogenic response of endothelial cells to FGF is modulated by changes in cell shape resulting from compositional alterations of the extracellular matrix.

While the clinical benefit of potential FGF antagonists for the manipulation and management of angiogenic events in dysfunctional organs, tissues, and solid tumors is promising, these benefits must await the development of such systems. Indeed, it is remarkable that no natural FGF antagonist has been identified to date. However, it is anticipated that FGF-mediated signaling must be regulated either by indirect mechanisms involving ligand availability or concurrently with direct mechanisms involving antagonistic signaling pathways. Thus, it is more likely that the clinical benefit of the FGF research effort will involve situations of organ/tissue repair including bone, spinal cord, and the numerous consequences of ischemia. Perhaps among these clinical situations, the control of myocardial ischemia by the induction of collateral coronary circulation through the administration of FGF gene family members appears to be most promising (Ware and Simons, 1997).

NOTE ADDED IN PROOF

While this chapter was in press, Ohbayashi and co-workers (Ohbayashi, N., Hoshikawa, M., Kimura, S., Yamasaki, M., Fukui, S., and Itoh, N. (1998). J. Biol. Chem. 273: 18161–18164) reported the cloning and expression of FGF-18.

REFERENCES

Amaya, E., Musci, T. J., and Kirschner, M. W. (1991). Expression of a dominant negative mutant of the FGF receptor disrupts mesoderm formation in Xenopus embryos. Cell 66: 257–270.

Aviezer, D., Hecht, D., Safran, M., Eisinger, M., David, G., and Yayon, A. (1994). Perlecan, basal lamina proteoglycan, promotes basic fibroblast growth factor-receptor binding, mitogenesis, and angiogenesis. Cell 79: 1005–1013.

Bonneh-Barkay, D., Shlissel, M., Berman, B., Shaoul, E., Admon, A., Vlodavsky, I., Carey, D. J., Asundi, V. K., Reich-Slotky, R., and Ron, D. (1997). Identification of glypican as a dual modulator of the biological activity of fibroblast growth factors. J. Biol. Chem. 272: 12415–12421.

Bouche, G., Gas, N., Prats, H., Baldin, V., Tauber, J.-P., Teiss, J., and Amalric, J. (1987). Basic fibroblast growth factor enters the nucleolus and stimulates the transcription of ribosomal genes in ABAE cells undergoing G_0–G_1 transition. Proc. Natl. Acad. Sci. USA 84: 6770–6774.

Brunner, G., Gabrilove, J., Rifkin, D. B., and Wilson, E. L. (1991). Phospholipase C release of basic fibroblast growth factor from human bone marrow cultures as a biologically active complex with a phosphatidylinositol-anchored heparan sulfate proteoglycan. J. Cell Biol. 114: 1275–1283.

Casscells, W., Speir, E., Sasse, J., Klagsbrun, M., Allen, P., Lee, M., Calvo, B., Chiba, M., Haggroth, L., Folkman, J., and Epstein, S. E. (1990). Isolation, characterization, and localization of heparin-binding growth factors in the heart. J. Clin. Invest. 85: 433–441.

Chernousov, M. A. and Carey, D. J. (1993). N-syndecan (syndecan 3) from neonatal rat brain binds basic fibroblast growth factor. J. Biol. Chem. 268: 16810–16814.

Coffin, J. D., Florkiewicz, R. Z., Neumann, J., Mort-Hopkins, T., Dorn, G. W. 2nd, Lightfoot, P., German, R., Howles, P. N., Kier, A., O'Toole, B. A., Sasse, J., Gonzalez, A. M., Baird, A. and Doetschman, T. (1995). Abnormal bone growth and selective translational regulation in basic fibroblast growth factor (FGF-2) transgenic mice. Mol. Biol. Cell 6: 1861–1873.

Coulier, F., Pontarotti, P., Roubin, R., Hartung, H., Goldfarb, M., and Birnbaum, D. (1997). Of worms and men: an evolutionary perspective on the fibroblast growth facor (FGF) and FGF receptor families. J. Mol. Evol. 44: 43–56.

Cuevas, P., Carceller, F., Ortega, S., Zazo, M., Nieto, I., and Gimenez-Gallego, G. (1991). Hypotensive activity of fibroblast growth factor. Science 254: 1208–1210.

Edelman, E. R., Nugent, M. A., Smith, L. T., and Karnovsky, M. J. (1992). Basic fibroblast growth factor enhances the coupling of intimal hyperplasia and proliferation of vasa vasorum in injured rat arteries. J. Clin. Invest. 89: 465–473.

Edelman, E. R., Nugent, M. A., and Karnovsky, M. (1993). Perivascular and intravenous administration of basic fibroblast growth factor: vascular and solid organ deposition. Proc. Natl. Acad. Sci. USA 30: 1513–1517.

Feres-Filho, E. J., Menassa, G. B., and Trackman, P. C. (1996). Regulation of lysyl oxidase by basic fibroblast growth factor in osteoblastic MC3T3-E1 cells. J. Biol. Chem. 271: 6411–6416.

Fernig, D. G. and Gallagher, J. T. (1994). Fibroblast growth factors and their receptors: an information network controlling tissue growth, morphogenesis and repair. Prog. Growth Factor Res. 5: 353–377.

Flamme, I. and Risau, W. (1992). Induction of vasculogenesis and hematopoiesis in vitro. Development 116: 435–439.

Florkiewicz, R. Z., Anchin, J., and Baird, A. (1998). The inhibition of fibroblast growth factor-2 export by cardenolides implies a novel function for the catalytic subunit of Na^+,K^+-ATPase. J. Biol. Chem. 273: 544–551.

Folkman, J. and Shing, Y. (1992). Angiogenesis. J. Biol. Chem. 267: 25803–25809.

Goldfarb, M. (1990). The fibroblast growth factor family. Cell Growth Differ. 1: 439–445.

Gualandris, A., Coltrini, D., Bergonzoni, L., Isacchi, A., Tenca, S., Ginelli, B., and Presta, M. (1993). The NH_2-terminal extension of high molecular weight forms of basic fibroblast growth factor (bFGF) is not essential for the binding of bFGF to nuclear chromatin in transfected NIH 3T3 cells. Growth Factors 8: 49–60.

Guo, L., Yu, Q. C., and Fuchs, E. (1993). Targeting expression of keratinocyte growth factor to keratinocytes elicits striking changes in epithelial differentiation in transgenic mice. EMBO J. 12: 973–986.

Herr, A. B., Ornitz, D. M., Sasisekharan, R., Venkataraman, G., and Waksman, G. (1997). Heparin-induced self-association of fibroblast growth factor-2. J. Biol. Chem. 272: 16382–16389.

Hsu, H. Y., Nicholson, A. C., and Hajjar, D. P. (1994). Basic fibroblast growth factor-induced low density lipoprotein receptor transcription and surface expression. J. Biol. Chem. 269: 9213–9220.

Hughes, S. E. and Hall, P. A. (1993). Immunolocalization of fibroblast growth factor receptor 1 and its ligands in human tissues. Lab. Invest. 69: 173–182.

Imamura, T., Engleka, K., Zhan, X., Tokita, Y., Forough, R., Roeder, D., Jackson, A., Maier, J. A. M., Hla, T., and Maciag, T. (1989). Recovery of mitogenic activity of a growth factor mutant with a nuclear translocation sequence. Science 249: 1567–1570.

Imamura, T., Friedman, S. A., Gamble, S., Tokita, Y., Opalenik, S. R., Thompson, J. A., and Maciag, T. (1995). Identification of the domain within fibroblast growth factor-1 responsible for heparin-dependence. Biochim. Biophys. Acta 1266: 124–130.

Jackson, A., Friedman, S., Zhan, X., Engleka, K. A., Forough, R., and Maciag, T. (1992). Heat shock induces the secretion of fibroblast growth factor-1. Proc. Natl. Acad. Sci. USA 89: 10691–10695.

Jaye, M., Schlessinger, J., and Dionne, C. A. (1992). Fibroblast growth factor receptor tyrosine kinases: molecular analysis and signal transduction. Biochim. Biophys. Acta 1135: 185–199.

Johnson, D. E. and Williams, L. T. (1993). Structural and functional diversity in the FGF receptor multigene family. Adv. Cancer Res. 60: 1–40.

Kan, M., Wang, F., Xu, J., Crabb, J. W., Hu, J., and McKeehan, W. L. (1993). An essential heparin-binding domain in the fibroblast growth factor receptor kinase. Science 259: 1918–1921.

Kan, M., Wang, F., Kan, M., To, B., Gabriel, J. L., and McKeehan, W. L. (1996). Divalent cations and heparin/heparan sulfate cooperate to control assembly and activity of the fibroblast growth factor receptor complex. J. Biol. Chem. 271: 26143.

Kardami, E. and Fandrich, R. R. (1989). Basic fibroblast growth factor in atria and ventricles of the vertebrate heart. J. Cell Biol. 109: 1865–1875.

Lee, F. S., Lane, T. F., Kuo, A., Shackleford, G. M., and Leder, P. (1995). Insertional mutagenesis identifies a member of the Wnt gene family as a candidate oncogene in the mammary epithelium of *int*-2/Fgf-3 transgenic mice. Proc. Natl. Acad. Sci. USA 92: 2268–2272.

Lin, X.-Z., Yao, S., and Hawiger, J. (1996). Role of the nuclear localization sequence in fibroblast growth factor-1-stimulated mitogenic pathways. J. Biol. Chem. 271: 5305–5308.

Lindner, V. and Reidy, M. A. (1991). Proliferation of smooth muscle cells after vascular injury is inhibited by an antibody against basic fibroblast growth factor. Proc. Natl. Acad. Sci. USA 88: 3739–3743.

Lindner, V. and Reidy, M. A. (1993). Expression of basic fibroblast growth factor and its receptor by smooth muscle cells and endothelium in injured rat arteries. An *en face* study. Circ. Res. 73: 589–595.

Lindner, V., Reidy, M. A., and Fingerle, J. (1989). Regrowth of arterial endothelium. Denudation with minimal trauma leads to complete endothelial cell regrowth. Lab. Invest. 61: 556–563.

Maher, P. A. (1996). Nuclear translocation of fibroblast growth factor (FGF) receptors in response to FGF-2. J. Cell Biol. 134: 529–536.

McKeehan, W. L. and Kan, M. (1994). Heparan sulfate fibroblast growth factor receptor complex: structure-function relationships. Mol. Reprod. Dev. 39: 69–81.

Mignatti, P., Morimoto, T., and Rifkin, D. B. (1992). Basic fibroblast growth factor, a protein devoid of secretory signal sequence, is released by cells via a pathway independent of the endoplasmic reticulum-Golgi complex. J. Cell. Physiol. 151: 81–93.

Miyamoto, S., Teramoto, H., Gutkind, J. S., and Yamada, K. M. (1996). Integrins can collaborate with growth factors for phosphorylation of receptor tyrosine kinases and MAP kinase activation: roles of integrin aggregation and occupancy of receptors. J. Cell Biol. 135: 1633–1642.

Muenke, M. and Schell, U. (1995). Fibroblast-growth-factor receptor mutations in human skeletal disorders. Trends Genet. 11: 308–313.

Nabel, E. G., Yang, Z., Plautz, G., Forough, R., Zhan, X., Haudenschild, C. C., Maciag, T., and Nabel, G. J. (1993). Recombinant fibroblast growth factor-1 promotes intimal hyperplasia and angiogenesis in arteries *in vivo*. Nature 362: 844–846.

Nakanishi, Y., Kihara, K., Mizuno, K., Masamune, Y., Yoshitake, Y., and Nishikawa, K. (1992). Direct effect of basic fibroblast growth factor on gene transcription in a cell-free system. Proc. Natl. Acad. Sci. USA 89: 5216–5220.

Neilson, K. M. and Friesel, R. E. (1995). Constitutive activation of fibroblast growth factor receptor-2 by a point mutation associated with Crouzon syndrome. J. Biol. Chem. 270: 26037–26040.

Nguyen, H. Q., Danilenko, D. M., Bucay, N., DeRose, M. L., Van, G. Y., Thomason, A., and Simonet, W. S. (1996). Expression of keratinocyte growth factor in embryonic liver of transgenic mice causes changes in epithelial growth and differentiation resulting in polycystic kidneys and other organ malformations. Oncogene 12: 2109–2119.

Nurcombe, B., Ford, M. D., Wildschut, J. A., and Bartlett, P. F. (1993). Developmental regulation of neuronal response to FGF-1 and FGF-2 by heparan sulfate proteoglycan. Science 260: 103–106.

Olson, N. E., Chao, S., Lindner, V., and Reidy, M. A. (1992). Intimal smooth muscle cell proliferation after balloon catheter injury. The role of basic fibroblast growth factor. Am. J. Pathol. 140: 1017–1023.

Padua, R. R., Sethi, R., Dhalla, N. S., and Kardami, E. (1995). Basic fibroblast growth factor is cardioprotective in ischemia-reperfusion injury. Mol. Cell. Biochem. 143: 129–135.

Parker, T. G., Chow, K. L., Schwartz, R. J., and Schneider, M. D. (1992). Positive and negative control of the skeletal alpha-actin promoter in cardiac muscle. A proximal serum response element is sufficient for induction by basic fibroblast growth factor (FGF) but not for inhibition by acidic FGF. J. Biol. Chem. 267: 3343–3350.

Patstone, G. and Maher, P. (1996). Copper and calcium binding motifs in the extracellular domains of fibroblast growth factor receptors. J. Biol. Chem. 271: 3343–3346.

Peters, K. G., Werner, S., Liao, X., Wert, S., Whitsett, J., and Williams, L. (1994). Targeted expression of a dominant negative FGF receptor blocks branching morphogenesis and epithelial differentiation of the mouse lung. EMBO J. 13: 3296–3301.

Plopper, G. E., McNamee, H. P., Dike, L. E., Bojanowski, K., and Ingber, D. E. (1995). Convergence of integrin and growth factor receptor signaling pathways within the focal adhesion complex. Mol. Biol. Cell. 6: 1349–1365.

Prudovsky, I. A., Savion, N., LaVallee, T. M., and Maciag, T. (1996). The nuclear trafficking of extracellular fibroblast growth factor (FGF)-1 correlates with the perinuclear association of the FGF receptor-1 alpha isoforms but not the FGF receptor-1 beta isoforms. J. Biol. Chem. 271: 14198–14205.

Robinson, M. L., MacMillan-Crow, L. A., Thompson, J. A., and Overbeek, P. A. (1995a). Expression of a truncated FGF receptor results in defective lens development in transgenic mice. Development 121: 3959–3967.

Robinson, M. L., Overbeek, P. A., Verran, D. J., Grizzle, W. E., Stockard, C. R., Friesel, R., Maciag, T., and Thompson, J. A. (1995b). Extracellular FGF-1 acts as a lens differentiation factor in transgenic mice. Development 121: 505–514.

Schneider, M. D., McLellan, W. R., Black, F. M., and Parker, T. G. (1992). Growth factors, growth factor response elements, and the cardiac phenotype. Basic Res. Cardiol. 87: 33–48.

Shi, J., Friedman, S., and Maciag, T. (1997). A carboxyl-terminal domain in fibroblast growth factor (FGF)-2 inhibits FGF-1 release in response to heat shock in vitro. J. Biol. Chem. 272: 1142–1147.

Shiang, R. T., Thompson, L. M., Zhu, Y.-Z., Church, D. M., Fielder, T. J., Bocian, M., Winokur, S. T., and Wasmuth, J. J. (1994). Mutations in the transmembrane domain of FGFR3 cause the most common genetic form of dwarfism, achondroplasia. Cell 78: 335–342.

Simonet, W. S., DeRose, M. L., Bucay, N., Nguyen, H. Q., Wert, S. E., Zhou, L., Ulich, T. R., Thomason, A., Danilenko, D. M., and Whitsett, J. A. (1995). Pulmonary malformation in transgenic mice expressing human keratinocyte growth factor in the lung. Proc. Natl. Acad. Sci. USA 92: 12461–12465.

Sosnowski, B. A., Gonzalez, A. M., Chandler, L. A., Buechler, Y. J., Pierce, G. F., and Baird, A. (1996). Targeting DNA to cells with basic fibroblast growth factor (FGF-2). J. Biol. Chem. 271: 33647–33653.

Stachowiak, M. K., Moffett, J., Joy, A., Puchacz, E., Florkiewicz, R., and Stachowiak, E. K. (1994). Regulation of bFGF gene expression and subcellular distribution of bFGF protein in adrenal medullary cells. J. Cell Biol. 127: 203–223.

Thompson, J. A., Anderson, K. D., DiPietro, J. M., Zwiebel, J. A., Zametta, M., Anderson, W. F., and Maciag, T. (1988). Site-directed neovessel formation *in vivo.* Science 241: 1349–1352.

Ueba, T., Nosaka, T., Takahashi, J. A., Shibata, F., Florkiewicz, R. Z., Vogelstein, B., Oda, Y., Kikuchi, H., and Hatanaka, M. (1994). Transcriptional regulation of basic fibroblast growth factor gene by p53 in human glioblastoma and hepatocellular carcinoma cells. Proc. Natl. Acad. Sci. USA 91: 9009–9013.

Vagner, S., Gensac, M. C., Maret, A., Bayard, F., Amalric, F., Prats, H., and Prats, A. C. (1995). Alternative translation of human fibroblast growth factor 2 mRNA occurs by internal entry of ribosomes. Mol. Cell Biol. 15: 35–44.

Vainikka, S., Paranen, J., Bellosta, P., Coulier, F., Basilico, C., Jaye, M., and Alitalo, K. (1992). Fibroblast growth factor receptor-4 shows novel features in genome structure, ligand binding, and signal transduction. EMBO J. 11: 4273–4280.

Wang, J.-K., Gao, G., and Goldfarb, M. (1994). Fibroblast growth factor receptors have different signaling and mitogenic potentials. Mol. Cell. Biol. 14: 181–188.

Ware, J. A. and Simons, M. (1997). Angiogenesis in ischemic heart disease. Nat. Med. 3: 158–164.

Weiner, H. L. and Swain, J. L. (1989). Acidic fibroblast growth factor mRNA is expressed by cardiac myocytes in culture and the protein is localized to the extracellular matrix. Proc. Natl. Acad. Sci. USA 86: 2683–2687.

Werner, S., Weinberg, W., Liao, X., Peters, K. G., Blessing, M., Yuspa, S. H., Weiner, R. L., and Williams, L. T. (1993). Targeted expression of a dominant-negative FGF receptor mutant in the epidermis of transgenic mice reveals a role of FGF in keratinocyte organization and differentiation. EMBO J. 12: 2635–2643.

Wiedlocha, A., Falnes, P. O., Rapak, A., Klingenberg, O., Munoz, R., and Olsnes, S. (1995). Translocation to cytosol of exogenous, CAAX-tagged acidic fibroblast growth factor. J. Biol. Chem. 270: 30680–30685.

Wiedlocha, A., Falnes, P. O., Rapak, A., Munoz, R., Klingenberg, O., and Olsnes, S. (1996). Stimulation of proliferation of a human osteosarcoma cell line by exogenous acidic fibroblast growth factor requires both activation of receptor tyrosine kinase and growth factor internalization. Mol. Cell. Biol. 16: 270–280.

Williams, E. J., Furness, J., Walsh, F. S., and Doherty, P. (1994). Activation of the FGF receptor underlies neurite outgrowth stimulated by L1, N-CAM, and N-cadherin. Neuron 13: 583–594.

Winkles, J. A., Friesel, R., Burgess, W. H., Howk, R., and Mehlman, T. (1987). Human vascular smooth muscle cells both express and respond to heparin-binding growth factor I (endothelial cell growth factor). Proc. Natl. Acad. Sci. USA 84: 7124–7128.

Zhan, X., Hu, X., Friedman, S., and Maciag, T. (1992). Analysis of endogenous and exogenous nuclear translocation of fibroblast growth factor-1 in NIH 3T3 cells. Biochem. Biophys. Res. Commun. 188: 982–991.

Zhan, X., Hu, X., Friesel, R., and Maciag, T. (1993). Long term growth factor exposure and differential tyrosine phosphorylation are required for DNA synthesis in BALB/c 3T3 cells. J. Biol. Chem. 268: 9611–9620.

Zuber, M. E., Zhou, Z., Dodge, N., and Olwin, B. B. (1997). Cysteine-rich FGF receptor regulates intracellular FGF-1 and FGF-2 levels. J. Cell. Physiol. 170: 217–227.

5

The Vascular Endothelial Growth Factor Family

NAPOLEONE FERRARA AND HANS PETER GERBER

The development of a vascular supply is a fundamental requirement for organ development and differentiation during embryogenesis as well as for wound healing and reproductive functions in the adult (Folkman, 1995). Angiogenesis is also implicated in the pathogenesis of a variety of disorders including proliferative retinopathies, age-related macular degeneration, tumors, rheumatoid arthritis, and psoriasis (Folkman, 1995).

This chapter discusses the molecular and biological properties of the vascular endothelial growth factor (VEGF) proteins. Work done by several laboratories over the last few years has elucidated the pivotal role of VEGF and its receptors in the regulation of normal and abnormal angiogenesis (Ferrara and Davis-Smyth, 1997). The finding that the loss of even a single VEGF allele results in embryonic lethality points to an irreplaceable role played by this factor in the development and differentiation of the vascular system. Furthermore, VEGF-induced angiogenesis results in a therapeutic effect in animal models of coronary or limb ischemia and, most recently, in a human patient affected by critical leg ischemia (Ferrara and Davis-Smyth, 1997).

BIOLOGICAL ACTIVITIES OF VEGF

VEGF is a mitogen for vascular endothelial cells derived from arteries, veins and lymphatics but does not have consistent appreciable mitogenic activity for other cell types (Ferrara and Davis-Smyth, 1997). VEGF promotes angiogenesis in tridimensional in vitro models, inducing confluent microvascular endothelial cells to invade collagen gels and form capillary-like structures (Pepper et al., 1992) and sprouting from rat aortic rings embedded in a collagen gel (Nicosia et al., 1994). VEGF also elicits a pronounced angiogenic response in a variety of in vivo models including the chick chorioallantoic membrane (Leung et al., 1989) and the primate iris (Tolentino et al., 1996).

VEGF induces expression of the serine proteases urokinase-type and tissue-type plasminogen activators (PA) and also PA inhibitor 1 (PAI-1) in cultured bovine microvascular endothelial cells (Pepper et al., 1991) and increases expression of the metalloproteinase interstitial collagenase in human umbilical vein endothelial cells but not in dermal fibroblasts (Unemori et al., 1992). Other studies have shown that VEGF promotes expression of urokinase receptor (uPAR) and stimulates hexose transport in cultured vascular endothelial cells (Pekala et al., 1990). (Mandriota et al., 1995).

VEGF is known also as vascular permeability factor (VPF) based on its ability to induce vascular leakage in the guinea pig skin. Dvorak and colleagues proposed that an increase in microvascular permeability is a crucial step in angiogenesis associated with tumors and wounds (Dvorak et al., 1995). According to this hypothesis, a major function of VPF/VEGF in the angiogenic process is the induction of plasma protein leakage. This effect would result in the formation of an extravascular fibrin gel, a substrate for endothelial and tumor cell growth. Recent studies have also suggested that VEGF may also induce fenestrations in endothelial cells (Roberts and Palade, 1997). Topical administration of VEGF acutely resulted in the development of fenestrations in the endothelium of small venules and capillaries, even in regions where endothelial cells are not normally fenestrated and was associated with increased vascular permeability (Roberts and Palade, 1997).

VEGF promotes expression of VCAM-1 and ICAM-1 in endothelial cells (Melder et al., 1996) This induction results in the adhesion of activated natural killer (NK) cells to endothelial cells, mediated by specific interaction of endothelial VCAM-1 and ICAM-1 with CD18 and VLA-4 on the surface of NK cells.

VEGF has certain regulatory effects on blood cells, including monocyte chemotaxis (Clauss et al., 1990); VEGF also induces colony formation by mature subsets of granulocyte-macrophage progenitor cells (Broxmeyer et al., 1995). These findings may be explained by the common origin of endothelial and hematopoietic cells and the presence of VEGF receptors in progenitor cells as early as hemangioblasts in blood islands in the yolk sac. Furthermore, VEGF may have an inhibitory effect on the maturation of host antigen-presenting cells such as dendritic cells (Gabrilovich et al., 1996). VEGF inhibits immature dendritic cells without having a significant effect on the function of mature cells. These findings led to the suggestion that one way that VEGF may facilitate tumor growth is by allowing the tumor to avoid the induction of an immune response (Gabrilovich et al., 1996).

VEGF induces vasodilation in vitro in a dose-dependent fashion (Ku et al., 1993; Yang et al., 1996) and produces transient tachycardia, hypotension, and a decrease in cardiac output when injected intravenously in conscious, instrumented rats (Yang et al., 1996). Such effects appear to be caused by a decrease in venous return, mediated primarily by endothelial cell-derived nitric oxide (NO), as assessed by the requirement for an intact endothelium and the prevention of the effects by N-methylarginine (Yang et al., 1996). Accordingly, VEGF has no direct effect on contractility or rate in isolated rat heart in vitro (Yang et al., 1996). These hemodynamic effects, however, are not unique to VEGF; other angiogenic factors such as FGF-1 and FGF-2 also have the ability to induce NO-mediated vasodilation and hypotension.

ORGANIZATION OF THE VEGF GENE AND CHARACTERISTICS OF THE VEGF PROTEINS

The human VEGF gene is organized in eight exons, separated by seven introns. The coding region spans approximately 14 kilobases (kb; Houck et al., 1991; Tischer et al., 1991) The human VEGF gene has been assigned to chromosome 6p21.3 (Vincenti et al., 1996). It is now well established that alternative exon splicing of a single VEGF gene results in the generation of four different molecular species, having 121, 165, 189, and 206 amino acids following signal sequence cleavage ($VEGF_{121}$, $VEGF_{165}$, $VEGF_{189}$, $VEGF_{206}$). $VEGF_{165}$ lacks the residues encoded by exon 6, while $VEGF_{121}$ lacks the residues encoded by exons 6 and 7. Compared to $VEGF_{165}$, $VEGF_{121}$ lacks 44 amino acids; $VEGF_{189}$ has an insertion of 24 amino acids highly enriched in basic residues and $VEGF_{206}$ has an additional insertion of 17 amino acids (Houck et al., 1991). Analysis of the VEGF gene promoter region reveals a single major transcription start which lies near a cluster of potential Sp1 factor binding sites.

$VEGF_{165}$ is the predominant molecular species produced by a variety of normal and transformed cells. Transcripts encoding $VEGF_{121}$ and $VEGF_{189}$ are detected in the majority of cells and tissues expressing the VEGF gene (Houck et al., 1991). In contrast, $VEGF_{206}$ is a very rare form, so far identified only in a human fetal liver cDNA library (Houck et al., 1991). The genomic organization of the murine VEGF gene has been also described (Shima et al., 1996). Similarly to the human gene, the coding region of the murine VEGF gene encompasses approximately 14 kb and is comprised of eight exons interrupted by seven introns. Analysis of exons suggests the generation of three isoforms, $VEGF_{120}$, $VEGF_{164}$ and $VEGF_{188}$. Therefore, murine VEGFs are shorter than human VEGF by one amino acid. A fourth isoform comparable to $VEGF_{206}$ is not predicted, however, since an in-frame stop codon is present in the region corresponding to the human $VEGF_{206}$ open reading frame. Analysis of the 3' untranslated region of the rat VEGF mRNA has revealed the presence of four potential polyadenylation sites (Levy et al., 1996). A frequently used site is about

1.9 kb further downstream from the previously reported transcription termination codon (Conn et al., 1990). The sequence within this 3' untranslated region reveals a number of sequence motifs that are known to regulate mRNA stability (Levy et al., 1996).

Native VEGF is a basic, heparin-binding, homodimeric glycoprotein of 45,000 daltons (Ferrara and Henzel, 1989). These properties are consistent with $VEGF_{165}$, the major VEGF isoform. $VEGF_{121}$ is a weakly acidic polypeptide that fails to bind to heparin. $VEGF_{189}$ and $VEGF_{206}$ are more basic and bind to heparin with greater affinity than does $VEGF_{165}$ (Houck et al., 1992). Such differences in the isoelectric point and in affinity for heparin may profoundly affect the bioavailability of VEGF. $VEGF_{121}$ is a freely diffusible protein; $VEGF_{165}$ is also secreted, although a significant fraction remains bound to the cell surface and the extracellular matrix (ECM). In contrast, $VEGF_{189}$ and $VEGF_{206}$ are almost completely sequestered in the ECM (Park et al., 1993). These isoforms may be released in a soluble form by heparin or heparinase, however, suggesting that their binding site is represented by proteoglycans containing heparin-like moieties. The long forms may be released also by plasmin following cleavage at the COOH terminus. This action generates a bioactive proteolytic fragment having molecular weight of ~34,000 daltons (Houck et al., 1992). Plasminogen activation and generation of plasmin have been shown to play an important role in the angiogenesis cascade. Thus, proteolysis of VEGF is likely to occur also in vivo. The bioactive product of plasmin action is comprised of the first 110 NH_2-terminal amino acids of VEGF (Keyt et al., 1996a). These findings suggest that the VEGF proteins may become available to endothelial cells by at least two different mechanisms: synthesis as freely diffusible proteins ($VEGF_{121}$, $VEGF_{165}$), or following protease activation and cleavage of the longer isoforms. Loss of heparin binding, whether it is due to alternative splicing of RNA or plasmin cleavage, results in a substantial loss of mitogenic activity for vascular endothelial cells; compared to $VEGF_{165}$, $VEGF_{121}$ or $VEGF_{110}$ demonstrates 50–100-fold reduced potency when tested in endothelial cell growth assay (Keyt et al., 1996a). The stability of VEGF–heparan sulfate–receptor complexes may contribute to effective signal transduction and stimulation of endothelial cell proliferation (Keyt et al., 1996a). Thus, VEGFs structural and functional heterogeneity has the potential to yield a graded and controlled biological response. Recently, evidence for the existence of an additional alternatively spliced molecular species of VEGF has been provided (Poltorak et al., 1997). A VEGF isoform containing exons 1–6 and 8 of the VEGF gene was found to be expressed as a major VEGF mRNA form in several cell lines derived from carcinomas of the female reproductive system. This mRNA is predicted to encode a VEGF form of 145 amino acids ($VEGF_{145}$). Recombinant $VEGF_{145}$ induced the proliferation of vascular endothelial cells, albeit at much lower potency than did $VEGF_{165}$. $VEGF_{145}$ binds to the KDR receptor on the surface of endothelial cells and also binds to heparin with an affinity similar to that of $VEGF_{165}$.

REGULATION OF VEGF GENE EXPRESSION

Oxygen Tension

Among the mechanisms that have been proposed to participate in the regulation of VEGF gene expression, oxygen tension is a particularly important mediator, both in vitro and in vivo. VEGF mRNA expression is rapidly and reversibly induced by exposure to low pO_2 in a variety of normal and transformed cultured cell types (Minchenko et al., 1994; Shima et al., 1995). Also, ischemia caused by occlusion of the left anterior descending coronary artery results in a dramatic increase in VEGF RNA levels in the pig and rat myocardium, suggesting the possibility that VEGF may mediate the spontaneous revascularization that follows myocardial ischemia (Hashimoto et al., 1994). Furthermore, hypoxic upregulation of VEGF mRNA in neuroglial cells, secondary to the onset of neuronal activity, has been proposed to play an important physiological role in the development of the retinal vasculature (Stone et al., 1995).

Similarities exist between the mechanisms leading to hypoxic regulation of VEGF and erythropoietin (Epo) (Goldberg and Schneider, 1994). Inducibility by hypoxia is conferred on both genes by homologous sequences. By deletion and mutation analysis, a 28-base sequence has been identified in the 5' promoter of the rat and human VEGF gene which mediated hypoxia-induced transcription (Levy et al., 1995; Liu et al., 1995). This sequence reveals a high degree of homology and protein-binding characteristics similar to the hypoxia-inducible factor 1 (HIF-1) binding site within the Epo gene (Madan and Curtin, 1993). HIF-1 has been identified as a mediator of transcriptional responses to hypoxia and is a basic, heterodimeric, helix-loop-helix protein (Wang and Semenza, 1995). When reporter constructs containing the VEGF sequences that mediate hypoxia-inducibility were cotransfected with expression vectors encoding HIF-1 subunits, reporter gene transcription was much greater than that observed in cells transfected with the reporter alone, both in hypoxic and normoxic conditions (Forsythe et al., 1996). Figure 5.1 provides a schematic representation of the putative signal transduction pathways resulting in increased transcription in response to hypoxia.

Transcriptional activation is not the only mechanism leading to VEGF upregulation in response to hypoxia, however (Ikeda et al., 1995; Levy et al., 1996). Increased mRNA stability has been identified as a significant factor as well. Sequences that mediate increased stability have been identified in the 3' untranslated region of the VEGF mRNA.

Cytokines

Various cytokines or growth factors may upregulate expression of VEGF mRNA. EGF, TGF-β, or KGF results in a marked induction of VEGF mRNA expression (Frank et al., 1995) EGF also stimulates VEGF release by cul-

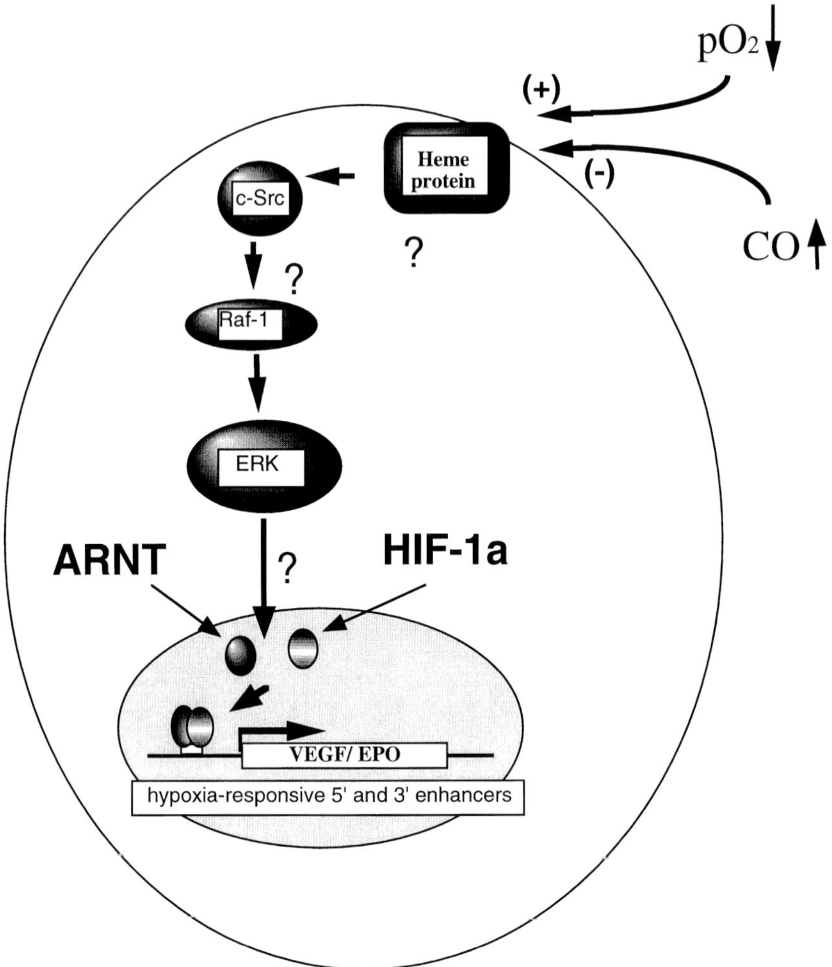

Figure 5.1. Putative signaling pathways involved in the regulation of VEGF and other genes inducible by hypoxia. Activation of the hypoxia signaling pathway can be initiated by low oxygen tension (pO_2) or $CoCl_2$. The presence of an oxygen-sensing molecule on the cell membrane has been postulated but not yet demonstrated. Events leading to the activation of c-Src kinase by the putative oxigen sensor remain to be characterized. C-Src and its downstream target Raf-1 were shown to be critically involved in the hypoxia signal transduction pathway. Raf-1 activation in turn leads to the activation of the extracellular signal-regulated kinases (ERKs). The processes leading to increased expression of the transcription factor subunits ARNT (aryl hydrocarbon receptor nuclear translocator) and HIF-1α forming the hypoxia inducible factor-1 (HIF-1) have not been identified yet. Hypoxia leads to increased expression of these subunits, which bind to their specific binding sites present in the regulatory regions of many hypoxia responsive genes, resulting in increased transcription.

tured glioblastoma cells (Goldman et al., 1993). In addition, treatment of quiescent cultures of epithelial and fibroblastic cell lines with TGF-β results in induction of VEGF mRNA and release of VEGF protein into the medium (Pertovaara et al., 1994). Based on these findings, it has been proposed that VEGF may function as a paracrine mediator for indirect-acting angiogenic agents such as TGF-β (Pertovaara et al., 1994). Furthermore, IL-1 β induces VEGF expression in aortic smooth muscle cells (Li et al., 1995). Both IL-1α and PGE_2 induce expression of VEGF in cultured synovial fibroblasts, suggesting the participation of such inductive mechanisms in inflammatory angiogenesis (Ben-Av et al., 1995). IL-6 also significantly induces VEGF expression in several cell lines (Cohen et al., 1996). IGF-1, a mitogen implicated in the growth of several malignancies, increases expression of VEGF mRNA and protein in cultured colorectal carcinoma cells (Warren et al., 1996). Such induction was mediated by a combined increase in transcriptional rate of the VEGF gene and in the stability of the mRNA.

Differentiation and Transformation

Cell differentiation regulates VEGF gene expression (Claffey et al., 1992). The VEGF mRNA is upregulated during the conversion of 3T3 preadipocytes into adipocytes and during the myogenic differentiation of C2C12 cells. Conversely, VEGF gene expression is repressed during the differentiation of the pheochromocytoma cell line PC12 into nonmalignant, neuron-like, cells.

Specific transforming events also induce VEGF gene expression. A mutated form of the murine p53 tumor suppressor gene increases VEGF mRNA expression in NIH 3T3 cells in transient transfection assays (Kieser et al., 1994). Likewise, oncogenic mutations or amplification of Ras leads to VEGF upregulation (Rak et al., 1995; Grugel et al., 1995). Interestingly, expression of oncogenic Ras, either constitutive or transient, potentiates the induction of VEGF by hypoxia (Mazure et al., 1996). Moreover, the von Hippel-Lindau (VHL) tumor suppressor gene has been implicated in the regulation of VEGF gene expression (Siemeister et al., 1996; Iliopoulos et al., 1996; Gnarra et al., 1996). The VHL tumor suppressor gene is inactivated in patients with von Hippel-Lindau disease and in most sporadic clear cell renal carcinomas. Human renal cell carcinoma cells either lacking endogenous wild-type VHL gene or expressing an inactive mutant demonstrate altered regulation of VEGF gene expression, which is corrected by introduction of wild-type VHL gene. Most of the endothelial cell mitogenic activity released by tumor cells expressing mutant VHL gene is neutralized by anti-VEGF antibodies (Siemeister et al., 1996). These findings suggest that VEGF is a key mediator of the abnormal vascular proliferation and solid tumors characteristic of the VHL syndrome. One function of the VHL protein is to regulate negatively a series of hypoxia-inducible genes, including those encoding VEGF, platelet derived growth factor B chain, and the glucose transporter GLUT1 (Iliopoulos et al., 1996). In the presence of a mutant VHL, mRNAs for such genes were produced both under normoxic and hypoxic conditions. Reintroduction of wild-type VHL resulted in inhibition of mRNA production under normoxic conditions and restored the characteristic hypoxia-inducibility of those genes (Iliopoulos et al., 1996). In addition, VHL regulates VEGF expression at a posttranscriptional level and its inactivation in target cells causes a loss of VEGF suppression, leading to formation of a vascular stroma (Gnarra et al., 1996). Interestingly, despite fivefold differences in VEGF mRNA levels, VHL overexpression did not affect VEGF transcription initiation.

THE VEGF RECEPTORS

Two classes of high-affinity VEGF binding sites were initially described on the surface of bovine endothelial cells, with K_d values of 10 pM and 100 pM, respectively (Vaisman et al., 1990; Plouet and Moukadiri, 1990). Lower-affinity binding sites on mononuclear phagocytes were subsequently described (Shen et al., 1993). Such binding sites may be involved in mediating VEGF's chemotactic effects for monocytes (Clauss et al., 1990).

Ligand autoradiography studies on fetal and adult rat tissue sections demonstrated that high-affinity VEGF binding sites are localized to the vascular endothelium of large or small vessels in situ (Jakeman et al., 1992; 1993). VEGF binding was apparent not only on proliferating but also on quiescent endothelial cells (Jakeman et al., 1992, 1993). Also, the earliest developmental identification of high-affinity VEGF binding was in the hemangioblasts in the blood islands in the yolk sac (Jakeman et al., 1993).

The Flt-1 and KDR/Flk-1 Tyrosine Kinases

Binding Characteristics

Two VEGF receptor tyrosine kinases (RTKs) have been identified. The Flt-1 (fms-like-tyrosine kinase) (de Vries et al., 1992) and KDR (kinase domain region) (Terman et al., 1992) receptors bind VEGF with high affinity. The murine homologue of KDR, Flk-1 (fetal liver kinase-1), shares 85% sequence identity with human KDR (Matthews et al., 1991). Both Flt-1 and KDR/Flk-1 have seven immunoglobulin (Ig)-like domains in the extracellular domain (ECD), a single transmembrane region and a consensus tyrosine kinase sequence that is interrupted by a kinase-insert domain (Shibuya et al., 1990; Terman et al., 1991; Matthews et al., 1991). Flt-1 has the highest affinity for $rhVEGF_{165}$, with a K_d of approximately 10-20 pM (de Vries et al., 1992). KDR has a somewhat lower affinity for VEGF; the K_d has been estimated to be approximately 75–125 pM (Terman et al., 1992).

A cDNA encoding an alternatively spliced soluble form of Flt-1 (sFlt-1), lacking the seventh Ig-like domain, transmembrane sequence, and the cytoplasmic domain, has been identified in human umbilical vein endothelial cells (Kendall et al., 1996). This sFlt-1 receptor binds VEGF with high affinity (K_d 10–20 pM) and inhibits VEGF-induced mitogenesis and thus may be a physiologically important negative regulator of VEGF action.

An additional member of the family of RTKs with seven Ig-like domains in the ECD is Flt-4 (Pajusola et al., 1992; Galland et al., 1992; Finnerty et al., 1993), which, however, is not a receptor for VEGF but rather binds a newly identified ligand called VEGF-C or VEGF-related peptide (VRP). Figure 5.2 illustrates the interaction of the members of the VEGF gene family with their tyrosine kinase receptors.

Recent studies have mapped the binding site for VEGF to the second immunoglobulin-like domain of Flt-1 and KDR. Deletion of the second domain of Flt-1 completely abolished the binding of VEGF. Introduction of the second domain of KDR into a Flt-1 mutant lacking the homologous domain restored VEGF binding. The ligand specificity, however, was characteristic of the KDR receptor. To test this hypothesis further, chimeric receptors in which the first three or just the second Ig-like domains of Flt-1 replaced the corresponding domains in Flt-4 were created. Either mutation conferred upon Flt-4 the ability to bind VEGF with an affinity nearly identical to that of wild-type Flt-1. Furthermore, transfected cells expressing these chimeric Flt-4 receptors exhibited increased DNA synthesis in response to VEGF or placental growth factor (PlGF) (Davis-Smyth

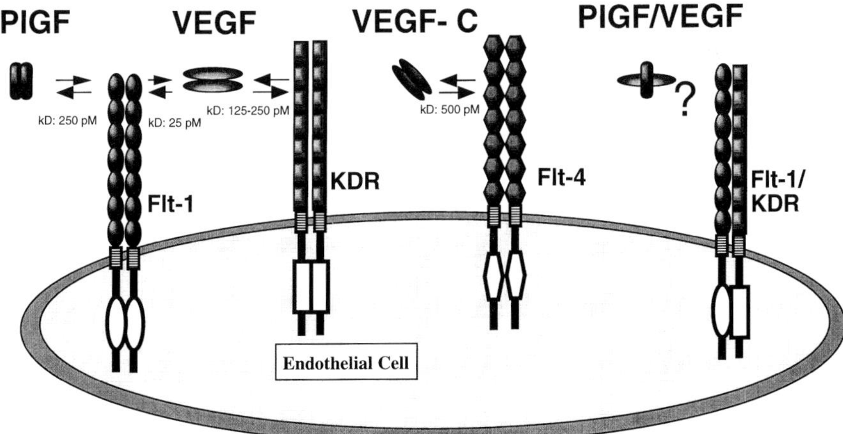

Figure 5.2. Interaction of VEGF and VEGF-related molecules (PlGF, VEGF-C) with the three members of the family of RTKs with seven Ig-like domains in the ECD (flt-1, KDR, Flt-4). VEGF interacts with Flt-1 and KDR; PlGF binds only Flt-1 and VEGF-C/VRP binds with high affinity to Flt-4. The possibility that Flt-1 and KDR form heterodimers is considered.

et al., 1996). One practical application of these structure–function studies is the generation of inhibitors of VEGF activity. The first three Ig-like domains of Flt-1 fused to a heavy-chain Fc potently inhibit VEGF bioactivity across species. The Fc may confer on the receptor portion sufficient half-life and stability when injected systemically (Chamow and Ashkenazi, 1996). Therefore this agent may a useful tool to determine the role of endogenous VEGF in several models in vivo.

Signal Transduction

Several studies have indicated that the signal transduction properties of Flt-1 and KDR differ (see also Chapter 2). (Waltenberger et al., 1994; Seetharam et al., 1995). Porcine aortic endothelial cells lacking endogenous VEGF receptors display chemotaxis and mitogenesis in response to VEGF when transfected with a plasmid encoding KDR (Waltenberger et al., 1994). In contrast, transfected cells expressing Flt-1 lack such responses (Waltenberger et al., 1994; Seetharam et al., 1995). Flk-1/KDR confers strong ligand-dependent tyrosine phosphorylation in intact cells, while Flt-1 reveals weak or undetectable responses (Waltenberger et al., 1994; Seetharam et al., 1995). Also, VEGF stimulation results in weak tyrosine phosphorylation that does not generate any mitogenic signal in transfected NIH 3T3 cells expressing Flt-1 (Seetharam et al., 1995). These findings agree with other studies showing that PlGF, which binds with high affinity to Flt-1 but not to Flk-1/KDR, lacks direct mitogenic or permeability-enhancing properties or the ability to stimulate tyrosine phosphorylation effectively in endothelial cells (Park et al., 1994). Therefore, interaction with Flk-1/KDR is a critical requirement to induce the full spectrum of VEGF biologic responses. In further support of this conclusion, VEGF mutants that bind selectively to Flk-1/KDR are fully active endothelial cell mitogens (Keyt et al., 1996b). These findings cast doubt on the role of Flt-1 as a truly signaling receptor. More recent evidence, however, indicates that Flt-1 induces signals, although our understanding of these events is fragmentary. An interaction between Flt-1 and the p85 subunit of phosphatidylinositol 3-kinase has been shown, suggesting that p85 couples Flt-1 to intracellular signal transduction systems and implicating elevated levels of PtdIns(3,4,5)P3 in this process (Cunningham et al., 1995). Also, members of the Src family, such as Fyn and Yes, show an increased level of phosphorylation following VEGF stimulation in transfected cells expressing Flt-1 but not KDR (Waltenberger et al., 1994). Furthermore, a specific biological response, the migration of monocytes in response to VEGF (or PlGF), is mediated by Flt-1(Barleon et al., 1996).

Regulation

The expression of Flt-1 and Flk-1/KDR genes is largely restricted to the vascular endothelium. The promoter region of Flt-1 has been cloned and characterized and a 1-kb fragment of the 5' flanking region essential for endothelial-specific expression was identified (Morishita et al., 1995). Likewise, a 4-kb 5' flanking sequence that confers endothelial cell specific activation has been identified in the promoter of KDR (Patterson et al., 1995).

Similarly to VEGF, hypoxia has been proposed to regulate VEGF receptor gene expression. Exposure of rats to acute or chronic hypoxia led to pronounced upregulation of both Flt-1 and Flk-1/KDR genes in the lung vasculature (Tuder et al., 1995). Also, Flk-1/KDR and Flt-1 mRNAs were substantially upregulated throughout the heart following myocardial infarction in the rat (Li et al., 1996). In vitro studies have yielded unexpected results, however. Hypoxia increases VEGF receptor number by 50% in cultured bovine retinal capillary endothelial cells but the expression of KDR is not induced: It paradoxically shows an initial downregulation (Takagi et al., 1996). The hypoxic upregulation of KDR observed in vivo may not be direct but may require the release of an unidentified paracrine mediator from ischemic tissues(Brogi et al., 1996). Recent studies have provided evidence for a differential transcriptional regulation of the Flt-1 and KDR genes by hypoxia (Gerber et al., 1997). When human umbilical vein endothelial cells (HUVEC) were exposed to hypoxic conditions in vitro, increased levels of Flt-1 expression were observed. In contrast, Flk-1/KDR mRNA levels were unchanged or slightly repressed. Promoter deletion analysis demonstrated a 430-bp region of the Flt-1 promoter to be required for transcriptional activation in response to hypoxia. This region includes a heptamer sequence matching the HIF-1 consensus binding site previously found in other genes inducible by hypoxia. The element mediating the hypoxia response was further defined as a 40-bp sequence including the putative HIF-1 binding site. Such an element was not found in the Flk-1/KDR promoter. These findings indicate that, unlike the KDR/Flk-1 gene, the Flt-1 receptor gene is directly upregulated by hypoxia via a hypoxia-inducible enhancer element located at position 976- to-937 of the Flt-1 promoter (Gerber et al., 1997). In addition both TNF-α (Patterson et al., 1996) and TGF-β (Mandriota et al., 1996) can inhibit the expression of the KDR gene in cultured endothelial cells.

ROLE OF VEGF AND ITS RECEPTORS IN PHYSIOLOGICAL ANGIOGENESIS

Distribution of VEGF, Flk-1/KDR, and Flt-1 mRNA

The proliferation of blood vessels is crucial for a wide variety of physiological processes such as embryonic development, normal growth and differentiation, wound healing and reproductive functions. During embryonic development, VEGF expression is first detected within the first few days following implantation in the giant cells of the trophoblast (Breier et al., 1992; Jakeman et al., 1993). At later developmental stages in the mouse or rat embryos, the VEGF mRNA is expressed in several organs, including heart, vertebral column, kidney, and along the surface of the spinal cord and brain. In the developing mouse brain, the highest levels of mRNA expression are associated with the choroid plexus and the ventricular epithelium (Breier et al., 1992). In the human fetus (16–22 weeks), VEGF mRNA expression is detectable in virtually all tissues and is most abundant in lung, kidney and spleen (Shifren et al., 1994).

In situ hybridization studies show that the Flk-1 mRNA is expressed in the yolk sac and intraembryonic mesoderm and later on in angioblasts, endocardium, and small and large vessel endothelium (Quinn et al., 1993; Millauer et al., 1993). These findings strongly suggest a role for Flk-1 in the regulation of vasculogenesis and angiogenesis. Expression of Flk-1 mRNA is first detected in the proximal-lateral embryonic mesoderm, which gives rise to the heart (Yamaguchi et al., 1993). Flk-1 is then detectable in endocardial cells of heart primordia and subsequently in the major embryonic and extraembryonic vessels (Yamaguchi et al., 1993). These studies have indicated that Flk-1 may be the earliest marker of endothelial cell precursors (for more details see Chapter 1.) The Flt-1 mRNA is selectively expressed in vascular endothelial cells, both in fetal and adult mouse tissues (Peters et al., 1993). Similar to the high affinity VEGF binding, the Flt-1 mRNA is expressed in both proliferating and quiescent endothelial cells, suggesting a role for Flt-1 in the maintenance of endothelial cells (Peters et al., 1993).

VEGF expression is also detectable around microvessels in areas in which endothelial cells are normally quiescent, such as the kidney glomerulus, pituitary, heart, lung, and brain (Ferrara et al., 1992; Monacci et al., 1993). These findings raise the possibility that VEGF may be required not only to induce active vascular proliferation but also, at least in some circumstances, for the maintenance of the differentiated state of blood vessels (Ferrara et al., 1992). In agreement with this hypothesis is the finding that VEGF acts as a survival factor, at least for the developing retinal vessels (Alon et al., 1995). Thus, hyperoxia-induced vascular regression in the retina of neonatal animals may be a consequence of inhibition of VEGF production by glial cells. Intraocular administration of VEGF to newborn rats at the onset of hyperoxia prevents apoptosis and regression of the retinal vasculature (Alon et al., 1995).

Role of VEGF in Corpus Luteum Angiogenesis

The development and endocrine function of the ovarian corpus luteum (CL) are dependent on the growth of new capillary vessels. Although several molecules have been implicated as mediators of CL angiogenesis, at present there is no direct evidence for the involvement of any. The VEGF mRNA is temporally and spatially related to the proliferation of blood vessels in the rat, mouse, and primate ovary and in the rat uterus, suggesting that VEGF is a mediator of the cyclical growth of blood vessels that occurs in the female reproductive tract (Phillips et al., 1990; Ravindranath et al., 1992). Recently, the hypothesis that VEGF is a mediator of CL angiogenesis has been examined in a rat model of hormonally induced ovulation (Ferrara et al., 1998). Treatment with a soluble VEGF receptor (Flt [1–3]-IgG) virtually completely suppresses CL angiogenesis, an effect associated with inhibition of CL development and progesterone release. Failure of maturation of the endometrium is also observed, as well areas of ischemic necrosis in the CL of treated animals. No effect on the preexisting ovarian vasculature was observed however. These findings demonstrate that, in spite of the redundancy of potential mediators, VEGF is essential for CL angiogenesis, and has implications for the control of fertility and the treatment of ovarian disorders characterized by hypervascularity and hyperplasia, such as polycystic ovary syndrome.

ROLE OF VEGF IN PATHOLOGIC ANGIOGENESIS

Tumor Angiogenesis

In 1945, Algire and Chalkley, based on microscopic observations of tumor xenografts in transparent chambers implanted in mice, proposed that the growth of solid tumors is dependent on the development of a new vascular supply derived from the host (Algire and Chalkley, 1945). In 1971, Folkman proposed inhibition of angiogenesis as a novel strategy to treat cancer (Folkman, 1971). Since then, extensive research has been devoted to the identification of tumor angiogenesis factor(s).

Many tumor cell lines secrete VEGF in vitro. (Ferrara et al., 1992). In situ hybridization studies have demonstrated that the VEGF mRNA is markedly upregulated in the vast majority of human tumors so far examined, including lung, breast, gastrointestinal tract, kidney, bladder, ovary, endometrium and uterine cervix, carcinomas, angiosarcoma, germ cell tumors, and several intracranial tumors including glioblastoma multiforme as well as hemangioblastoma associated with the VHL syndrome. In glioblastoma multiforme and other tumors with significant necrosis, the expression of VEGF mRNA is highest in hypoxic tumor cells adjacent to necrotic areas. A correlation exists between the degree of vascularization of the malignancy and VEGF mRNA expression. In virtually all specimens examined, VEGF mRNA was expressed in tumor cells but not in endothelial cells. In contrast, the mRNAs for Flt-1 and KDR were upregulated in the endothelial cells associated with the tumor. These findings are consistent with the hypothesis that VEGF is primarily a paracrine mediator. Immunohistochemical studies have localized the VEGF protein not only to the tumor cells but also to the vasculature. This localization indicates that tumor-secreted VEGF accumulates in the target cells.

Elevations in VEGF levels have been detected in the serum of some cancer patients (Kondo et al., 1994). Also, a correlation has been noted between VEGF expression and microvessel density in primary breast cancer sections (Toi et al., 1996).

The availability of specific monoclonal antibodies capable of inhibiting VEGF-induced angiogenesis in vivo and in vitro (Kim et al., 1992) made it possible to generate direct evidence for a role of VEGF in tumorigenesis. Such antibodies exert a potent inhibitory effect ranging from 70% to >95% on the growth of three human tumor cell lines injected subcutaneously in nude mice, the SK-LMS-1 leiomyosarcoma, the G55 glioblastoma multiforme, and the A673 rhabdomyosarcoma (Kim et al., 1993). Subsequently, other tumor cell lines were found to be inhibited in vivo by this treatment. In agreement with the hypothesis that inhibition of neovascularization is the mechanism of tumor suppression, the density of blood vessels was significantly lower in sections of tumors from antibody-treated animals compared with controls. Furthermore, neither the antibodies nor VEGF had any effect on the in vitro growth of the tumor cells (Kim et al., 1993). Noninvasive imaging of the vasculature by intravital videomicroscopy revealed a nearly complete suppression of tumor angiogenesis in anti-VEGF treated animals as compared with controls, at all time points examined (Borgstrom et al., 1996).

In addition to changes in the number of vessels, their properties can be affected by blocking VEGF as well. Treatment with anti-VEGF monoclonal antibodies initiated when tumor xenografts were already established and vascularized results in time-dependent reductions in vascular permeability (Yuan et al., 1996). These effects were accompanied by striking changes in the morphology of vessels, with dramatic reduction in diameter and tortuosity. Such a reduction in diameter eventually stops flow in the tumor vascular network. Regression of blood vessels is observed after repeated administrations of anti-VEGF antibody. Thus, tumor vessels require constant stimulation with VEGF to maintain not only their proliferative properties but also some key morphological features.

An independent verification of the hypothesis that the VEGF action is required for tumor angiogenesis has been provided by the finding that retrovirus-mediated expression of a dominant negative Flk-1 mutant, which inhibits signal transduction through wild-type Flk-1 receptor, suppresses the growth of glioblastoma multiforme as well as other tumor cell lines in vivo (Millauer et al., 1994).

Angiogenesis Associated With Other Pathological Conditions

Diabetes mellitus, occlusion of central retinal vein, or prematurity with subsequent exposure to oxygen can all be associated with intraocular neovascularization. The new blood vessels may lead to vitreous hemorrhage, retinal detachment, neovascular glaucoma, and eventual blindness. All of these conditions are associated with retinal ischemia. VEGF, by virtue of its diffusible nature and hypoxia-inducibility, is an attractive candidate for a mediator of intraocular neovascularization. Accordingly, elevations of VEGF levels in the aqueous and vitreous of eyes with proliferative retinopathy have been described (Aiello et al., 1994; Adamis et al., 1994). A strong correlation is found between levels of immunoreactive VEGF in the aqueous and vitreous humors and active proliferative retinopathy. VEGF levels were undetectable or very low (<0.5 ng/ml) in the eyes of patients affected by nonneovascular disorders or diabetes without proliferative retinopathy (Aiello et al., 1994). In contrast, the VEGF levels are in the range of 3–10 ng/ml in the presence of active proliferative retinopathy associated with diabetes, occlusion of central retinal vein, or prematurity. In agreement with these findings, in situ hybridization studies have demonstrated upregulation of VEGF mRNA in the retina of patients with proliferative retinopathies secondary to diabetes, central retinal vein occlusion, retinal detachment, or intraocular tumors (Pe'er et al., 1996).

More direct evidence for a role of VEGF as a mediator of intraocular neovascularization has been generated in a primate model of iris neovascularization and in a murine model of retinopathy of prematurity (Miller et al., 1994; Pierce et al., 1995). In the former, intraocular administration of anti-VEGF antibodies dramatically inhibits the neovascularization that follows occlusion of central retinal veins (Adamis et al., 1996). Likewise, soluble Flt-1 or Flk-1 fused to an IgG antibody suppresses retinal angiogenesis in the mouse model (Aiello et al., 1995).

Neovascularization is a major cause of visual loss also in age-related macular degeneration (AMD), the overall leading cause of blindness. A role for VEGF in the progression of AMD-related choroidal neovascularization has been suggested (Lopez et al., 1996; Kvanta et al., 1996), raising the possibility that a pharmacological treatment with monoclonal antibodies or other VEGF inhibitors may constitute a therapy for this condition.

Two independent studies have suggested that VEGF is involved in the pathogenesis of rheumatoid arthritis (RA), an inflammatory disease in which angiogenesis plays a significant role (Koch et al., 1994; Fava et al., 1994). Levels of immunoreactive VEGF are high in the synovial fluid of RA patients while they are very low or undetectable in the synovial fluid of patients affected by other forms of arthritis or by degenerative joint disease. Furthermore, anti-VEGF antibodies significantly reduced the endothelial cell chemotactic activity of the RA synovial fluid (Koch et al., 1994).

Other diseases characterized by increased vascularity and permeability in which VEGF expression is increased include psoriasis (Detmar et al., 1994). (McLaren et al., 1996; Shifren et al., 1996), and Stein-Leventhal syndrome (Kamat et al., 1995) and it has been proposed that VEGF may be responsible for the characteristic hypervascularity of Graves' disease (Sato et al., 1995).

VEGF-RELATED MOLECULES

Over the last few years, several VEGF-related genes have been identified from mammalian sources. The encoded factors are known as placenta growth factor (PlGF), VEGF-B, and VEGF-C/VRP. In addition, two sequences in the genome of the parapoxvirus *orf* virus show homology to VEGF. Although the biological role of these factors is still largely unclear, their structural homology to VEGF suggests that they may regulate blood vessel growth. The first VEGF-related factor identified was PlGF. This molecule has 53% identity with the PDGF-like region of VEGF. The encoded protein was expected to have 149 amino acids, including the signal peptide (Maglione et al., 1991). Subsequently, a longer form characterized by a 21-amino-acid insertion was identified (Maglione et al., 1993). Similar to the 24-amino-acid insertion in the longer forms of VEGF, this insertion was highly enriched in basic residues. These two isoforms, which arise from alternative splicing of mRNA, are known as PlGF-1 and PlGF-2 or $PlGF_{131}$ and $PlGF_{152}$, respectively. Similar to VEGF, these molecules are dimeric glycoproteins. PlGF binds with high affinity (K_d ~250 pM) to Flt-1 but not to KDR (Park et al., 1994). Purified PlGF has minimal activity in vascular endothelial cell growth and vascular permeability assays, suggesting that binding to KDR is a requirement for both activities (Park et al., 1994). Naturally occurring heterodimers between VEGF and PlGF have been identified in the conditioned medium of a rat glioma cell line (DiSalvo et al., 1995; Cao et al., 1996). In agreement with previous studies, the PlGF homodimer demonstrated minimal mitogenic activity on endothelial cells. The VEGF: PlGF heterodimer was active, however, although its potency was lower than the VEGF homodimer (DiSalvo et al., 1995; Cao et al., 1996).

As previously described, Flt-4 is a RTK with seven Ig-like domains and with significant structural homology to the VEGF receptors. The expression of Flt-4 mRNA, which is initially localized to angioblasts and venules in the early embryo, becomes restricted to lymphatic endothelium at later stages of development. This expression pattern suggests that Flt-4 may regulate lymphangiogenesis (Kaipainen et al., 1995). A ligand selective for Flt-4 has been recently identified by two groups and named both VEGF-C (Joukov et al., 1996) and VEGF-related peptide (VRP) (Lee et al., 1996). VEGF-C/VRP is a secreted protein with 399 amino acid residues and has a 32% identity to VEGF. Its terminal half contains a 180-amino-acid region that is not found in VEGF. VEGF-C/VRP stimulates the growth of human lung endothelial cells, albeit with 100-fold less potency than does $VEGF_{165}$. VEGF-C appears to be a specific regulator of the growth of lymphatic vessels. Overexpression of VEGF-C in the skin of transgenic mice produces lymphatic hyperplasia but not vascular endothelial proliferation (Jeltsch et al., 1997).

A newly identified member of the VEGF gene family is VEGF-B (Olofsson et al., 1996). This molecule consists of 188 amino acids, including the signal peptide. VEGF-B stimulates the growth of human and bovine vascular endothelial cells (Olofsson et al., 1996). VEGF-B is distributed primarily in the skeletal muscle and myocardium and is coexpressed with VEGF. Similar to the long forms of VEGF, VEGF-B is expressed as a membrane-bound protein that can be released in a soluble form following addition of heparin. These findings led to the hypothesis that VEGF-B may also regulate angiogenesis, particularly in muscle (Olofsson et al., 1996).

Two sequences having homology to VEGF have been identified in the genome of two different strains of *orf* virus, a parapoxvirus that affects goats, sheep, and occasionally humans. It is noteworthy that the lesions of goats and humans following *orf* virus infection are characterized by extensive microvascular proliferation in the skin, raising the possibility that the product of the viral VEGF-like gene is responsible for such lesions (Lyttle et al., 1994).

CONCLUSIONS

The recent findings that heterozygous mutations inactivating the VEGF gene result in profound deficits in vasculogenesis and blood island formation, leading to early intrauterine death, emphasize the pivotal role played by this molecule in the development of the vascular system (see Chapter 1). The use of technology to delete genes on an inducible basis should be valuable not only in determining the timing when the embryo is most vulnerable to VEGF deficiency but also in assessing the role of VEGF and its receptors in the adult animal.

The elucidation of the signal transduction properties of the Flt-1 and KDR receptors holds the promise to dissect the pathways leading to such fundamental biological events as endothelial cell differentiation, morphogenesis, and angiogenesis. Furthermore, a more complete understanding of the signaling events involving other endothelial cell specific tyrosine kinases as well as cell adhesion molecules and their interrelation with the VEGF/VEGF receptor system should provide a more integrated view of the biology of the endothelial cell, both in normal and abnormal circumstances.

An attractive possibility is that recombinant VEGF or gene therapy with the VEGF gene may be used to promote endothelial cell growth and collateral vessel formation (see Chapter 13). This represents a novel therapeutic option for conditions that frequently are refractory to conservative measures and unresponsive to pharmacological therapy. rhVEGF is already in clinical trials for the treatment of myocardial ischemia resulting from coronary artery disease.

The high expression of VEGF mRNA in human tumors and the presence of the VEGF protein in ocular fluids of individuals with opthalmologic disorders and in the synovial fluid of RA patients strongly support the hypothesis that VEGF is a key mediator of angiogenesis associated with various disorders. Therefore, anti-VEGF antibodies or other inhibitors of VEGF used alone or in combination with other agents may be of therapeutic value for a variety of malignancies as well as for other disorders. Recently, a humanized version of a high-affinity anti-VEGF monoclonal antibody, which retains the same affinity and efficacy as the original murine antibody, has been generated (Presta et al., 1997) and is being tested in humans as a treatment for solid tumors.

In conclusion, although many factors are potentially involved in angiogenesis, one specific factor, VEGF, appears to be a key mediator in a variety of physiological and pathological circumstances.

REFERENCES

Adamis, A. P., Miller, J. W., Bernal, M. T., D'Amico, D. J., Folkman, J., Yeo, T. K., and Yeo, K. T. (1994). Increased vascular endothelial growth factor levels in the vitreous of eyes with proliferative diabetic retinopathy. Am. J. Ophthalmol. 118: 445–450.

Adamis, A. P., Shima, D. T., Tolentino, M. J., Gragoudas, E. S., Ferrara, N., Folkman, J., D'Amore, P. A., and Miller, J. W. (1996). Inhibition of vascular endothelial growth factor prevents retinal ischemia-associated iris neovascularization in a nonhuman primate. Arch. Ophthalmol. 114: 66–71.

Aiello, L. P., Avery, R. L., Arrigg, P. G., Keyt, B. A., Jampel, H. D., Shah, S. T., Pasquale, L. R., Thieme, H., Iwamoto, M. A., Park, J. E., Nguyen, H., Aiello, L. M., Ferrara, N., and King, G. L. (1994). Vascular endothelial growth factor in ocular fluid of patients with diabetic retinopathy and other retinal disorders. N. Engl. J. Med. 331: 1480–1487.

Aiello, L. P., Pierce, E. A., Foley, E. D., Takagi, H., Chen, H., Riddle, L., Ferrara, N., King, G. L., and Smith, L. E. (1995). Suppression of retinal neovascularization in vivo by inhibition of vascular endothelial growth factor (VEGF) using soluble VEGF-receptor chimeric proteins. Proc. Natl. Acad. Sci. USA 92: 10457–10461.

Algire, G. H. and Chalkley, H. W. (1945). Vascular reactions of normal and malignant tissues in vivo. I. Vascular reactions of mice to wounds and to normal and neoplastic transplants. J. Natl. Cancer Inst., 6, 73–85.

Alon, T., Hemo, I., Itin, A., Pe'er, J., Stone, J., and Keshet, E. (1995). Vascular endothelial growth factor acts as a survival factor for newly formed retinal vessels and has implications for retinopathy of prematurity. Nat. Med. 1: 1024–1028.

Barleon, B., Sozzani, S., Zhou, D., Weich, H. A., Mantovani, A., and Marme, D. (1996). Migration of human monocytes in response to vascular endothelial growth factor (VEGF) is mediated via the VEGF receptor flt-1. Blood 87: 3336–3343.

Ben-Av, P., Crofford, L. J., Wilder, R. L., and Hla, T. (1995). Induction of vascular endothelial growth factor expression in synovial fibroblasts. FEBS Lett. 372: 83–87.

Borgstrom, P., Hillan, K. J., Sriramarao, P., and Ferrara, N. (1996). Complete inhibition of angiogenesis and growth of microtumors by anti-vascular endothelial growth factor neutralizing antibody: novel concepts of angiostatic therapy from intravital videomicroscopy. Cancer Res. 56: 4032–4039.

Breier, G., Albrecht, U., Sterrer, S., and Risau, W. (1992). Expression of vascular endothelial growth factor during embryonic angiogenesis and endothelial cell differentiation. Development 114: 521–532.

Brogi, E., Schatteman, G., Wu, T., Kim, E. A., Varticovski, L., Keyt, B., and Isner, J. M. (1996). Hypoxia-induced paracrine regulation of vascular endothelial growth factor receptor expression. J. Clin. Invest. 97: 469–476.

Broxmeyer, H. E., Cooper, S., Li, Z. H., Lu, L., Song, H. Y., Kwon, B. S., Warren, R. E., and Donner, D. B. (1995). Myeloid progenitor cell regulatory effects of vascular endothelial cell growth factor. Int. J. Hematol. 62: 203–215.

Cao, Y., Chen, H., Zhou, L., Chiang, M. K., Anand Apte, B., Weatherbee, J. A., Wang, Y., Fang, F., Flanagan, J. G., and Tsang, M. L. (1996). Heterodimers of placenta growth factor/vascular endothelial growth factor. Endothelial activity, tumor cell expression, and high affinity binding to Flk-1/KDR. J. Biol. Chem. 271: 3154–3162.

Chamow, S. M. and Ashkenazi, A. (1996). Immunoadhesins: principles and applications. Trends Biotechnol. 14: 52–60.

Claffey, K. P., Wilkison, W. O., and Spiegelman, B. M. (1992). Vascular endothelial growth factor. Regulation by cell differentiation and activated second messenger pathways. J. Biol. Chem. 267: 16317–16322.

Clauss, M., Gerlach, M., Gerlach, H., Brett, J., Wang, F., Familletti, P. C., Pan, Y. C., Olander, J. V., Connolly, D. T., and Stern, D. (1990). Vascular permeability factor: a tumor-derived polypeptide that induces endothelial cell and monocyte procoagulant activity, and promotes monocyte migration. J. Exp. Med. 172: 1535–1545.

Cohen, T., Nahari, D., Cerem, L. W., Neufeld, G., and Levi, B. Z. (1996). Interleukin 6 induces the expression of vascular endothelial growth factor. J. Biol. Chem. 271: 736–741.

Conn, G., Bayne, M. L., Soderman, D. D., Kwok, P. W., Sullivan, K. A., Palisi, T. M., Hope, D. A., and Thomas, K. A. (1990). Amino acid and cDNA sequences of a vascular endothelial cell mitogen that is homologous to platelet-derived growth factor. Proc. Natl. Acad. Sci. USA 87: 2628–2632.

Cunningham, S. A., Waxham, M. N., Arrate, P. M., and Brock, T. A. (1995). Interaction of the Flt-1 tyrosine kinase receptor with the p85 subunit of phosphatidylinositol 3-kinase. Mapping of a novel site involved in binding. J. Biol. Chem. 270: 20254–20257.

Davis-Smyth, T., Chen, H., Park, J., Presta, L. G., and Ferrara, N. (1996). The second immunoglobulin-like domain of the VEGF tyrosine kinase receptor Flt-1 determines ligand binding and may initiate a signal transduction cascade. EMBO J. 15: 4919–4927.

de Vries, C., Escobedo, J. A., Ueno, H., Houck, K., Ferrara, N., and Williams, L. T. (1992). The fms-like tyrosine kinase, a receptor for vascular endothelial growth factor. Science 255: 989–991.

Detmar, M., Brown, L. F., Claffey, K. P., Yeo, K. T., Kocher, O., Jackman, R. W., Berse, B., and Dvorak, H. F. (1994). Overexpression of vascular permeability factor/vascular endothelial growth factor and its receptors in psoriasis. J. Exp. Med. 180: 1141–1146.

DiSalvo, J., Bayne, M. L., Conn, G., Kwok, P. W., Trivedi, P. G., Soderman, D. D., Palisi, T. M., Sullivan, K. A., and Thomas, K. A. (1995). Purification and characterization of a naturally occurring vascular endothelial growth factor.placenta growth factor heterodimer. J. Biol. Chem. 270: 7717–7723.

Dvorak, H. F., Brown, L. F., Detmar, M., and Dvorak, A. M. (1995). Vascular permeability factor/vascular endothelial growth factor, microvascular hyperpermeability, and angiogenesis. Am. J. Pathol. 146: 1029–1039.

Fava, R. A., Olsen, N. J., Spencer-Green, G., Yeo, K. T., Yeo, T. K., Berse, B., Jackman, R. W., Senger, D. R., Dvorak, H. F., and Brown, L. F. (1994). Vascular permeability factor/endothelial growth factor (VPF/VEGF): accumulation and expression in human synovial fluids and rheumatoid synovial tissue. J. Exp. Med. 180: 341–346.

Ferrara, N. and Davis-Smyth, T. (1997). The biology of vascular endothelial growth factor. Endocr. Rev. 18: 4–25.

Ferrara, N. and Henzel, W. J. (1989). Pituitary follicular cells secrete a novel heparin-binding growth factor specific for vascular endothelial cells. Biochem. Biophys. Res. Commun. 161: 851–858.

Ferrara, N., Houck, K., Jakeman, L., and Leung, D. W. (1992). Molecular and biological properties of the vascular endothelial growth family of proteins. Endocr. Rev. 13: 18–32.

Ferrara, N., Chen, H., Davis-Smyth, T., Gerber, H.-P., Nguyen, T.-N., Peers, D., Chisholm, V., Hillan, K. J., and Schwall, R. H.(1998). Vascular endothelial growth factor is essential for corpus luteum angiogenesis. Nat. Med. 3: 336–340.

Finnerty, H., Kelleher, K., Morris, G. E., Bean, K., Merberg, D. M., Kriz, R., Morris, J. C., Sookdeo, H., Turner, K. J., and Wood, C. R. (1993). Molecular cloning of murine FLT and FLT4. Oncogene 8: 2293–2298.

Folkman, J. (1971). Tumor angiogenesis: therapeutic implications. N. Engl. J. Med. 285: 1182–1186.

Folkman, J. (1995). Angiogenesis in cancer, vascular, rheumatoid and other disease. Nat. Med. 1: 27–31.

Forsythe, J. A., Jiang, B. H., Iyer, N. V., Agani, F., Leung, S. W., Koos, R. D., and Semenza, G. L. (1996). Activation of vascular endothelial growth factor gene transcription by hypoxia-inducible factor 1. Mol. Cell. Biol. 16: 4604–4613.

Frank, S., Hubner, G., Breier, G., Longaker, M. T., Greenhalg, D. G., and Werner, S. (1995). Regulation of VEGF expression in cultured keratinocytes. Implications for normal and impaired wound healing. J. Biol. Chem. 270: 12607–12613.

Gabrilovich, D. I., Chen, H. L., Girgis, K. R., Cunningham, H. T., Meny, G. M., Nadaf, S., Kavanaugh, D., and Carbone, D. P. (1996). Production of vascular endothelial growth factor by human tumors inhibits the functional maturation of dendritic cells. Nat. Med. 2: 1096–1103.

Galland, F., Karamysheva, A., Mattei, M. G., Rosnet, O., Marchetto, S., and Birnbaum, D. (1992). Chromosomal localization of FLT4, a novel receptor-type tyrosine kinase gene. Genomics 13: 475–478.

Gerber, H. P., Condorelli, F., Park, J., and Ferrara, N. (1997). Differential transcriptional regulation of the two VEGF receptor genes. Flt-1, but not Flk-1/KDR, is up-regulated by hypoxia. J. Biol. Chem., 272: 23659–23667.

Gnarra, J. R., Zhou, S., Merrill, M. J., Wagner, J. R., Krumm, A., Papavassiliou, E., Oldfield, E. H., Klausner, R. D., and Linehan, W. M. (1996). Post-transcriptional regulation of vascular endothelial growth factor mRNA by the product of the VHL tumor suppressor gene. Proc. Natl. Acad. Sci. USA 93: 10589–10594.

Goldberg, M. A. and Schneider, T. J. (1994). Similarities between the oxygen-sensing mechanisms regulating the expression of vascular endothelial growth factor and erythropoietin. J. Biol. Chem. 269: 4355–4361.

Goldman, C., Kim, J., Wonf, W.-L., King, V., Brock, T., and Gillespie, Y. (1993). Epidermal growth factor stimulates vascular endothelial growth factor production by malignant glioma cells. A model of glioblastoma multiforme pathophysiology. Mol. Biol. Cell 4: 121–133.

Grugel, S., Finkenzeller, G., Weindel, K., Barleon, B., and Marme, D. (1995). Both v-Ha-Ras and v-Raf stimulate expression of the vascular endothelial growth factor in NIH 3T3 cells. J. Biol. Chem. 270: 25915–25919.

Hashimoto, E., Ogita, T., Nakaoka, T., Matsuoka, R., Takao, A., and Kira, Y. (1994). Rapid induction of vascular endothelial growth factor expression by transient ischemia in rat heart. Am. J. Physiol 267: H1948–H1954.

Houck, K. A., Ferrara, N., Winer, J., Cachianes, G., Li, B., and Leung, D. W. (1991). The vascular endothelial growth factor family: identification of a fourth molecular species and characterization of alternative splicing of RNA. Mol. Endocrinol. 5: 1806–1814.

Houck, K. A., Leung, D. W., Rowland, A. M., Winer, J., and Ferrara, N. (1992). Dual regulation of vascular endothelial growth factor bioavailability by genetic and proteolytic mechanisms. J. Biol. Chem. 267: 26031–26037.

Ikeda, E., Achen, M. G., Breier, G., and Risau, W. (1995). Hypoxia-induced transcriptional activation and increased mRNA stability of vascular endothelial growth factor in C6 glioma cells. J. Biol. Chem. 270: 19761–19766.

Iliopoulos, O., Levy, A. P., Jiang, C., Kaelin, W. G., Jr., and Goldberg, M. A. (1996). Negative regulation of hypoxia-inducible genes by the von Hippel-Lindau protein. Proc. Natl. Acad. Sci. USA 93: 10595–10599.

Jakeman, L. B., Winer, J., Bennett, G. L., Altar, C. A., and Ferrara, N. (1992). Binding sites for vascular endothelial growth factor are localized on endothelial cells in adult rat tissues. J. Clin. Invest. 89: 244–253.

Jakeman, L. B., Armanini, M., Philips, H. S., and Ferrara, N. (1993). Developmental expression of binding sites and mRNA for vascular endothelial growth factor suggests a role for this protein in vasculogenesis and angiogenesis. Endocrinology 133: 848–859.

Jeltsch, M., Kaipainen, A., Joukov, V., Meng, X., Lakso, M., Rauvala, H., Awartz, M., Fukumura, D., Jain, R. K., and Alitalo, K. (1997). Hyperplasia of lymphatic vessels in VEGF-C transgenic mice. Science 276: 1423–1425.

Joukov, V., Pajusola, K., Kaipainen, A., Chilov, D., Lahtinen, I., Kukk, E., Saksela, O., Kalkkinen, N., and Alitalo, K. (1996). A novel vascular endothelial growth factor, VEGF-C, is a ligand for the Flt4 (VEGFR-3) and KDR (VEGFR-2) receptor tyrosine kinases. EMBO J. 15: 1751.

Kaipainen, A., Korhonen, J., Mustonen, T., van Hinsbergh, V. W., Fang, G. H., Dumont, D., Breitman, M., and Alitalo, K. (1995). Expression of the fms-like tyrosine kinase 4 gene becomes restricted to lymphatic endothelium during development. Proc. Natl. Acad. Sci. USA 92: 3566–3570.

Kamat, B. R., Brown, L. F., Manseau, E. J., Senger, D. R., and Dvorak, H. F. (1995). Expression of vascular permeability factor/vascular endothelial growth factor by human granulosa and theca lutein cells. Role in corpus luteum development. Am. J. Pathol. 146: 157–165.

Kendall, R. L., Wang, G., and Thomas, K. A. (1996). Identification of a natural soluble form of the vascular endothelial growth factor receptor, FLT-1, and its heterodimerization with KDR. Biochem. Biophys. Res. Commun. 226: 324–328.

Keyt, B. A., Berleau, L. T., Nguyen, H. V., Chen, H., Heinsohn, H., Vandlen, R., and Ferrara, N. (1996a). The carboxyl-terminal domain (111–165) of vascular endothelial growth factor is critical for its mitogenic potency. J. Biol. Chem. 271: 7788–7795.

Keyt, B. A., Nguyen, H. V., Berleau, L. T., Duarte, C. M., Park, J., Chen, H., and Ferrara, N. (1996b). Identification of vascular endothelial growth factor determinants for binding KDR and FLT-1 receptors. Generation of receptor-selective VEGF variants by site-directed mutagenesis. J. Biol. Chem. 271: 5638–5646.

Kieser, A., Weich, H., Brandner, G., Marme, D., and Kolch, W. (1994). Mutant p53 potentiates protein kinase C induction of vascular endothelial growth factor expression. Oncogene 9: 963–969.

Kim, K. J., Li, B., Houck, K., Winer, J., and Ferrara, N. (1992). The vascular endothelial growth factor proteins: identification of biologically relevant regions by neutralizing monoclonal antibodies. Growth Factors 7: 53–64.

Kim, K. J., Li, B., Winer, J., Armanini, M., Gillett, N., Phillips, H. S., and Ferrara, N. (1993). Inhibition of vascular endothelial growth factor-induced angiogenesis suppresses tumor growth in vivo. Nature 362: 841–844.

Koch, A. E., Harlow, L., Haines, G. K., Amento, E. P., Unemori, E. N., Wong, W.-L., Pope, R. M., and Ferrara, N. (1994). Vascular endothelial growth factor: a cytokine modulating endothelial function in rheumatoid arthritis. J. Immunol. 152: 4149–4156.

Kondo, S., Asano, M., Matsuo, K., Ohmori, I., and Suzuki, H. (1994). Vascular endothelial growth factor/vascular permeability factor is detectable in the sera of tumor-bearing mice and cancer patients. Biochim. Biophys. Acta 1221: 211–214.

Ku, D. D., Zaleski, J. K., Liu, S., and Brock, T. A. (1993). Vascular endothelial growth factor induces EDRF-dependent relaxation in coronary arteries. Am. J. Physiol. 265: H586–H592.

Kvanta, A., Algvere, P. V., Berglin, L., and Seregard, S. (1996). Subfoveal fibrovascular membranes in age-related macular degeneration express vascular endothelial growth factor. Invest. Ophthalmol. Vis. Sci. 37: 1929–1934.

Lee, J., Gray, A., Yuan, J., Luoh, S. M., Avraham, H., and Wood, W. I. (1996). Vascular endothelial growth factor-related protein: a ligand and specific activator of the tyrosine kinase receptor Flt4. Proc. Natl. Acad. Sci. USA 93: 1988–1992.

Leung, D. W., Cachianes, G., Kuang, W. J., Goeddel, D. V., and Ferrara, N. (1989). Vascular endothelial growth factor is a secreted angiogenic mitogen. Science 246: 1306–1309.

Levy, A. P., Levy, N. S., Wegner, S., and Goldberg, M. A. (1995). Transcriptional regulation of the rat vascular endothelial growth factor gene by hypoxia. J. Biol. Chem. 270: 13333–13340.

Levy, A. P., Levy, N. S., and Goldberg, M. A. (1996). Post-transcriptional regulation of vascular endothelial growth factor by hypoxia. J. Biol. Chem. 271: 2746–2753.

Li, J., Perrella, M. A., Tsai, J. C., Yet, S. F., Hsieh, C. M., Yoshizumi, M., Patterson, C., Endego, W. O., Zhou, F., and Lee, M. (1995). Induction of vascular endothelial growyh factor gene expression by interleukin-1 beta in rat aortic smooth muscle cells. J. Biol. Chem. 270: 308–312.

Li, J., Brown, L. F., Hibberd, M. G., Grossman, J. D., Morgan, J. P., and Simons, M. (1996). VEGF, flk-1, and flt-1 expression in a rat myocardial infarction model of angiogenesis. Am. J. Physiol. 270: H1803–H1811.

Liu, Y., Cox, S. R., Morita, T., and Kourembanas, S. (1995). Hypoxia regulates vascular endothelial growth factor gene expression in endothelial cells. Identification of a 5' enhancer. Circ. Res. 77: 638–643.

Lopez, P. F., Sippy, B. D., Lambert, H. M., Thach, A. B., and Hinton, D. R. (1996). Transdifferentiated retinal pigment epithelial cells are immunoreactive for vascular endothelial growth factor in surgically excised age-related macular degeneration-related choroidal neovascular membranes. Invest. Ophthalmol. Vis. Sci. 37: 855–868.

Lyttle, D. J., Fraser, K. M., Flemings, S. B., Mercer, A. A., and Robinson, A. J. (1994). Homologs of vascular endothelial growth factor are encoded by the poxvirus orf virus. J. Virol. 68: 84–92.

Madan, A. and Curtin, P. T. (1993). A 24-base-pair sequence 3' to the human erythropoietin gene contains a hypoxia-responsive transcriptional enhancer. Proc. Natl. Acad. Sci. USA 90: 3928–3932.

Maglione, D., Guerriero, V., Viglietto, G., Delli-Bovi, P., and Persico, M. G. (1991). Isolation of a human placenta cDNA coding for a protein related to the vascular permeability factor. Proc. Natl. Acad. Sci. USA 88: 9267–9271.

Maglione, D., Guerriero, V., Viglietto, G., Ferraro, M. G., Aprelikova, O., Alitalo, K., Del Vecchio, S., Lei, K. J., Chou, J. Y., and Persico, M. G. (1993). Two alternative mRNAs coding for the angiogenic factor, placenta growth factor (PlGF), are transcribed from a single gene of chromosome 14. Oncogene 8: 925–931.

Mandriota, S. J., Seghezzi, G., Vassalli, J. D., Ferrara, N., Wasi, S., Mazzieri, R., Mignatti, P., and Pepper, M. S. (1995). Vascular endothelial growth factor increases urokinase receptor expression in vascular endothelial cells. J. Biol. Chem. 270: 9709–9716.

Mandriota, S. J., Menoud, P. A., and Pepper, M. S. (1996). Transforming growth factor beta 1 down-regulates vascular endothelial growth factor receptor 2/flk-1 expression in vascular endothelial cells. J. Biol. Chem. 271: 11500–11505.

Matthews, W., Jordan, C. T., Gavin, M., Jenkins, N. A., Copeland, N. G., and Lemischka, I. R. (1991). A receptor tyrosine kinase cDNA isolated from a population of enriched primitive hematopoietic cells and exhibiting close genetic linkage to c-kit. Proc. Natl. Acad. Sci. USA 88: 9026–9030.

Mazure, N. M., Chen, E. Y., Yeh, P., Laderoute, K. R., and Giaccia, A. J. (1996). Oncogenic transformation and hypoxia synergistically act to modulate vascular endothelial growth factor expression. Cancer Res. 56: 3436–3440.

McLaren, J., Prentice, A., Charnock-Jones, D. S., and Smith, S. K. (1996). Vascular endothelial growth factor (VEGF) concentrations are elevated in peritoneal fluid of women with endometriosis. Hum. Reprod. 11: 220–223.

Melder, R. J., Koenig, G. C., Witwer, B. P., Safabakhsh, N., Munn, L. L., and Jain, R. K. (1996). During angiogenesis, vascular endothelial growth factor and basic fibroblast growth factor regulate natural killer cell adhesion to tumor endothelium. Nat. Med. 2: 992–997.

Millauer, B., Wizigmann Voos, S., Schnurch, H., Martinez, R., Moller, N. P., Risau, W., and Ullrich, A. (1993). High affinity VEGF binding and developmental expression suggest Flk-1 as a major regulator of vasculogenesis and angiogenesis. Cell 72: 835–846.

Millauer, B., Shawver, L. K., Plate, K. H., Risau, W., and Ullrich, A. (1994). Glioblastoma growth inhibited in vivo by a dominant-negative Flk-1 mutant. Nature 367: 576–579.

Miller, J. W., Adamis, A. P., Shima, D. T., D'Amore, P. A., Moulton, R. S., O'Reilly, M. S., Folkman, J., Dvorak, H. F., Brown, L. F., Berse, B., Yeo, T-K and Yeo K-T. (1994). Vascular endothelial growth factor/vascular permeability factor is temporally and spatially correlated with ocular angiogenesis in a primate model. Am. J. Pathol. 145: 574–584.

Minchenko, A., Bauer, T., Salceda, S., and Caro, J. (1994). Hypoxic stimulation of vascular endothelial growth factor expression in vivo and in vitro. Lab. Invest. 71: 374–379.

Monacci, W. T., Merrill, M. J., and Oldfield, E. H. (1993). Expression of vascular permeability factor/vascular endothelial growth factor in normal rat tissues. Am. J. Physiol. 264: C995–1002.

Morishita, K., Johnson, D. E., and Williams, L. T. (1995). A novel promoter for vascular endothelial growth factor receptor (flt-1) that confers endothelial-specific gene expression. J. Biol. Chem. 270: 27948–27953.

Nicosia, R., Nicosia, S. V., and Smith, M. (1994). Vascular endothelial growth factor, platelet-derived growth factor and insulin-like growth factor stimulate angiogenesis in vitro. Am. J. Pathol. 145: 1023–1029.

Olofsson, B., Pajusola, K., Kaipainen, A., von Euler, G., Joukov, V., Saksela, O., Orpana, A., Pettersson, R. F., Alitalo, K., and Eriksson, U. (1996). Vascular endothelial growth factor B, a novel growth factor for endothelial cells. Proc. Natl. Acad. Sci. USA 93: 2576–2581.

Pajusola, K., Aprelikova, O., Korhonen, J., Kaipainen, A., Pertovaara, L., Alitalo, R., and Alitalo, K. (1992). FLT4 receptor tyrosine kinase contains seven immunoglobulin-like loops and is expressed in multiple human tissues and cell lines. Cancer Res. 52: 5738–5743.

Park, J. E., Keller, H.-A., and Ferrara, N. (1993). The vascular endothelial growth factor isoforms (VEGF): differential deposition into the subepithelial extracellular matrix and bioactivity of extracellular matrix-bound VEGF. Mol. Biol. Cell 4: 1317–1326.

Park, J. E., Chen, H. H., Winer, J., Houck, K. A., and Ferrara, N. (1994). Placenta growth factor. Potentiation of vascular endothelial growth factor bioactivity, in vitro and in vivo, and high affinity binding to Flt-1 but not to Flk-1/KDR. J. Biol. Chem. 269: 25646–25654.

Patterson, C., Perrella, M. A., Hsieh, C. M., Yoshizumi, M., Lee, M. E., and Haber, E. (1995). Cloning and functional analysis of the promoter for KDR/flk-1, a receptor for vascular endothelial growth factor. J. Biol. Chem. 270: 23111–23118.

Patterson, C., Perrella, M. A., Endege, W. O., Yoshizumi, M., Lee, M. E., and Haber, E. (1996). Downregulation of vascular endothelial growth factor receptors by tumor necrosis factor-alpha in cultured human vascular endothelial cells. J. Clin. Invest. 98: 490–496.

Pe'er, J., Folberg, R., Itin, A., Gnessin, H., Hemo, I., and Keshet, E. (1996). Upregulated expression of vascular endothelial growth factor in proliferative diabetic retinopathy. Br. J. Ophthalmol. 80: 241–245.

Pekala, P., Marlow, M., Heuvelman, D., and Connolly, D. (1990). Regulation of hexose transport in aortic endothelial cells by vascular permeability factor and tumor necrosis factor-alpha, but not by insulin. J. Biol. Chem. 265: 18051–18054.

Pepper, M. S., Ferrara, N., Orci, L., and Montesano, R. (1991). Vascular endothelial growth factor (VEGF) induces plasminogen activators and plasminogen activator inhibitor-1 in microvascular endothelial cells. Biochem. Biophys. Res. Commun. 181: 902–906.

Pepper, M. S., Ferrara, N., Orci, L., and Montesano, R. (1992). Potent synergism between vascular endothelial growth factor and basic fibroblast growth factor in the induction of angiogenesis in vitro. Biochem. Biophys. Res. Commun. 189: 824–831.

Pertovaara, L., Kaipainen, A., Mustonen, T., Orpana, A., Ferrara, N., Saksela, O., and Alitalo, K. (1994). Vascular endothelial growth factor is induced in response to transforming growth factor-beta in fibroblastic and epithelial cells. J. Biol. Chem. 269: 6271–6274.

Peters, K. G., De Vries, C., and Williams, L. T. (1993). Vascular endothelial growth factor receptor expression during embryogenesis and tissue repair suggests a role in endothelial differentiation and blood vessel growth. Proc. Natl. Acad. Sci. USA 90: 8915–8919.

Phillips, H. S., Hains, J., Leung, D. W., and Ferrara, N. (1990). Vascular endothelial growth factor is expressed in rat corpus luteum. Endocrinology 127: 965–967.

Pierce, E. A., Avery, R. L., Foley, E. D., Aiello, L. P., and Smith, L. E. (1995). Vascular endothelial growth factor/vascular permeability factor expression in a mouse model of retinal neovascularization. Proc. Natl. Acad. Sci. USA 92: 905–909.

Plouet, J. and Moukadiri, H. J. (1990). Characterization of the receptors for vasculotropin on bovine adrenal cortex-derived capillary endothelial cells. J. Biol. Chem. 265: 22071–22075.

Poltorak, Z., Cohen, T., Sivan, R., Kandelis, Y., Spira, G., Vlodavsky, I., Keshet, E., and Neufeld, G. (1997). VEGF145, a secreted vascular endothelial growth factor isoform that binds to extracellular matrix. J. Biol. Chem. 272: 7151–7158.

Presta, L. G., Chen, H., O'Connor, S. J., Chisholm, V., Meng, Y. G., Krummen, L., Winkler, M., and Ferrara, N. (1997) Humanization of an anti-VEGF monoclonal antibody for the therapy of solid tumors and other disorders. Cancer Res. 57: 4593–99.

Quinn, T. P., Peters, K. G., De Vries, C., Ferrara, N., and Williams, L. T. (1993). Fetal liver kinase 1 is a receptor for vascular endothelial growth factor and is selectively expressed in vascular endothelium Proc. Natl. Acad. Sci. USA 90: 7533–7537.

Rak, J., Mitsuhashi, Y., Bayko, L., Filmus, J., Shirasawa, S., Sasazuki, T., and Kerbel, R. S. (1995). Mutant ras oncogenes upregulate VEGF/VPF expression: implications for induction and inhibition of tumor angiogenesis. Cancer Res. 55: 4575–4580.

Ravindranath, N., Little-Ihrig, L., Phillips, H. S., Ferrara, N., and Zeleznik, A. J. (1992). Vascular endothelial growth factor messenger ribonucleic acid expression in the primate ovary. Endocrinology 131: 254–260.

Risau, W. (1997). Mechanisms of angiogenesis. Nature 386: 671–674.

Roberts, W. G. and Palade, G. E. (1997). Neovasculature induced by vascular endothelial growth factor is fenestrated. Cancer Res. 57: 765–772.

Sato, K., Yamazaki, K., Shizume, K., Kanaji, Y., Obara, T., Ohsumi, K., Demura, H.,

Yamaguchi, S., and Shibuya, M. (1995). Stimulation by thyroid-stimulating hormone and Graves' immunoglobulin G of vascular endothelial growth factor mRNA expression in human thyroid follicles in vitro and flt mRNA expression in the rat thyroid in vivo. J. Clin. Invest. 96: 1295–1302.

Seetharam, L., Gotoh, N., Maru, Y., Neufeld, G., Yamaguchi, S., and Shibuya, M. (1995). A unique signal transduction from FLT tyrosine kinase, a receptor for vascular endothelial growth factor VEGF. Oncogene 10: 135–147.

Shen, H., Clauss, M., Ryan, J., Schmidt, A. M., Tijburg, P., Borden, L., Connolly, D., Stern, D., and Kao, J. (1993). Characterization of vascular permeability factor/vascular endothelial growth factor receptors on mononuclear phagocytes. Blood 81: 2767–2773.

Shibuya, M., Yamaguchi, S., Yamane, A., Ikeda, T., Tojo, A., Matsushime, H., and Sato, M. (1990). Nucleotide sequence and expression of a novel human receptor-type tyrosine kinase (flt) closely related to the fms family. Oncogene 8: 519–527.

Shifren, J. L., Doldi, N., Ferrara, N., Mesiano, S., and Jaffe, R. B. (1994). In the human fetus, vascular endothelial growth factor is expressed in epithelial cells and myocytes, but not vascular endothelium: implications for mode of action. J. Clin. Endocrinol. Metab. 79: 316–322.

Shifren, J. L., Tseng, J. F., Zaloudek, C. J., Ryan, I. P., Meng, Y. G., Ferrara, N., Jaffe, R. B., and Taylor, R. N. (1996). Ovarian steroid regulation of vascular endothelial growth factor in the human endometrium: implications for angiogenesis during the menstrual cycle and in the pathogenesis of endometriosis. J. Clin. Endocrinol. Metab. 81: 3112–3118.

Shima, D. T., Adamis, A. P., Ferrara, N., Yeo, K. T., Yeo, T. K., Allende, R., Folkman, J., and D'Amore, P. A. (1995). Hypoxic induction of endothelial cell growth factors in retinal cells: identification and characterization of vascular endothelial growth factor (VEGF) as the mitogen. Mol. Med. 1: 182–193.

Shima, D. T., Kuroki, M., Deutsch, U., Ng, Y. S., Adamis, A. P., and D'Amore, P. A. (1996). The mouse gene for vascular endothelial growth factor. Genomic structure, definition of the transcriptional unit, and characterization of transcriptional and post-transcriptional regulatory sequences. J. Biol. Chem. 271: 3877–3883.

Siemeister, G., Weindel, K., Mohrs, K., Barleon, B., Martiny Baron, G., and Marme, D. (1996). Reversion of deregulated expression of vascular endothelial growth factor in human renal carcinoma cells by von Hippel-Lindau tumor suppressor protein. Cancer Res. 56: 2299–2301.

Stone, J., Itin, A., Alon, T., Pe'er, J., Gnessin, H., Chan Ling, T., and Keshet, E. (1995). Development of retinal vasculature is mediated by hypoxia-induced vascular endothelial growth factor (VEGF) expression by neuroglia. J. Neurosci. 15: 4738–4747.

Takagi, H., King, G. L., Ferrara, N., and Aiello, L. P. (1996). Hypoxia regulates vascular endothelial growth factor receptor KDR/Flk gene expression through adenosine A2 receptors in retinal capillary endothelial cells. Invest. Ophthalmol. Vis. Sci. 37: 1311–1321.

Terman, B. I., Carrion, M. E., Kovacs, E., Rasmussen, B. A., Eddy, R. L., and Shows, T. B. (1991). Identification of a new endothelial cell growth factor receptor tyrosine kinase. Oncogene 6: 1677–1683.

Terman, B. I., Dougher Vermazen, M., Carrion, M. E., Dimitrov, D., Armellino, D. C., Gospodarowicz, D., and Bohlen, P. (1992). Identification of the KDR tyrosine kinase as a receptor for vascular endothelial cell growth factor. Biochem. Biophys. Res. Commun. 187: 1579–1586.

Tischer, E., Mitchell, R., Hartman, T., Silva, M., Gospodarowicz, D., Fiddes, J. C., and Abraham, J. A. (1991). The human gene for vascular endothelial growth factor. Multiple protein forms are encoded through alternative exon splicing. J. Biol. Chem. 266: 11947–11954.

Toi, M., Kondo, S., Suzuki, H., Yamamoto, Y., Inada, K., Imazawa, T., Taniguchi, T., and Tominaga, T. (1996). Quantitative analysis of vascular endothelial growth factor in primary breast cancer. Cancer 77: 1101–1106.

Tolentino, M. J., Miller, J. W., Gragoudas, E. S., Chatzistefanou, K., Ferrara, N., and Adamis, A. P. (1996). Vascular endothelial growth factor is sufficient to produce iris neovascularization and neovascular glaucoma in a nonhuman primate. Arch. Ophthalmol. 114: 964–970.

Tuder, R. M., Flook, B. E., and Voelkel, N. F. (1995). Increased gene expression for VEGF and the VEGF receptors KDR/Flk and Flt in lungs exposed to acute or to chronic hypoxia. Modulation of gene expression by nitric oxide. J. Clin. Invest. 95: 1798–1807.

Unemori, E. N., Ferrara, N., Bauer, E. A., and Amento, E. P. (1992). Vascular endothelial growth factor induces interstitial collagenase expression in human endothelial cells. J. Cell. Physiol. 153: 557–562.

Vaisman, N., Gospodarowicz, D., and Neufeld, G. (1990). Characterization of the receptors for vascular endothelial growth factor. J. Biol. Chem. 265: 19461–19466.

Vincenti, V., Cassano, C., Rocchi, M., and Persico, G. (1996). Assignment of the vascular endothelial growth factor gene to human chromosome 6p21.3. Circulation 93: 1493–1495.

Waltenberger, J., Claesson Welsh, L., Siegbahn, A., Shibuya, M., and Heldin, C. H. (1994). Different signal transduction properties of KDR and Flt1, two receptors for vascular endothelial growth factor. J. Biol. Chem. 269: 26988–26995.

Wang, G. L. and Semenza, G. L. (1995). Purification and characterization of hypoxia-inducible factor 1. J. Biol. Chem. 270: 1230–1237.

Warren, R. S., Yuan, H., Matli, M. R., Ferrara, N., and Donner, D. B. (1996). Induction of vascular endothelial growth factor by insulin-like growth factor 1 in colorectal carcinoma. J. Biol. Chem. 271: 29483–29488.

Yamaguchi, T. P., Dumont, D. J., Conlon, R. A., Breitman, M. L., and Rossant, J. (1993). flk-1, an flt-related receptor tyrosine kinase, is an early marker for endothelial cell precursors. Development 118: 489–498.

Yang, R., Thomas, G. R., Bunting, S., Ko, A., Ferrara, N., Keyt, B., Ross, J., and Jin, H. (1996). Effects of vascular endothelial growth factor on hemodynamics and cardiac performance. J. Cardiovasc. Pharmacol. 27: 838–844.

Yuan, F., Chen, Y., Dellian, M., Safabakhsh, N., Ferrara, N., and Jain, R. K. (1996). Time-dependent vascular regression and permeability changes in established human tumor xenografts induced by an anti-vascular endothelial growth factor/vascular permeability factor antibody. Proc. Natl. Acad. Sci. USA 93: 14765–14770.

6

Platelet-Derived Growth Factor and Other Modulators of Angiogenesis

THOMAS F. DEUEL

Understanding the complexity of the formation of the vascular system and its regulation has been exceedingly difficult since this is also the study of organogenesis. Remarkable advances in the identification and characterization of factors capable of inducing new blood vessel growth have recently made study of the important processes of neovascularization and maintenance of blood vessels at the molecular level possible. These advances have assumed additional importance since it is now apparent that new therapies can be developed that effectively modify disease processes that depend upon angiogenesis for progression.

In this chapter, several angiogenic factors that are less well known in comparison with the fibroblastic growth factor and vascular endothelial growth factor families, described elsewhere in the book, will be discussed. The extraordinary complexity of the angiogenic process and the ability of different factors to influence it in diverse ways will be illustrated. Although progress in the field is both rapid and remarkable, major challenges remain. The integration of the functions of the multiple factors that promote angiogenesis/vasculogenesis is not yet understood, and the key regulatory points in these systems are only beginning to be identified.

PLATELET-DERIVED GROWTH FACTOR (PDGF)

PDGF is a family of proteins that are composed of two closely related A- and B-polypeptide chains that are expressed as heterodimers in platelets and as homodimers of the PDGF A-and B-chains (PDGF-AB, -AA, -BB) in other cell types. The PDGF isoforms are independently expressed and differentially regulated in different cell types. Each of the PDGF isoforms binds with essentially equal affinity to the PDGF receptor alpha (Rα) but only PDGF-BB binds effectively to PDGF-R beta (Rβ). PDGF was first described as a mitogen in serum for mesenchymal cells. PDGF is now known to promote cell survival, apoptosis, malignant transformation, and chemotaxis (Bejcek et al., 1989; Deuel, 1987; Deuel et al., 1982; Heldin, 1992; Kim et al., 1995; Raff et al., 1988; Ross et al., 1974; Waterfield et al., 1983). It stimulates production of extracellular matrix components (Bauer et al., 1985) and contraction of smooth-muscle cells (Berk et al., 1986; Gullberg et al., 1990). It is expressed in endothelial cells, monocytes, smooth-muscle cells, fibroblasts, placental cytotrophoblasts, neurons, and glial cells (reviewed, Heldin, 1992; Heldin and Westermark). During development, the PDGF genes are expressed in a cell-type specific and temporally specific manner (Holmgren et al., 1991; Schatterman et al., 1992; Yeh et al., 1991). Their expression is required for embryogenesis to proceed normally. Mice with homozygous loss of PDGF-A exhibit developmental abnormalities in the kidney and deficits in the development of lung alveolar myofibroblasts and associated elastin fiber deposits (Bostrom et al., 1996). Mice with homozygous loss of PDGF-B (Leveen et al., 1994) and of PDGF-R (Soriano, 1994) are deficient in hematopoiesis and cardiovascular development.

With the exception of the nervous system in adults, the PDGF genes are expressed in a self-limited and cell type specific manner that results from functional activation, such as in inflammation and wound healing (Pierce et al., 1987, 1988, 1989). However, in pathological conditions such as atherosclerosis and restenosis (Ross, 1993), and tumors such as glioblastoma, osteosarcoma, and rhabdomyosarcoma (Bejcek et al., 1989; Beltsholtz et al., 1986; Eva et al., 1982; Heldin, 1992; Waterfield et al., 1983), expression of the endogenous PDGF genes is constitutively high, suggesting that the continuous expression of PDGF, and the inability of its expression to be self-limiting may be causally responsible for aspects of the lesions that characterize these conditions. In each of these conditions, significant abnormal cell migration, proliferation, and neovascularization are characteristically found, suggesting that the inappropriate and continuous expression of PDGF may directly contribute to these lesions, and, indirectly, through its ability to upregulate a number of inducible genes, including genes to encode cytokines, transcription factors, and other important factors that themselves may contribute to the pathological conditions through constitutive expression. Some of these upregulated genes appear to be important in angiogenesis.

Evidence that implicates PDGF in angiogenesis includes its expression in sites of new blood vessel formation and the fact that it induces an angiogenic response both in vitro and in vivo (Folkman and Klagsburn, 1987; Klagsbrun and D'Amore, 1991; Risau et al., 1992; Sato et al., 1993). Recombinant PDGF-BB alone, when injected into skeletal muscle (Brown et al., 1995), induces new vessel formation, indicating that it is strongly angiogenic in an appropriate context; components of the vessel wall, such as fibroblasts and smooth-muscle cells, are induced to migrate (Senior et al., 1983) and proliferate by exogenous PDGF, (Grotendorst et al., 1981; Ross et al., 1974) and PDGF is synthesized and secreted by many cell types, including endothelial cells (DiCorleto and Bowen-Pope, 1983; Kavanaugh et al., 1988; Starksen et al., 1987) and the macrophage, a cell that also chemotactically responds to PDGF (Senior et al., 1983). Both of the PDGF receptors are expressed in endothelial cells (Kavanaugh et al., 1988; Starksen et al., 1987). Other growth factors and cytokines are upregulated locally by receptor-mediated PDGF responses, (Joseph-Silverstein and Rifkin, 1987; Pierce, 1990; Pierce et al., 1989) suggesting that the effects of PDGF in angiogenesis may be synergistic, and that PDGF functions both in the paracrine recruitment of angiogenesis-inducing cells to the vessel wall and as an autocrine regulator of endothelial cell growth.

The patterns of expression of PDGF and its receptors support the potential of PDGF to function in both a paracrine and autocrine fashion in angiogenesis; however, a number of apparently conflicting results have challenged these views. These conflicting results are most likely resolved by recognizing that both ligand and receptor expression levels are highly regulated, and thus it is the conditions of study that often dictate whether expression levels of the PDGF isoforms are sufficient for ready detection. As examples, in the developing human placenta, capillaries express the mRNA for PDGF-B and the PDGF receptor (Dumont et al., 1995), but significant levels of expression of these genes are not seen in larger vessels (Shinbrot et al., 1994). Endothelial cells in the foci of new blood vessels that develop in high density at the margins of cortical infarcts following ischemic brain injury strongly express the PDGF-A-chain gene whereas the microvasculature of nonischemic, uninjured cortex fails to express detectable levels of the PDGF-A-chain gene (Yeh et al., 1998). Bovine aortic endothelial cells that spontaneously form tubes when cultured in vitro are positive for PDGF-α receptor expression but monolayers of endothelial cells that overlay these tube-forming cells lack detectable expression of the PDGF-β receptor (Battegay et al., 1994). The results support the importance of the induction of the PDGF isoforms and their receptors during angiogenesis and suggest that PDGF is essential to the formation of vessels through both paracrine and autocrine regulation. Both PDGF-A and PDGF-B-null mice die early in neonatal life. Both PDGF-β and the PDGF (receptor null mice lack mesangial cells in the kidney and develop aneurysmal sacs in capillary tufts in the renal glomerulus (Leveen et al., 1994; Soriano, 1994). The aneurysmal sacs are lined by endothelium but appear to lack pericytes, suggesting that loss of supporting cells in the vessel wall may result in capillary aneurysms. The defects in the PDGF-B- or β receptor-deficient mice are confined to the microvasculature. PDGF-A-null mice also appear to fail to appropriately recruit pericytes, but the primary developmental problem appears to be the failure to recruit the smooth muscle cell to the vessel wall. The Patch mouse has homozygous loss of the PDGFα receptor gene locus. In these mice, fewer layers of smooth muscle cells are observed in the vessel wall, despite a normal vascular endothelium (Schatteman et al., 1995). These interpretations fit well with earlier observations that PDGF-A is more active with the smooth-muscle cell than it is with the pericyte (D'Amore and Smith, 1993).

The PDGF-inducible cytokine genes (Kawahara and Deuel, 1989; Oppenheim et al., 1991; Rollins et al., 1988) constitute a subfamily of PDGF-inducible genes whose products have been shown to influence important aspects of inflammatory responses and wound repair, including angiogenesis. The PDGF-inducible cytokine genes have also been found to be constitutively expressed in pathological sites at which PDGF is also expressed (Heldin, 1992; Nelken et al., 1991; Ross, 1993). As an example, constitutively high levels of expression of the PDGF-inducible gene JE (MCP-1) (Nelken et al., 1991) are found in those atherosclerotic lesions in which high levels of the PDGF-A-chain gene are constitutively expressed. Furthermore, the pleiotrophin (see below) and the PDGF-A-chain genes (both PDGF inducible) are expressed at high levels in cells transformed by v-sis, the viral counterpart of the PDGF B-chain gene.

The complexity of the PDGF response can perhaps be illustrated in experiments in which PDGF was applied as a single dose to experimentally induced wounds (Pierce et al., 1987, 1988, 1989). In these experiments, the application of PDGF accelerated all aspects of healing, including the repair of tissues not previously thought to be influenced by PDGF and beyond the time at which PDGF can be demonstrated in the wounds. These results may suggest that single application of PDGF induced a sequential activation of cytokines and other genes that are required to orchestrate the wound healing response, which results in exuberant neovascularization. The wound healing response is highly regulated, and it is likely that continued expression of the cytokine genes would most likely lead to serious pathological consequences. Thus, the distinction between self-limiting and constitutive expression of PDGF and the PDGF-inducible cytokine genes may be lost in chronic inflammatory states, such as atherosclerosis, restenosis, pulmonary fibrosis, tumor stromal formation and tumor angiogenesis, thus the constitutive expression of the PDGF-inducible genes may lead to a number of the pathological consequences that are characteristic of these abnormalities.

Pleiotrophin

Pleiotrophin (PTN) is a heparin-binding protein of 168 amino acids that includes a 32-amino-acid signal sequence. It was recently purified and characterized as a weak mitogen in bovine uterus (Milner et al., 1989) and as a neurite outgrowth-promoting factor in neonatal rat brain (Li et al., 1990; Rauvala, 1989). The human, bovine, rat, and mouse Ptn cDNAs have been cloned and encode proteins with >98% conservation of amino acid sequence once the 32-amino-acid signal peptide is removed from consideration (Rauvala, 1989). Both the N-and C-terminal domains of

PTN are exceptionally rich in lysine, which is likely to account for the ability of PTN to bind tightly to heparin and to extracellular matrix (Kinnunen, 1996; Li et al., 1990). PTN has nearly 50% amino acid sequence identity with a retinoic-acid-induced differentiation protein termed MK (for midkine, in mouse) (Kadomatsu et al., 1988; Muramatsu, 1994; Muramatsu et al., 1993)/RIHB (for retinoic-acid-inducible heparin binding, in chicken). MK also binds tightly to heparin, has weak growth-promoting activity, and, together with PTN, constitutes a family of growth/differentiation factors (Kadomatsu et al., 1988; Li et al., 1990; Muramatsu, 1994; Muramatsu et al., 1993).

The transcripts of the PTN gene are regulated in a temporally and cell-type-specific manner in developing mouse (Silos-Santiago et al., 1996). PTN is widely expressed in early mesoderm and in developing bone and brain (Guillerman, 1991; Silos-Santiago et al., 1996; Tamura et al., 1995). The PTN gene is upregulated in cells stimulated by PDGF (Li et al., 1992). Its 5' promoter region has a functional serum response element (SRE) (Li et al., 1992). and thus PTN is a member of the PDGF inducible gene family. PTN is upregulated in endothelial cells and macrophages at sites of injury. Increased expression of the PTN gene follows that of the PDGF-A-chain gene, consistent with the view that PDGF-A upregulates PTN gene expression and suggesting the possibility that PDGF may be angiogenic in part through its ability to induce expression of PTN.

PTN has mitogenic activity for fibroblasts (Milner et al., 1989), for brain capillary endothelial cells (Courty et al., 1991), and for SW-13 cells in soft agar culture (Hoschuetzky et al., 1994). It is angiogenic in the rabbit corneal pocket assay (Courty et al., 1991). PTN also is required for maintenance of the tube-like structures that form when microvascular endothelial cells are cultured on matrigel surfaces (Yeh et al.—unpublished observations). PTN also accelerates differentiation of primary cultures of oligodendrocyte progenitor cells; the endogenous PTN gene is also required for the spontaneous differentiation of these cells which occurs when the oligodendrocyte cultures are cultured without PDGF, suggesting the possibility that one role of PTN in angiogenesis is that of a differentiation factor.

Overexpression of PTN transforms NIH 3T3 cells (Chauhan et al., 1993), and these transformed cells elicit a striking neovascular response when injected into the flanks of nude mice (Chauhan et al., 1993) suggesting that the unregulated expression of PTN is sufficient to signal a vascular response. The endogenous PTN gene is constitutively expressed in a number of cell lines that are derived from human tumors, and its mRNA levels are high in specimens of a number of human tumors, raising the possibility that PTN may contribute to the initiation and maintenance of transformation in these tumors. Ptn expression in tumor cell lines correlates directly with degree of tumor angiogenesis when these cell lines are implanted in the nude mouse, indicating that PTN signaling may be angiogenic. Furthermore, significant levels of FGF-2 are found in proximity to the tumors formed at sites of injection of PTN transformed cells, indicating that FGF-2 may be released from cells in response to PTN signaling.

The importance of PTN gene expression to angiogenesis is further suggested by experiments in which the expression of the PDGF-A and PTN genes is examined by in situ hybridization 24, 72, and 168 hours after a 90-minute ligation of the middle cerebral artery in rat. In this model, a cortical infarct results. The area of the infarct and surrounding tissues can be examined using the contralateral hemisphere as control. At 6 hours after ligation of the middle cerebral artery, neither the PDGF-A nor the PTN mRNAs are detected in the infarct or in the surrounding tissues. At day 1, however, a substantial increase in expression of the PDGF-A-chain gene is seen in endothelial cells, macrophages, and astrocytes within and in immediate proximity to the infarct but not on the contralateral site. Expression of the PTN gene is barely detectable at day 1. At day 3, the PDGF-A-chain gene continues to be expressed at high levels. A striking upregulation of the PTN gene is now seen in endothelial cells, macrophages, and astrocytes at sites of neovascularization both within and in immediate proximity to the infarct itself. At day 7, large numbers of PTN-positive endothelial cells and macrophages are present within numerous hyperplastic blood vessels within the infarct and immediate contiguous areas. The results clearly demonstrate that the PTN gene is expressed in vascular endothelial cells and in activated macrophages and astrocytes at sites of neovascularization in response to ischemic injury. Expression of the PTN gene follows expression of the PDGF-A-chain gene in temporal sequence by ~24–48 hours, further supporting the view that the PTN gene product may be induced by PDGF-A and that PTN may be a downstream effector of PDGF (Yeh et al., 1998).

PTN (50 ng/ml) stimulates a twofold increase in cell number and a 2.4-fold increase in bromodeoxyuridine (BrdU) incorporation into DNA of cultured bovine capillary endothelial cells (BCECs) over a 48-hour period. When BCECs were cultured on a Matrigel surface, tube-like structures formed spontaneously; the tube-like structures were not seen when Matrigel was not included in cultures. The tube-like structures that are formed in the absence of PTN are fragile and fail to maintain the tube-like (differentiated-like) morphology over the 2–7 days of observation. In contrast, tube-like structures formed in the presence of PTN maintain their appearance over a 7-day period and do not collapse. PTN thus directly influences endothelial cells, presumably contributing to an aspect of its differentiation.

OTHER ANGIOGENIC FACTORS

Transforming Growth Factor-β (TGF-β)

The TGF-β family is composed of homodimeric polypeptides that act as growth regulators of different cell types. They reduce endothelial and smooth muscle cell growth (Battegay et al., 1991; D'Amore and Smith, 1993; Heinmark et al., 1986) and migration (Sato and Rifkin, 1989) and are the primary factors that contribute to the mass and composition of extracellular matrix (Basson et al., 1992). Nearly 50% of TGF-β null mice die during embryogenesis with defective hematopoiesis and vasculogenesis (Dicksom et al., 1995). These mice have abnormalities of extraembryonic yolk sac vessel development, defective contacts between endothelial and mesothelial layers, and distended capillary structures (Dicksom et al., 1995). TGF-β regulates integrin function, integrin gene expression, and matrix accumulation. TGF-β receptor type 2 null mice also are embryonic lethals with striking abnormalities in hematopoiesis and vasculogenesis (Oshima et al., 1996).

Hereditary hemorrhagic telangiectasia results from mutations in the endoglin and the activin receptor kinase genes (Johnson et al., 1996; McAllister et al., 1994). Both endoglin and the activin receptor kinases are expressed by vascular endothelial cells. Although uncleur, endoglin may bind TGF-β and present it to its receptors. The activin receptor-like kinase-1 gene encodes a serine-threonine kinase receptor similar to that for TGF-β.

Epithelial–mesenchymal interactions in developing vessels may influence the development of the vessels themselves. Cell contact between endothelial cells and undifferentiated mesenchymal cells or smooth-muscle cells activates TGF-β (Antonelli-Orlidge et al., 1989; Rohovski et al., 1996), suggesting a role of TGF-β in the inhibition of endothelial cell growth and migration and perhaps in differentiation of vessels (Orlidge and D'Amore, 1987; Rohovsky et al., 1996; Sato and Rifkin 1989).

Thc tic Receptor Family and Angiopoietin

The tie receptor tyrosine kinases are first expressed in angioblasts of mesenchyme, in endothelial cells of the developing dorsal aorta, and in blood islands of the yolk sac (Korhonen et al., 1994). Tie-1-null animals lack integrity of the vessels (Sato et al., 1995) and for this reason have subcutaneous hemorrhages and edema and early lcthatity.

Tie-2 (also known as tek) is expressed in endocardium and dorsal aortae (Sato et al., 1993). It is minimally expressed in endothelium in adults with the exception of the adult heart (Dumont et al., 1994). When tie-2 gene expression is deleted, the tie-2 null embryos demonstrated distended yolk sac vessel, disorganized trabeculae within the heart, and lack the chu-arts-istic capillary sprouts in neuroectoderm, suggesting that vascular remodeling is deficient.

tie-2 Ligands

The two identifiable ligands for tie-2 appear to have very different functions. Angiopoietin-1 activates tyrosine phosphorylation whereas angiopoietin-2 antagonizes the effects of angiopoietin-1. Angiopoietin-1 is expressed most prominently in the myocardium in areas that surround the endocardium and in association with the mesenchyme adjacent to developing vessels; angiopoietin-1 null mice phenotypes are essentially identical to tie-2 null mice (Suri et al., 1996); they have immature endocardium and trabeculae and the vascular plexes have not remodeled adequately.

A definitive association of tie-2 with the vascular system has been recently established by the observation that a dominantly inherited syndrome of venous malformation is localized to the tie-2 locus (Vikkula et al., 1996). An interesting feature of this mutation is that when the mutated protein is expressed by recombinant means, a six-to 10-fold increase in autophosphory to time is seen. The venous malformations include a paucity of vascular smooth muscle cells, and decreased migration, proliferation, and differentiation (Folkman and D'Amore, 1996).

REFERENCES

Antonelli-Orlidge, A. M., Saunders, K. B., Smith, S. R., and A'more, P. A. (1989). An activated form of transforming growth factor (is produced by cocultures of endothelial cells and peiocytes. Proc. Natl. Acad. Sci. USA 86: 4544–4548.

Bauer, E. A., Cooper, T. W., Huang, J. S., Altman, J., and Deuel, T. F. (1985). Stimulation of in vitro human skin collagenase expression by platelet-derived growth factor. Proc. Natl. Acad. Sci. USA 82: 4132–4136.

Basson, C. T., Kocher, O., Basson, M. D., Asis, A., and Madri, J. A. (1992). Differential modulation of vascular cell integrin and extracellular matrix expression in vitro by TGF-(1 correlates with reciprocal effects on cell migration J. Cell. Physiol. 153: 118–128.

Battegay, E. J., Raines, E. W., Seifert, R. A., Bowen-Pope, D. F., and Ross, R. (1991). TGF-β induces bimodal proliferation of connective tissue cells via control of an autocrinn PDGF loop. Cell 63: 515–524.

Battegay, E. J., Rupp, J., Iruela-Arispe, L., Sage, E. H, and Oech, M. (1994). PDGF-BB modulates endothelial proliferation and angiogenesis in vitro via PDGF α-receptors. J. Cell Biol. 125: 917–928.

Bejcek, B. E., Li, D. Y., and Deuel, T. F. (1989). Transformation by v-sis occurs by an internal autocrine mechanism. Science 245: 1496–1499.

Berk, B. C., Alexander, R. W., Brock, T. A., Gimbrone, M. A., Jr., and Webb, R. C. (1986). Vasoconstriction: a new activity for platelet-derived growth factor. Science 232: 87–90.

Betsholtz, C., Johnsson, A., Heldin, C.-H., Westermark, B., Lind, P., Urdea, M. S., Eddy, R., Shows, T. B., Philpott, K., Mellor, A. L., Knott, T. J., and Scott, J. (1986). cDNA sequence and chromosomal localization of human platelet-derived growth factor and its expression in tumor cell lines. Nature 320: 695–699.

Bostrom, H., Willetts, K., Pekny, M., Leveen, P., Lindahl, P., Hedstrand, H., Pekna, M., Hellstrom, M., Gebre-Medhin, S., Schalling, M., Nilsson, M., Kurland, S., Tornell, J., Heath, JK., Betsholtz, C. (1996). PDGF-A signaling is a critical event in lung alveolar myofibroblast development and alveogenesis. Cell 85: 863–873.

Brown, D. M., Hong, S. P., Farrell, C. L. Pierce, G. F. and Khouri, R. K. (1995). Platelet derived growth fctor induces functional vascular anastomosis in vivo. Proc. Natl. Acad. Sci. USA 92: 5920–5924.

Chauhan, A. K., Li, Y.-S., and Deuel, T. F. (1993). Pleiotrophin transforms NIH 3T3 cells and induces tumors in nude mice. Proc. Natl. Acad. Sci. USA 90: 679–682.

Courty, J., Dauchel, M. C., Caruelle, D., Perderiset, M., and Barritault, D. (1991). Mitogenic properties of a new endothelial cell growth factor related to pleiotrophin. Biochem. Biophys. Res. Commun. 180: 145–151.

D'Amore, P. A. and Smith, S. R. (1993). Growth factor effects on cells of the vascular wall: a survey. Growth Factors 8: 61–75.

Deuel, T. F. (1987). Polypeptide growth factors: roles in normal and abnormal cell growth. Annu. Rev. Cell. Biol. 3: 443–492.

Deuel, T. F., Senior, R. M., Huang, J. S., and Griffin, G. L. (1982). Chemotaxis of monocytes and neutrophils to platelet-derived growth factor. J. Clin. Invest. 69: 1046–1049.

Dicksom, M. C. Martin, J. S. Cousins, F. M. Kulkarni, A. B., Karlsson, S., and Akhurst, R. J. (1995). Defective haematopoiesis and vasculogeneisis in transforming growth factor-(1 knock-out mice. Development 121: 1845–1854.

DiCorleto, P. E., and Bowen-Pope, D. F. (1983). Cultured endothelial cells produce a platelet-derived growth factor-like protein. Proc. Natl. Acad. Sci. USA 80 (7): 1919–1923.

Dumont, D. J., Gradwohl, G., Fong., G.-H., Puri, M. C., Gerttsenstein, M., Auerbach, A., and Breitman, M. L. (1994). Dominant-negative and targeted null mutations in the endothelial receptor tyrosine kinase, tek, reveal a critical role in vasculogenesis of the embryo. Genes Dev. 8: 1897–1907.

Dumont, D. J., Fong, G. H., Puri, M. C., Gradwohl, G., Alitalo, K., and Breitman, M. L. (1995). Vascularization of the embryo: a study of flk-1, teck tie, and vascular endothelial growth factor expression during development. Dev. Dyn. 203: 80–92.

Eva, A., Robbins, K. C., Amdersen, P. R., Srinivasan, A., Tronick, S. R., Aaronson, S. A., Reddy, E. P., Ellemore, N. W., Galen, A. T., Lautenberger, J. A., and Papas, T. S. (1982). Cellular genes analogous to retroviral oncogenes are transcribed in human tumour cells. Nature 295: 116–119.

Fang, W., Hartmann, N., Chow, D. T., Riegel, A-T., and Wellstein, A. (1992). Pleiotrophin stimulates fibroblasts and endothelial and epithelial cells and is expressed in human cancer. J. Biol. Chem. 262: 25889–25897.

Folkman, J. and D'Amore, P. A. (1996). Blood vessel formation: what is its molecular basis? Cell 87: 1153–1155.

Folkman, J. and Klagsburn, M. (1987). Angiogenic factors. Science. 235 (4787): 442–447.

Grotendorst, G. R., Seppa, H. E., Kleinman, H. K., and Martin, G. R. (1981). Attachment of smooth muscle cells to collagen and their migration toward platelet-derived growth factor. Proc. Natl. Acad. Sci. USA 78 (6): 3669–3672.

Guillerman, P. (1991). Masters thesis. Washington University, St. Louis.

Gullberg, D., Tingstrom, A., Thuresson, A.-C., Olsson, L., Terracio, L., Borg, T. K., and Rubin, K. (1990). (1 Integrin-mediated collagen gel contraction is simulated by PDGF. Exp. Cell. Res. 186: 264–272.

Heimark, R. L., Twardzik, D. R., and Schwarts, S. M. (1986). Inhibition of endothelial regeneration by type-beta transforming growth factor from platelets. Science 233: 1078–1080.

Heldin, C.-H. (1992). Structural and functional studies on platelet-derived growth factor. EMBO J. 12: 4251–4259.

Heldin, C.-H. and Westermark, B. (1990). Platelet-derived growth factor: mechanism of action and possible in vivo function. Cell Regul. 1: 555–566.

Holmgren, L., Glaser, A., Pfeifer-Ohlsson, S., and Ohlsson, R. (1991). Angiogenesis during human extraembryonic development involves the spatiotemporal control of PDGF ligand and receptor gene expression. Development 113: 749–754.

Hom, D. B., Baker, S. R., Graham, L. M., and McClatchey, K. D. (1988). Utilizing angiogenic agents to expedite the neovascularization process in skin flaps. Laryngoscope 98 (5):521–526.

Hoschuetzky, H., Aberle, A., and Kemler, R. C. (1994). Beta-catenin mediates the interaction of the cadherin-catenin complex with epidermal growth factor. J. Cell Biol. 127: 1375–1380.

Johnson, D. W., Berg, J. N., Baldwin, M. A., Gallione, C. J., Marondel, L., Uoon, S. J., Stenzel, T. T., Speer, M., Pericak-Vance, M. A., Diamond, A., Guttmacher, A. E., Jackson, C. E., Atisano, L., Kucherlapati, R., Porteous, M. E. M., and Marchuk, D. A. (1996). Mutations in the activan receptor like kinase 1 gene in hereditary haemorrhagic telegiactasic type 2. Nat. Genet. 13: 189–195.

Joseph-Silverstein, J. and Rifkin, D. B. (1987). Endothelial cell growth factors and the vessel wall. Semin. Thromb. Hemost. 13 (4): 504–513.

Kadomatsu, K., Tomomura, M., and Muramatsu, T. (1988). cDNA cloning and sequence of a new gene intensely expressed in early differentiation stages of embryonal carcinoma cells and in mid-gestation period of mouse embryogenesis. Biochem. Biophys. Res. Commun. 151: 1312–1318.

Kavanaugh, W. M., Harsh, G. R. T., Starksen, N. F., Rocco, C. M., and Williams, L. T. (1988). Transcriptional regulation of the A and B chain genes of platelet-derived growth factor in microvascular endothelial cells. J. Biol. Chem. 263 (17): 8470–8472.

Kawahara, R. S. and Deuel, T. F. (1989). Platelet-derived growth factor inducible gene JE is a member of a family of small inducible genes related to platelet factor 4. J. Biol. Chem. 264: 679–682.

Khouri, R. K., Brown, D. M., Leal-Khouri, S. M., Tark, K. C., and Shaw, W. W. (1991). The effect of basic fibroblast growth factor on the neovascularisation process: skin flap survival and staged flap transfers. Br. J. Plast. Surg. 44 (8): 585–588.

Kim, H.-R. C., Upadhyay, S., Li, G., Palmer, K. C., and Deuel, T. F. (1995). Platelet-derived growth factor induces apoptosis in growth-arrested murine fibroblasts. Proc. Natl. Acad. Sci. USA 92: 9500–9504.

Kinnunen, T. (1996). Neurite outgrowth in brain neurons induced by heparin-binding growth-associated molecule (HB-GAM) depends on the specific interaction of HB-GAM with heparan sulfate at the cell surface. J. Biol. Chem. 271: 2243–2248.

Klagsbrun, M. and D'Amore, P. A. (1991). Regulators of angiogenesis. Annu. Rev. Physiol. 53: 217–239.

Korhonen, J., Polvi, A., Partanen, K. M, and Alitalo, K. (1994). The mouse tie receptor tyrosine kinase gene: expression during embryonic angiogenesis. Oncogene 9: 395–403.

Leveen, P., Pekny, M., Gebre-Medhin, S., Swolin, B., Larsson, E., Betsholtz, C.

(1994). Mice deficient for PDGF B show renal, cardiovascular, and hematological abnormalities. Genes Dev. 8: 1875–1887.

Li, Y.-S., Milner, P. G., Chauhan, A. K., Watson, M. A., Hoffman, R. M., Kodner, C. M., Milbrandt, J., and Deuel, T. F. (1990). Cloning and expression of a developmentally regulated protein that induces mitogenic and neurite outgrowth activity. Science 250: 1690–1694.

Li, Y.-S., Gurrieri, M., and Deuel, T. F. (1992). Pleiotrophin gene expression is highly restricted and is regulated by platelet-derived growth factor. Biochem. Biophys. Res. Commun. 184: 427–432.

Li, Y.-S., Hoffman, R. M., LeBeau, M. M., Espinosa, R., III, Jenkins, N. A., Gilgert, D. J., Copeland, N. G., and Deuel, T. F. (1992). Characterization of the human pleiotrophin gene promoter region and chromosomal localization. J. Biol. Chem. 267: 26011–26016.

McAllister, K., Grogg K. M., Johnson, D. W., Gallione, C. J., Baldwin, M. A., Jackson, C. E., Hembold, E. A., Markel, D. S., McKinnon, W. C., Murrell., J., McCormick, M. K., Pericak-Vance, M. A., Heutink, P., Oostra, B., A., Haitjema, T., Westerman, C. J. J. Porteous, M. E., Guttmacher, A. E., Letarte, M., and Marchuk, D. A. (1994). Endoglin, a TGF-β binding protein of endothelial cells, is the gene for hereditary haemorrhagic telangiectasia type 1. Nat. Genet. 8: 345–351.

Milner, P. G., Li, Y.-S., Hoffman, R. M., Kodner, C. M., Siegel, N. R., and Deuel, T. F. (1989). A novel 17 kD heparin-binding growth factor (HBGF-8) in bovine uterus: purification and N-terminal amino acid sequence. Biochem. Biophys. Res. Commun. 165: 1096–1103.

Muramatsu, M. (1994). The Midkine family of growth/differentiation factors. Cell Growth/Differ. 36: 1–8.

Muramatsu, H., Shirahama, H., Yonezawa, S., Maruta, H., and Muramatsu, T. (1993). Midkine, a retinoic acid-inducible growth/differentiation factor: immunochemical evidence for the function and distribution. Dev. Biol. 159: 392–402.

Naunheim, K. S., Fiore, A. C., Wadley, J. J., McBride, L. R., Kanter, K. R., Pennington, D. G., Barner, H. B., Kaiser, G. C., and Willman, V. L., (1988). The changing profile of the patient undergoing coronary artery bypass surgery. J. Am. Coll. Cardiol. 11 (3): 494–498.

Nelken, N. A., Coughlin, S. R., Gordon, D., and Wilcox, J. N. (1991). Properties of the novel proinflammatory supergene "intercrene" cytokine family. Annu. Rev. Immunol. 9: 617–648.

Oppenheim, J. J., Zacharian, C. O., Mukaide, N., MaksUshima, K. (1991). Properties of the novel proinflammatory supergene "intercrine" cytokine family. Annu. Rev. Immunol. 9: 617–648.

Orlidge, A. and D'Amore, P. A. (1987). Inhibition of capillary endothelial cell growth pericytes and smooth muscle cells. J. Cell Biol, 105: 1455–1462.

Oshima, M., Oshima, H., and Taketo, M. M. (1996). TGF-β receptor type II deficiency results in defects in yolk sac hematopoiesis and vasculogenesis. Dev. Biol. 179: 297–302.

Pierce, G. F. (1990). Macrophages: important physiologic and pathologic sources of polypeptide growth factors [comment]. Am. J. Respir. Cell Mol. Biol. 2 (3): 233–234.

Pierce, G. F., Mustoe, T. A., Thomason, A., Senior, R. M., and Deuel, T. F. (1987). Recombinant platelet-derived growth factor induced augmentation of healing in rat incisional wounds. Clin. Res. 35: 602A.

Pierce, G. F., Mustoe, T. A., Senior, R. M., Reed, J., Griffin, G. L., Thomason, A., and Deuel, T. F. (1988). In vivo incisional wound healing augmented by platelet-derived growth factor and recombinant c-sis gene homodimeric proteins. J. Exp. Med. 167: 974–987.

Pierce, G. F., Mustoe, T. A., Lingelbach, J., Masakowski, V. R., Griffin, G. L., Senior, R. M., and Deuel, T. F. (1989). Platelet-derived growth factor and transforming growth factor-beta enhance tissue repair activities by unique mechanisms. J. Cell Biol. 109 (1): 429–440.

Pu, L. Q., Sniderman, A. D., Brassard, R., Lachapelle, K. J., Graham, A. M., Lisbona, R., Symes, J. F. (1993). Enhanced revascularization of the ischemic limb by angiogenic therapy. Circulation 88: 208–214.

Raff, M. C., Lillien, L. E., Richardson, W. D., Burne, J. F., and Noble, M. D. (1988). Platelet-derived growth factor from astrocytes drives the clock that times oligodendrocyte development in culture. Nature 333: 562–565.

Rauvala, H. (1989). An 18 kd heparin-binding protein of developing brain that is distinct from fibroblast growth factors. EMBO J. 8: 2933–2941.

Risau, W., Drexler, H., V. Mironov, Smits, A., Siegbahn, A., Funa, K., and Heldin, C. H. (1992). Platelet-derived growth factor is angiogenic in vivo. Growth Factors 7 (4):261–266.

Rohovsky, S. A., Hirschi, K. K. and D'Amore, P. A. (1996). Growth factor effects on a model of vessel formation. Surg. Forum 47: 390–391.

Rollins, B. J., Morrison, E. D., and Stiles, C. D. (1988). Cloning and expression of JE, a gene inducible by PDGF and whose product has cytokine-like properties. Proc. Natl. Acad. Sci. USA 85: 3738–3742.

Ross, R. (1993). The pathogenesis of atherosclerosis: a perspective for the 1990s. Nature 362: 801–809.

Ross, R., Glomset, J., Kariya, B., and Harker, L. (1974). A platelet-dependent serum factor that stimulates the proliferation of arterial smooth muscle cells in vitro. Proc. Nat. Acad. Sci. USA 71 (4): 1207–1210.

Rutherford, R. B. and Ross, R. (1976). Platelet factors stimulate fibroblasts and smooth muscle cells quiescent in plasma serum to proliferate. J. Cell Biol. 69 (1): 196–203.

Sato, Y. and Rifkin, D. B. (1989). Inhibition of endothelial cell movement by pericytes and smooth muscle cells: activation of latent transformation growth factor-beta 1-like molecule by plasmin during co-culture. J. Cell Biol. 109: 309–315.

Sato, T. N., Qin, Y., Kozak, C., and Audus, K. L. (1993). tie tie-1 and tie-2 define another class of putative receptor tyrosine kinase gfenes expressed in early embryonic vascular system. Proc. Natl. Acad. Sci. USA 90: 9355–9358.

Sato, N., Beitz, J. G., Kato, J., Yamamoto, M., Clark, J. W., Calabresi, P., Raymond, A., and Frackelton, A. R., Jr. (1993). Platelet-derived growth factor indirectly stimulates angiogenesis in vitro. Am. J. Pathol. 142 (4): 1119–1130.

Sato, T., Tozawa, Y., Deutsch, U., Wolburg-Buchholz, K., Fujiwara, Y., Gendron-Magure, M., Gridley, T., Wolburg, H., Risau, W., and Qin, Y. (1995). Distinct roles of the receptor tyrosine kinases tie-1 and tie-2 in blood vessel formation. Nature 376: 70.

Schatterman, G. C., Morrison-Graham, K., van Koppen, A., Weston, J. A., and Bowen-Pope, D. F. (1992). Regulation and role of PDGF receptor (-subunit expression during embryogenesis. Development 115: 125–131.

Schatteman, G. C., Motley, S. T., Effmann, E. L., and Bowen-Pope, D. F. (1995).

Platelet-derived growth factor receptor alpha subunit deleted patch mouse exhibits severe cardiovascular dysmorphogenesis. Teratololgy 51: 351–366.

Senior, R. M., Griffin, G. L., Huang, J. S., Walz, D. A., and Deuel, T. F. (1983). Chemotactic activity of platelet alpha granule proteins for fibroblasts. J. Cell Biol. 96 (2): 382–385.

Shinbrot, E., Peter, K. G., and Williams, L. T. (1994). Expression of platelet-growth factorβ receptor during organogenesis and tissue differentiation in the mouse embryo. Dev. Dyn. 199: 169–175.

Silos-Santiago, I., Yeh, H.-J., Gurrieri, M., Guillerman, R. P., Li, Y.-S., Snider, W., and Deuel, T. F. (1996). The localization of pleiotrophin and its mRNA in subpopulations of neurons and their corresponding axonal tracts suggests important roles in neural-glial interactions during development and in maturity. J. Neurobiol. 31 (3): 283–296.

Soriano, P. (1994). Abnormal kidney development and hematological disorders in PDGFβ-receptor mutant mice. Genes Dev. 8: 1888–1896.

Starksen, N. F., Harsh, G. R. T., Gibbs, V. C., and Williams, L. T. (1987). Regulated expression of the platelet-derived growth factor A chain gene in microvascular endothelial cells. J. Biol. Chem. 262 (30): 14381–14384.

Suri, C., Jones, P. F., Patan, S., Bartunkova, S., Maisonpierre, P. C., Davis, S., Sato, T. N., and Yancopoulos, G. D. (1996). Requisite role of angiopoietin-1, a ligand for the TIE2 receptor, during embryonic angiogenesis Cell. 87: 1171–1180.

Tamura, M., Ichikawa, F., Guillerman, R. P., Deuel, T. F., and Noda, M. (1995).β1, 25 Dihydroxyvitamin D3 down-regulates pleiotrophin messenger RNA expression in osteoblast-like cells. Endocrine 3: 21–24.

Teoh, K. H., Christakis, G. T., Weisel, R. D., Katz, A. M., Tong, C. P., Mickleborough, L. L., Scully, H. E., Baird, R. J., and Goldman, B. S. (1987). Increased risk of urgent revascularization. J. Thorac. Cardiovasc. Surg. 93 (2):291–9.

Vikkula, M., Boon, L. M., Carraway, K. L., Calvert, J. T., Diamonti, A. J. Goumnerov, B., Pasyk, K. A., Marchuk, D. A., Warman, M. L, Cantley, L. C., Mulliken, J. B., and Olsen, B. R. (1996). Vascular dysmorphogenesis caused by an activating mutation in the receptor tyrosine kinase TIE2 Cell. 87: 1181–1190.

Waterfield, M. D., Scrace, G. T., Whittle, N., Stroobant, P., Johnsson, A., Wasteson, A., Westermark, B., Heldin, C.-H., Huang, J. S., and Deuel, T. F. (1983). Platelet-derived growth factor is structurally related to the putative transforming protein p28sis of simian sarcoma virus. Nature 304: 35–39.

Yeh, H.-J., He, Y. Y., Xu, J., Hsu, C. Y., Deuel, T. F. (1998). Upregulation of pleiotrophin gene expression in developing microvasculature, macrophages, and astrocytes after acute ischemic brain injury. J. Neurosci. 18: 3699–3707.

Yeh, H.-J., Ruit, K. G., Wang, Y.-X., Parks, W. C., Snider, W. D., and Deuel, T. F. (1991). PDGF A-chain gene is expressed by mammalian neurons during development and in maturity. Cell 64: 209–216.

II

ANGIOGENESIS IN THE PATHOPHYSIOLOGY AND TREATMENT OF ISCHEMIC VASCULAR DISEASE

7

Angiogenesis in Atherosclerosis and Restenosis

MARK POST AND J. ANTHONY WARE

Small arteries and arterioles that penetrate the adventitia and the media provide the blood supply of the wall of medium and large-size arteries. The intima and the lumenal part of the media are usually avascular; the thickness of this avascular layer is surprisingly constant (approximately 0.5 mm) even when the arterial wall thickens with age and seems to be determined by the diffusion coefficient of oxygen (Wolinsky and Glagov, 1967). Thus, the thickened arterial wall seen during adulthood is supported by new blood vessels that grow into the media.

Despite this adaptive angiogenesis, parts of the arterial wall may become ischemic, either acutely as a result of mural thrombus formation or chronically as a result of atherogenesis or neointima formation (Zemplenyi et al., 1989), eventually leading to the necrotic cores that are found in a majority of advanced lesions. As is the case with other tissues, ischemia of the vessel may itself be a stimulator of angiogenesis (Shweiki et al., 1992). In addition, inflammatory cells are frequently found in the shoulders and the fibrotic cap of the atherosclerotic plaque (Hansson et al., 1989; van der Wal et al., 1989), and such cells are often associated with, and potentially are required for, initiation of angiogenesis (Barger et al., 1984). Another contributory cause to angiogenesis in the arterial wall is iatrogenic damage. Current intervention techniques for percutaneous recanalization of arteries inevitably damage the arterial wall and elicit a healing response, the hallmark of which is intimal hyperplasia (Forrester et al., 1991). This leads to wall thickening and provokes angiogenesis. Thus, the major pathophysiologic conditions for promotion of angiogenesis are derived from factors already present in the normal arterial wall or those that occur with the atherogenic process or its treatment. It remains to be seen to what extent the mechanism by which angiogenesis occurs in the atherosclerotic plaque differs from that in other tissues. The concomitant presence of atherosclerosis, as well as certain anatomic and physiologic characteristics of the environment of the vascular wall, provides additional considerations, however, and the clinical implications of plaque angiogenesis are likely to differ from those of angiogenesis elsewhere.

VASA VASORUM AND NEOVASCULARIZATION OF ATHEROSCLEROTIC PLAQUE

Several morphologic studies in human cadavers and in other species have focused on the anatomy of the vasa vasorum of normal and atherosclerotic arteries (Geiringer, 1951; Bo et al., 1989). Most of the vasa vasorum originate outside the adventitia, which then enter the adventitia and then penetrate the media of large arteries, and usually end at the internal elastic membrane. In cases of severe intimal thickening, these vasa may actually penetrate the internal elastic membrane and enter the intima. In atherosclerotic carotid (Bo et al., 1989) and coronary arteries (Zamir and Silver, 1985; Kumamoto et al., 1995) some vasa vasorum, albeit a minority, were shown to communicate with the lumen of the main artery; it seems most likely that this communication resulted from exuberant growth of the vasa, rather than from outgrowth from the lumen of the main artery. It is about 30 times more likely for plaque vessels to originate in or near the adventitia than it is for them to originate in the lumen. During atherogenesis and intimal thickening, the vasa vasorum increase in number and can form plexi in either the adventitia or media (Fig. 7.1) (Winternitz et al., 1938; Barger et al., 1984; Zamir and Silver, 1985).

The strong association of atherosclerotic plaques with neovascularization by vasa vasorum has triggered hypotheses regarding the role of these newly formed vessels in the pathogenesis of atherosclerosis itself (Martin et al., 1990) and of its complications, such as intraplaque hemorrhage (Alpern-Elran et al., 1989) and vascular spasm at the site of the arterial stenosis (Barger et al., 1984). Plaque angiogenesis occurs only in complicated atherosclerotic plaques, but does not necessarily correlate with degree of stenosis. Although atherosclerosis is closely associated with neovascularization by vasa vasorum, the evidence that the vasa have a role in the early stages of atherosclerosis is largely circumstantial. Most standard theories on atherogenesis postulate that endothelial dysfunction or damage allows for initiation of atherosclerosis and neglect the possibility that atherogenic stimuli might enter the damaged artery through the adventitia, via the vasa vasorum. One possibility is that, since in many cases angiogenesis occurs in response to the growth of tissue (intimal mass in the case of atherosclerosis), as the neointima grows during progression of atherosclerosis, increasing oxygen demand or concomitant inflammation triggers angiogenesis.

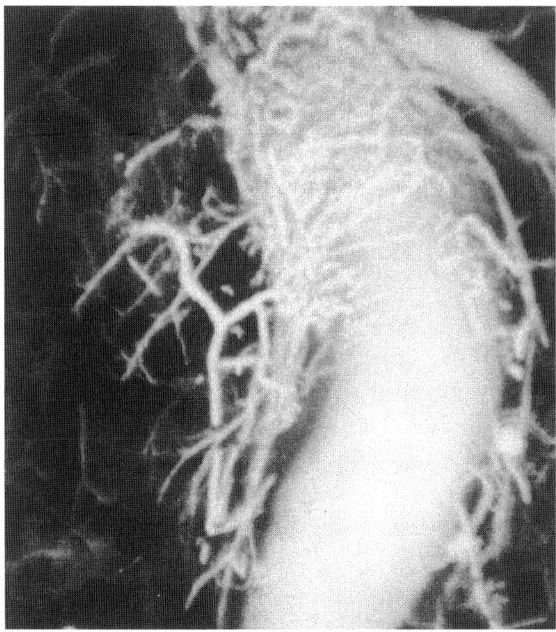

Figure 7.1. Vasa vasorum of atherosclerotic human coronary artery. The vasa are filled with a silicone polymer. The area of dense vascular network colocalizes with calcified plaque [From New Engl J Med 1984; 310: 175–177].

Experiments with perivascular cuffs (Martin et al., 1991; Dashwood et al., 1993) or adventitial stripping (Barker et al., 1994) have shown that disruption of the adventitial blood supply results in neointima formation even though the endothelial lining remains intact. Thus, it is at least plausible that hypoxia of the vessel wall caused by such disruption of the adventitial blood supply promotes one of the central pathophysiologic features of atherosclerosis. The question then arises as to whether some event could initiate arterial wall hypoxia in the absence of substantial intimal thickening, as would be expected in the early stages of atherosclerosis. Although newly formed vessels are usually thin walled, the vasa vasorum in atherosclerotic monkey coronary arteries have been shown to respond to vasoactive substances such as phenylephrine and serotonin (Williams et al., 1988), which demonstrates that they have functional smooth muscle. These vasa also express endothelin-1 receptors and may therefore constrict in the presence of that peptide (Dashwood et al., 1993). Thus, release of substances that cause vasoconstriction of the vasa vasorum may be an initiating event that leads to arterial wall hypoxia, necrosis, and a subsequent healing response that is indistinguishable from neointima formation during atherogenesis.

An alternative hypothesis that relates vasa vasorum to the etiology of atherosclerosis emphasizes the increased permeability of newly formed vessels to macromolecules like albumin and fibrinogen (Zhang et al., 1993; Dvorak et al., 1995). Leakage of proinflammatory and proangiogenic (Senger, 1996) cytokines into the arterial wall by this mechanism could promote further neovascularization of the plaque as well as intimal hyperplasia and matrix deposition. These two models, of course, are not mutually exclusive.

In addition to the possible roles of the vasa vasorum in the early stages of atherosclerosis, the importance of plaque angiogenesis in later stages of the disease, such as intraplaque hemorrhage, plaque rupture, or local vasospasm, has been considered (Fig. 7.2). A propensity for vasospasm at the site of an atherosclerotic plaque, even when the stenosis is not hemodynamically significant, has been noted, and the major pathogenetic mechanism for this phenomenon is endothelial dysfunction (Yamagishi et al., 1994). Although loss or damage of luminal endothelium is likely to be an important contributor to focal vasospasm, it has been proposed that the vasa vasorum might contribute because of the greater abundance of nerve endings near the vascular plexus (Barger et al., 1984), but no additional direct evidence has been obtained to support this hypothesis.

The idea that the presence of abundant microvasculature near an area of inflammation is a risk for sudden intraplaque hemorrhages or rupture of the plaque cap is attractive. Indeed, hemorrhages in the vicinity of vessels in the plaque have frequently been identified (Kumamoto et al., 1995). These vessels are prone to such hemorrhage, because, as noted above, neovascularization of the intima is most prominent at sites of chronic inflammation, as marked by the presence of lymphocytes and macrophages. At those sites, matrix degradation by proteases released by macrophages or the endothelial cells themselves is high, and the vessels may therefore be fragile and susceptible to injury. Newly formed vessels that originate from the lumen of the atherosclerotic artery are more frequently associated with intimal hemorrhage than are adventitial and medial vasa vasorum; whether this observation reflects a difference in pressure gradient or in local cellular context is not clear. Angiogenesis and inflammation is much more extensive in the walls of aneurysmal abdominal aortas than in atherosclerotic control aortas (Thompson et al., 1996), thus suggesting that new vessel formation weakens the arterial wall and may predispose it to rupture. Hypercholesterolemia is, of course, a leading cause of atherosclerosis; paradoxically, angiogenesis may actually be inhibited by hypercholesterolemia, perhaps due to its ability to cause endothelial dysfunction (Henry, 1993). In aortic explants from hypercholesterolemic rabbits, endothelial outgrowth and tube formation is reduced compared to normocholesterolemic controls (Chen et al., 1997). This effect can be simulated in normocholesterolemic controls by adding neutralizing antibodies against FGF-2; additional exogenous FGF-2 to explants from hypercholesterolemic rabbits stimulates endothelial outgrowth. Measurement of FGF-2 in the culture medium of hypercholesterolemic specimens shows marked reduction of FGF-2 levels. These findings have been

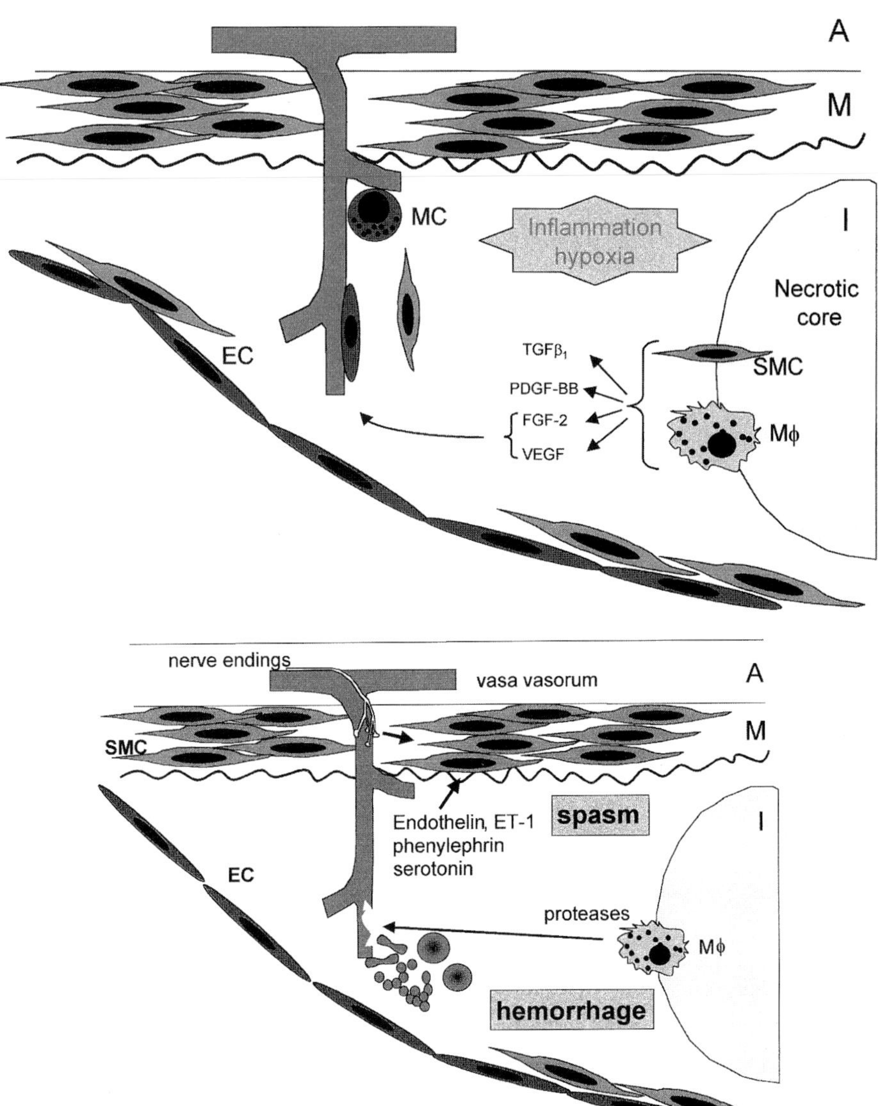

Figure 7.2. (Top) Schematic drawing of atherosclerotic plaque with neovascularization from vasa vasorum. Inflammation and hypoxia of the arterial wall are the main triggers of angiogenesis in the atherosclerotic plaque. Growth factors are released from smooth muscle cells (SMC), macrophages (Mϕ), mast cells (MC), and endothelial cells (EC). The growth factors activate receptors on endothelial cells and smooth muscle cells of the newly forming vessel.

(Bottom) Schematic drawing of the atherosclerotic plaque with neovascularization from vasa vasorum. The abundant presence of small arteries with nerve endings and vasoactive substances may trigger vasospasm of the atherosclerotic artery. Inflammatory processes in atherosclerotic plaques are associated with a high level of protease activity which potentially initiates hemorrhage from already-fragile newly formed vessels in the plaque (A: adventitia, M: media, I: intima, SMC: smooth muscle cell, EC: endothelial cells, Mϕ: macrophage).

confirmed in endothelial cells from human coronary arteries (Chen et al., 1995). Expression of mRNA encoding FGF-2 can be reduced by oxidized low-density lipoprotein (LDL) in a dose-dependent manner, suggesting that this reduction is mediated by an effect on gene expression. These observations suggest that hypercholesterolemia (and especially oxidized LDL) reduces angiogenesis in atherosclerotic plaques by reducing FGF-2 expression. Thus, factors favoring plaque angiogenesis are sufficient to overcome an antiangiogenic effect of LDL.

MEDIATORS OF ANGIOGENESIS

The growth factors that promote angiogenesis are reviewed in various chapters elsewhere in this book. Four major growth factors that have been associated with angiogenesis are transforming growth factor β-1 (TGF-β_1), platelet-derived growth factor (PDGF), basic fibroblast growth factor (FGF-2), and vascular endothelial growth factor, initially discovered and described as vascular permeability factor (VEGF/VPF). Although all of these factors and others are likely to be present in an atherosclerotic plaque, a careful comparison of these growth factors and their receptors during individual stages of atherogenesis needs to be performed before their importance in atherosclerosis-associated neovascularization can be established.

Plaque material itself has angiogenic activity in standard in vivo assays, such as the chick chorioallantoic membrane assay (CAM) (Bo et al., 1992) and the rabbit cornea assay (Alpern-Elran et al., 1989). The specific factors present in plaque that mediate angiogenesis have not been identified. Plaques containing only fibrous material are as angiogenic as are plaques with organized thrombus and calcifications, suggesting that those factors are not the key mediators. Furthermore, cell-rich plaques have the same angiogenic activity as do cell-poor, matrix-rich plaques. This observation suggests that intrinsic matrix components or factors stored in the matrix exert angiogenic activity. Boiling of the plaque results in loss of angiogenic potential, implying that heat sensitive proteins in the plaque are responsible for its angiogenic activity.

The major sources of TGF-β_1 in the vascular wall are platelets, macrophages, and lymphocytes (Björkerud, 1991), although TGF-β_1 is produced by smooth muscle cells in culture (Kirschenlohr et al., 1993) and in pericytes. In situ hybridization studies show that TGF-β_1 is expressed in atherosclerotic tissue and to an even greater extent in restenotic tissue (Nikol et al., 1992). The effect of TGF-β_1 on angiogenesis is complicated. In a CAM assay, TGF-β_1 prevents angiogenesis, probably by inhibiting endothelial cell migration (Madri et al., 1989). In contrast, TGF-β_1 stimulates the formation of cords by endothelial cells cultured on collagen I gel in the presence of plasminogen (Sueishi et al., 1990). Most evidence suggests that TGF-β_1 has roles during the maturation of new blood vessels from endothelial cords (Colville-Nash et al., 1995), and in the recruitment and consolidation of pericytes, concomitant with inhibition of endothelial cell proliferation (Folkman 1996). TGF-β_1's effects in established arteries, in contrast, are directed primarily at matrix proteins; it facilitates the incorporation of fibronectin into the matrix, the secretion of collagen (Ignotz and Massague, 1986), and the upregulation of biglycan (Riessen et al., 1994). Because of these effects, TGF-β_1 enhances neointima formation after arterial injury, not by increasing cell number but by increasing extracellular matrix production, further emphasizing its ability to stimulate matrix protein secretion (Kanzaki et al., 1995). In addition to these direct effects, TGF-β_1 is chemotactic for monocytes and stimulates monocytes to produce other growth factors like FGF-2 (McCartney Francis et al., 1990; Colville-Nash et al., 1995). TGF-β_1 also stimulates production of VEGF in the rat heart (Li et al., 1997). The local activity of TGF-β_1 is regulated in at least two ways: First, TGF-β_1 is secreted as a latent protein and needs to be activated to exert its angiogenic effect. Once released, TGF-β_1 binds to various matrix proteins like decorin, biglycan, and fibromodulin (Hildebrand et al., 1994), thus creating a reservoir of growth factor in the matrix that can be released by local mediators. These effects of TGF-β_1 on vessel maturation and matrix production are probably more important than are its direct angiogenic effects in promoting angiogenesis in atherosclerotic plaques.

Basic fibroblast growth factor (FGF-2) is a potent mitogen for endothelial cells, smooth muscle cells, and fibroblasts (Thomas and Gimenez-Gallego, 1986) and promotes endothelial cord formation in collagen gels in vitro as well as vessel formation in vivo (Passaniti et al., 1992). FGF-2 and its receptor FGFR-1 are present in healthy arteries, predominantly in medial smooth muscle cells and adventitial blood vessels, but not in the luminal endothelium. In all stages of atherosclerosis, both FGF-1 and FGF-2 are expressed in macrophages and smooth muscle cells (Hughes et al., 1993). Increased expression of FGF-2 is correlated with neovascularization of the plaque and also with the presence of monocytes in the vicinity of newly formed blood vessels. FGFR-1 is present almost exclusively in adventitial vessels, although a small number of monocytes and smooth muscle cells in fibro-fatty plaques expressed the receptor as well. Increased expression of FGF-2 also accompanies accelerated atherogenesis in human cardiac transplants (Isik et al., 1991). These observations suggest that FGF-2 may mediate angiogenesis in the atherosclerotic plaque.

Many studies have investigated the role of FGF-2 in arterial healing after balloon injury. In the rat carotid artery injury model, FGF-2 and the FGFR-1 receptor are expressed at the leading edge of regenerating endothelium (Lindner and Reidy, 1993) and exogenous FGF-2 enhances reendothelialization (Lindner et al., 1991). Interestingly, when exogenous FGF-2 is administered to the adventitia of injured arteries, intimal hyperplasia is enhanced and correlates with the growth of adventitial vasa vasorum (Cuevas et al., 1991; Edelman et al., 1992). Thus, FGF-2 may participate in the accelerated arteriopathy following arterial damage.

Another major angiogenic growth factor, VEGF/VPF, acts synergistically with FGF-2 to induce angiogenesis (Goto et al., 1993) and its release is, under some circumstances, induced by FGF-2 (Stavri et al., 1995). Its importance in angiogenesis is illustrated by the fact that administration of VEGF in an adenoviral vector expressing the growth factor induces angiogenesis in the absence of hypoxia or inflammation (Magovern et al., 1997). Recently, the expression of VEGF/VPF protein and mRNA in normal and atherosclerotic arteries has been compared to that in normal arteries (Couffinhal et al., 1997). VEGF expression is increased in atherosclerotic specimens, mainly in the smooth muscle cells. VEGF expression did not correlate the presence of macrophages, nor did these cells demonstrate enhanced expression of the cytokine. An important source for VEGF may be vascular smooth muscle cells, which release mitogens of several kinds for endothelial cells. When treated with smooth muscle cell-conditioned medium, cultured endothelial cells adopt angiogenic phenotypes, that is, they invade collagen and form cords. This effect can be blocked by antibodies that block VEGF but not by FGF-2 antibodies (Kuzuya et al., 1995). After injury of rat carotid and baboon arteries, VEGF levels in the arterial wall and in the intima (Lindner and Reidy, 1996; Ruef et al., 1997) are increased. Together, these data suggest that smooth muscle cells in atherosclerotic plaques may promote angiogenesis by releasing VEGF/VPF. The intensity of VEGF/VPF immunostaining does not correlate, however, with the number of vessels counted using CD31 immunostaining. Furthermore, exogenous VEGF does not promote endothelial regrowth in damaged arteries (Lindner and Reidy, 1996). Thus, the in vivo angiogenic effect of VEGF/VPF in atherosclerosis is still not certain despite the suggestive evidence.

In addition to these growth factors, PDGF (especially BB isoform) and IGF-1 induce angiogenesis in rat aorta explants and are potential candidates for mediators of angiogenesis in atherosclerotic vessels (Nicosia et al., 1994). PDGF-BB induces cord formation by endothelial cells in vitro either by a direct effect via the PDGF-β receptor that is present on these endothelial cells (Battegay et al., 1994; Marx et al., 1994) or indirectly by stimulating macrophages (Sato et al., 1993) or pericytes (Sundberg et al., 1993). In an vivo CAM assay, PDGF-BB, and not PDGF-AA, induces angiogenesis (Risau et al., 1992). No direct evidence exists for the involvement of PDGF in atherosclerosis-associated angiogenesis, but both PDGF-BB and the PDGF-β receptor have been observed in the microvasculature, specifically the pericytes, of healing skin wounds, and PDGF-AA and the PDGF-β receptor have been found in carotid (Majesky et al., 1990) and coronary arteries (Scott et al., 1996) during healing following balloon denudation. In arterial tissue, PDGF is mainly expressed in or near smooth muscle cells in the adventitia, media, and intima, where it is thought to promote smooth muscle cell migration. Another mechanism by which PDGF-BB may act is by promoting expression of the integrin αvβ3; PDGF-BB's stimulation of endothelial migration and proliferation is enhanced when endothelial cells are plated on αvβ3 binding matrices (Schneller et al., 1997). This member of the integrin family is abundant in microvessels in the adventitia of atherosclerotic arteries (Hoshiga et al., 1995) and appears to be essential for endothelial cell adhesion and prevention of apoptosis. (See elsewhere in this book.) Therefore, although PDGF-BB is primarily secreted by smooth muscle cells and pericytes, its effect on endothelial cells may have pathophysiologic significance.

A potential source of these growth factors, in addition to macrophages, smooth muscle cells, and the endothelial cells themselves, is mast cells, which are often found near microvessels and appear to contribute to angiogenesis in tumors. A number of mast-cell-derived mediators are candidates to promote angiogenesis in atherosclerotic arteries, including TNF-α, interleukin-8, FGF-2, the prostaglandins PGD_2 and PGE_2, leukotrienes, platelet activating factor (PAF), and TGF-β (Norrby, 1997). As part of a potential paracrine or autocrine loop, FGF-2, VEGF, and PDGF-AB promote migration and chemotaxis of mast cells (Gruber et al., 1995). The adventitia of aorta and coronary arteries contains abundant mast cells and their numbers are increased at stages of atherosclerosis that are more advanced (Atkinson et al., 1994). Although mast cells have received relatively little attention in the pathogenesis and pathology of atherosclerosis, they should be considered as potentially important cellular mediators of this vascular disease and the associated angiogenesis.

MATRIX COMPONENTS IN THE ATHEROSCLEROTIC PLAQUE THAT FAVOR ANGIOGENESIS

Matrix proteins are clearly important in supporting, regulating, and directing angiogenesis. In addition to glycosaminoglycans, and a host of other matrix components, atherosclerotic plaques and thrombi adherent to the lesion contain relatively large amounts of fibronectin, collagen, fibrinogen, and fibrin. These matrix proteins, especially fibronectin, support angiogenesis by promoting the adhesion and migration of endothelial and smooth muscle cells (Yamada, 1983). Collagens, especially types I and III, are abundant in the arterial wall and can affect angiogenesis in many ways. Both collagen degradation and collagen synthesis are necessary for angiogenesis. Substances that interfere with synthesis, such as proline analogs, or with crosslinking of collagen, inhibit angiogenesis (Eisenstein, 1991). On the other hand, degradation of collagen XVIII, a component of basement membranes, results in the release of endostatin, a potent inhibitor of angiogenesis (O'Reilly et al., 1997). Expression of matrix metalloproteinases is increased in atherosclerotic plaques, and correlates with the degree of infiltrate, hemorrhage, and granulation tissue.

Fibrinogen, fibrin, and fibrin degradation products are all present in the atherosclerotic plaque as a result of recurrent thrombosis (Clagett et al., 1986) and leakage from newly formed, and thus hyperpermeable, vessels (Zhang et al., 1993). These proteins induce adhesion and spreading of endothelial cells (Eisenstein, 1991; Thompson et al., 1991). Thus, many of the matrix proteins can contribute to endothelial growth and can further the inflammatory response that accompanies angiogenesis in the atherosclerotic plaque. Inhibitory functions of certain matrix components suggest that this is one mechanism by which angiogenesis is tightly regulated in the atherosclerotic plaque.

ARTERIAL INJURY, RESTENOSIS, AND ANGIOGENESIS

Accelerated forms of atherosclerosis are seen following mechanical injury of arteries, such as occurs during the course of therapeutic coronary recanalization procedures. Arterial healing is associated with intimal hyperplasia, which is the result of smooth muscle cell proliferation, migration, and matrix protein synthesis. In addition to the angiogenic stimulus of increasing wall thickness with resulting intramural ischemia, specific direct stimulators of angiogenesis may be related to injury. After balloon injury in the rabbit aorta, inflammatory cells including macrophages and T-lymphocytes remain activated up to 30 days after injury (Tanaka et al., 1993). When activated, macrophages appear to be important cellular mediators of angiogenesis accompanying wound healing in the skin (Hunt et al., 1984), and are plausible mediators of the angiogenesis that occurs in limb ischemia (Ito et al., 1997). Also, as noted previously, arterial injury augments the expression of VEGF (Lindner and Reidy, 1996) and FGF-2 (Lindner et al., 1991), and adventitial application of FGF-2 increases the number of vasa vasorum after arterial injury. Interestingly, the enlarged area of vasa vasorum was proportional to the area of intimal hyperplasia resulting from the balloon denudation injury (Edelman et al., 1992). One might suppose that balloon dilation damages or even ruptures vasa vasorum, thus leading to necrosis and intimal hyperplasia. Instead, balloon angioplasty causes reactive hyperemia of the arterial wall by increasing the number of vasa vasorum (Cragg et al., 1983),. Thus, in addition to the role of angiogenesis in atherogenesis, angiogenesis also is a necessary component of arterial healing and neointima formation after injury.

SUMMARY

A plethora of evidence has emerged that angiogenesis occurs in the atherosclerotic plaque and in accelerated atherosclerotic diseases such as restenosis after balloon angioplasty. The mechanism by which angiogenesis develops in atherosclerotic plaque shares many features with that seen elsewhere; however, such vessel formation has specific consequences of clinical importance, such as hemorrhage and other events that may promote acute coronary obstruction. Direct evidence for the role of plaque angiogenesis in plaque instability is lacking, although many observations suggest such a mechanism. Plaque angiogenesis might be promoted or inhibited by agents designed for these purposes in diseases other than atherosclerosis and thus may be a potential side effect of their use. Observations of the consequences of enhanced or diminished plaque vascularity in atherosclerosis will further our understanding of the relationships between angiogenesis and the complications of atherosclerosis.

REFERENCES

Alpern-Elran, H., Morog, N., Robert, F., Hoover, G., Kalant N., and Brem, S. (1989). Angiogenic activity of the atherosclerotic carotid artery plaque. J. Neurosurg. 70: 942–945.

Atkinson, J. B., Harlan, C. W., Harlan, G. C., and Virmani, R. (1994). The association of mast cells and atherosclerosis: a morphologic study of early atherosclerotic lesions in young people. Hum. Pathol. 25: 154–159.

Barger, A. C., Beeuwkes, R., 3rd, Lainey, L. L., and Silverman, K. J. (1984). Hypothesis: vasa vasorum and neovascularization of human coronary arteries. A possible role in the pathophysiology of atherosclerosis. N. Engl. J. Med. 310: 175–177.

Barker, S. G., Tilling, L. C., Miller, G. C., Beesley, J. E., Fleetwood, G., Stavri, G. T., Baskerville, P. A., and Martin, J. F. (1994). The adventitia and atherogenesis: removal initiates intimal proliferation in the rabbit which regresses on generation of a 'neoadventitia.' Atherosclerosis 105: 131–144.

Battegay, E. J., Rupp, J., Iruela-Arispe, L., Sage, E. H., and Pech, M. (1994). PDGF-BB modulates endothelial proliferation and angiogenesis in vitro via PDGF beta-receptors. J. Cell Biol. 125: 917–928.

Björkerud, S. (1991). Effects of transforming growth factor-beta 1 on human arterial smooth muscle cells in vitro. Arterioscler. Thromb. 11: 892–902.

Bo, W. J., McKinney, W. M., and Bowden, R. L. (1989). The origin and distribution of vasa vasorum at the bifurcation of the common carotid artery with atherosclerosis. Stroke 20: 1484–1487.

Bo, W. J., Mercuri, M., Tucker, R., and Bond, M. G. (1992). The human carotid atherosclerotic plaque stimulates angiogenesis on the chick chorioallantoic membrane. Atherosclerosis 94: 71–78.

Chen, C. H., Nguyen, H. H., Weilbaecher, D., Luo, S., Gotto, A. M., Jr., and Henry P. D. (1995). Basic fibroblast growth factor reverses atherosclerotic impairment of human coronary angiogenesis-like responses in vitro. Atherosclerosis 116: 261–268.

Chen, C. H., Cartwright, J., Jr., Li, Z., Lou, S., Nguyen, H. H., Gotto, A. M., Jr., and Henry, P. D. (1997). Inhibitory effects of hypercholesterolemia and ox-LDL on angiogenesis-like endothelial growth in rabbit aortic explants. Essential role of basic fibroblast growth factor. Arterioscler. Thromb. Vasc. Biol. 17: 1303–1312.

Clagett, G. P., Robinowitz, M., Youkey, J. R., Fisher, D. F., Jr., Fry, R. E., Myers S. I.,

Lee, E. L., Collins, G. J., Jr., and Virmani, R. (1986). Morphogenesis and clinicopathologic characteristics of recurrent carotid disease. J. Vasc. Surg. 3: 10–23.

Colville-Nash, P. R., Alam, C. A., Appleton, I., Brown, J. R., Seed, M. P., and Willoughby, D. A. (1995). The pharmacological modulation of angiogenesis in chronic granulomatous inflammation. J. Pharmacol. Exp. Ther. 274: 1463–1472.

Couffinhal, T., Kearney, M., Witzenbichler, B., Chen, D., Murohara, T., Losordo, D. W., Symes, J., and Isner, J. M. (1997). Vascular endothelial growth factor/vascular permeability factor (VEGF/VPF) in normal and atherosclerotic human arteries. Am. J. Pathol. 150: 1673–1685.

Cragg, A. H., Einzig, S., Rysavy, J. A., Castaneda-Zuniga, W. R., Borgwardt, B., and Amplatz, K. (1983). The vasa vasorum and angioplasty. Radiology 148: 75–80.

Cuevas, P., Gonzalez, A. M., Carceller, F., and Baird, A. (1991). Vascular response to basic fibroblast growth factor when infused onto the normal adventitia or into the injured media of the rat carotid artery. Circ. Res. 69: 360–369.

Dashwood, M. R., Barker, S. G., Muddle, J. R., Yacoub, M. H., and Martin, J. F. (1993). [125I]-endothelin-1 binding to vasa vasorum and regions of neovascularization in human and porcine blood vessels: a possible role for endothelin in intimal hyperplasia and atherosclerosis. J. Cardiovasc. Pharmacol. 22 Suppl. 8: S343–S347.

Dvorak, H. F., Brown, L. F., Detmar, M., and Dvorak, A. M. (1995). Vascular permeability factor/vascular endothelial growth factor, microvascular hyperpermeability, and angiogenesis. Am. J. Pathol. 146: 1029–1039.

Edelman, E. R., Nugent, M. A., Smith, L. T., and Karnovsky, M. J. (1992). Basic fibroblast growth factor enhances the coupling of intimal hyperplasia and proliferation of vasa vasorum in injured rat arteries. J. Clin. Invest. 89: 465–473.

Eisenstein, R. (1991). Angiogenesis in arteries: review. Pharmacol.Ther. 49: 1–19.

Folkman, J. and Pa, D. A. (1996). Blood vessel formation: what is its molecular basis? [comment]. Cell 87: 1153–1155.

Forrester, J. S., Fishbein, M. C., Helfant, R., and Fagin, J. A. (1991). A paradigm for restenosis based on cell biology: clues for the development of new preventive therapies. J. Am. Coll. Cardiol. 17: 758–769.

Geiringer, E. (1951). Intimal vascularization and atherosclerosis. J. Pathol. Bact. 63: 201–211.

Goto, F., Goto, K., Weindel, K., and Folkman, J. (1993). Synergistic effects of vascular endothelial growth factor and basic fibroblast growth factor on the proliferation and cord formation of bovine capillary endothelial cells within collagen gels [see comments]. Lab. Invest. 69: 508–517.

Gruber, B. L., Marchese, M. J., and Kew, R. (1995). Angiogenic factors stimulate mast-cell migration. Blood 86: 2488–2493.

Hansson, G. K., Jonasson, L., Seifert, P. S., and Stemme, S. (1989). Immune mechanisms in atherosclerosis. Arteriosclerosis 9: 567–578.

Henry, P. D. (1993). Hypercholesterolemia and angiogenesis. Am. J. Cardiol. 72: 61C–64C.

Hildebrand, A., Romaris, M., Rasmussen, L. M., Heinegard, D., Twardzik, D. R., Border, W. A., and Ruoslahti, E. (1994). Interaction of the small interstitial proteoglycans biglycan, decorin and fibromodulin with transforming growth factor beta. Biochem. J. 302(Pt 2): 527–534.

Hoshiga, M., Alpers, C. E., Smith, L. L., Giachelli, C. M., and Schwartz, S. M. (1995). Alpha-v beta-3 integrin expression in normal and atherosclerotic artery. Circ. Res. 77: 1129–1135.

Hughes, S. E., Crossman, D., and Hall, P. A. (1993). Expression of basic and acidic fibroblast growth factors and their receptor in normal and atherosclerotic human arteries. Cardiovasc. Res. 27: 1214–1219.

Hunt, T. K., Knighton, D. R., Thakral, K. K., Goodson, W. H., 3rd, and Andrews, W. S. (1984). Studies on inflammation and wound healing: angiogenesis and collagen synthesis stimulated in vivo by resident and activated wound macrophages. Surgery 96: 48–54.

Ignotz, R. A. and Massague, J. (1986). Transforming growth factor-beta stimulates the expression of fibronectin and collagen and their incorporation into the extracellular matrix. J. Biol. Chem. 261: 4337–4345.

Isik, F. F., Valentine, H. A., McDonald, T. O., Baird, A., and Gordon, D. (1991). Localization of bFGF in human transplant coronary atherosclerosis. Ann. N.Y. Acad. Sci. 638: 487–488.

Ito, W. D., Arras, M., Winkler, B., Scholz, D., Schaper, J., and Schaper, W. (1997). Monocyte Chemotactic Protein-1 increases collateral and peripheral conductance after femoral artery occlusion. Circ. Res. 80: 829–837.

Kanzaki, T., Tamura, K., Takahashi, K., Saito, Y., Akikusa, B., Oohashi, H., Kasayuki, N., Veda, M., and Morisaki, N. (1995). In vivo effect of TGF-β1—enhanced intimal thickening by administration of TGF-β1 in rabbit arteries injured with a balloon catheter. Arterioscler. Thromb. Vasc. Biol. 15: 1951–1957.

Kirschenlohr, H. L., Metcalfe, J. C., Weissberg, P. L., and Grainger, D. J. (1993). Adult human aortic smooth muscle cells in culture produce active TGF-β. Am. J. Physiol. 265: C571–C576.

Kumamoto, M., Nakashima, Y., and Sueishi, K. (1995). Intimal neovascularization in human coronary atherosclerosis: its origin and pathophysiological significance. Hum. Pathol. 26: 450–456.

Kuzuya, M., Satake, S., Esaki, T., Yamada, K., Hayashi, T., Naito, M., Asai, K., and Iguchi, A. (1995). Induction of angiogenesis by smooth muscle cell-derived factor: possible role in neovascularization in atherosclerotic plaque. J. Cell Physiol. 164: 658–667.

Li, J., Hampton, T., Morgan, J. P., and Simons, M. (1997). Stretch-induced VEGF expression in the heart. J. Clin. Invest. 100: 18–24.

Lindner, V. and Reidy, M. A. (1993). Expression of basic fibroblast growth factor and its receptor by smooth muscle cells and endothelium in injured rat arteries: an en face study. Circ. Res. 73: 589–595.

Lindner, V. and Reidy, M. A. (1996). Expression of VEGF receptors in arteries after endothelial injury and lack of increased endothelial regrowth in response to VEGF. Arterioscler. Thromb. Vasc. Biol. 16: 1399–1405.

Lindner, V., Lappi, D. A., Baird, A., Majack, R. A., and Reidy, M. A. (1991). Role of basic fibroblast growth factor in vascular lesion formation. Circ. Res. 68: 106–113.

Madri, J. A., Reidy, M. A., Kocher, O., and Bell, L. (1989). Endothelial cell behavior after denudation injury is modulated by transforming growth factor-beta1 and fibronectin. Lab. Invest. 60: 755–765.

Magovern, C. J., Mack, C. A., Zhang, J., Rosengart, T. K., Isom, O. W., and Crystal, R. G. (1997). Regional angiogenesis induced in nonischemic tissue by an adenoviral vector expressing vascular endothelial growth factor. Hum. Gene Ther. 8: 215–227.

Majesky, M. W., Reidy, M. A., Bowen Pope, D. F., Hart, C. E., Wilcox, J. N., and Schwartz, S. M. (1990). PDGF ligand and receptor gene expression during repair of arterial injury. J. Cell Biol. 111: 2149–2158.

Martin, J. F., Booth, R. F., and Moncada, S. (1990). Arterial wall hypoxia following hypoperfusion through the vasa vasorum is an initial lesion in atherosclerosis. Eur. J. Clin. Invest. 20: 588–592.

Martin, J. F., Booth, R. F. G., and Moncada, S. (1991). Arterial wall hypoxia following thrombosis of the vasa vasorum is an initial lesion in atherosclerosis. Eur. J. Clin. Invest. 21: 355–359.

Marx, M., Perlmutter, R. A., and Madri, J. A. (1994). Modulation of platelet-derived growth factor receptor expression in microvascular endothelial cells during in vitro angiogenesis. J. Clin. Invest. 93: 131–9.

McCartney Francis, N., Mizel, D., Wong, H., Wahl, L., and Wahl, S. (1990). TGF-beta regulates production of growth factors and TGF-beta by human peripheral blood monocytes. Growth Factors 4: 27–35.

Nicosia, R. F., Nicosia, S. V., and Smith, M. (1994). Vascular endothelial growth factor, platelet-derived growth factor, and insulin-like growth factor-1 promote rat aortic angiogenesis in vitro. Am. J. Pathol. 145: 1023–1029.

Nikol, S., Isner, J. M., Pickering, J. G., Kearney, M., Leclerc, G., and Weir, L. (1992). Expression of transforming growth factor-β1 is increased in human vascular restenosis lesions. J. Clin. Invest. 90: 1582–1592.

Norrby, K. (1997). Mast cells and de novo angiogenesis: angiogenic capability of individual mast-cell mediators such as histamine, TNF, IL-8 and bFGF. Inflamm. Res. 46 Suppl. 1: S7–8.

O'Reilly, M. S., Boehm, T., Shing, Y., Fukai, N., Vasios, G., Lane, W. S., Flynn, E., Birkhead, J. R., Olsen B. R., and Folkman, J. (1997). Endostatin: an endogenous inhibitor of angiogenesis and tumor growth. Cell 88: 277–285.

Passaniti, A., Taylor, R. M., Pili, R., Guo, Y., Long, P. V., Haney, J. A., Pauly, R. R., Grant, D. S., and Martin, G. R. (1992). A simple, quantitative method for assessing angiogenesis and antiangiogenic agents using reconstituted basement membrane, heparin, and fibroblast growth factor. Lab. Invest. 67: 519–528.

Riessen, R., Isner, J. M., Blessing, E., Loushin, C., Nikol, S., and Wight, T. N. (1994). Regional differences in the distribution of the proteoglycans biglycan and decorin in the extracellular matrix of atherosclerotic and restenotic human coronary arteries. Am. J. Pathol. 144: 962–974.

Risau, W., Drexler, H., Mironov, V., Smits, A., Siegbahn, A., Funa, K., and Heldin, C. H. (1992). Platelet-derived growth factor is angiogenic in vivo. Growth Factors 7: 261–266.

Ruef, J., Hu, Z. Y., Yin, L. Y., Wu, Y., Hanson, S. R., Kelly, A. B., Harker L. A., Rao, G. N., Runge, M. S., and Patterson, C. (1997). Induction of vascular endothelial growth factor in balloon-injured baboon arteries. A novel role for reactive oxygen species in atherosclerosis. Circ. Res. 81:24–33.

Sato, N., Beitz, J. G., Kato, J., Yamamoto, M., Clark, J. W., Calabresi, P., Raymond, A., and Frackelton, A. R., Jr. (1993). Platelet-derived growth factor indirectly stimulates angiogenesis in vitro. Am. J. Pathol. 142: 1119–1130.

Schneller, M., Vuori, K., and Ruoslahti, E. (1997). Alphavbeta3 integrin associates with activated insulin and PDGFbeta receptors and potentiates the biological activity of PDGF. Embo J. 16: 5600–5607.

Scott, N. A., Cipolla, G. D., Ross, C. E., Dunn, B., Martin, F. H., Simonet, L., and Wilcox, J. N. (1996). Identification of a potential role for the adventitia in vascular lesion formation after balloon overstretch injury of porcine coronary arteries. Circulation 93: 2178–2187.

Senger, D. R. (1996). Molecular framework for angiogenesis: a complex web of interactions between extravasated plasma proteins and endothelial cell proteins induced by angiogenic cytokines [comment]. Am. J. Pathol. 149: 1–7.

Shweiki, D., Itin, A., Soffer, D., and Keshet, E. (1992). Vascular endothelial growth factor induced by hypoxia may mediate hypoxia-initiated angiogenesis. Nature 359: 843–845.

Stavri, G. T., Zachary, J. C., Baskerville, P. A., Martin, J. F. and Erusalimsky, J. D. (1995). Basic fibroblast growth factor upregulates the expression of vascular endothelial growth factor in vascular smooth muscle cells. Synergistic interaction with hypoxia. Circulation 92: 11–14.

Sueishi, K., Yasunaga, C., Castellanos, E., Kumamoto, M., and Tanaka, K. (1990). Sustained arterial injury and progression of atherosclerosis. Ann. N.Y. Acad. Sci. 598: 223–231.

Sundberg, C., Ljungstrom, M., Lindmark, G., Gerdin, B., and Rubin, K. (1993). Microvascular pericytes express platelet-derived growth factor-beta receptors in human healing wounds and colorectal adenocarcinoma. Am. J. Pathol. 143: 1377–1388.

Tanaka, H., Sukhova, G. K., Swanson, S. J., Clinton, S. K., Ganz, P., Cybulsky, M. I., and Libby, P. (1993). Sustained activation of vascular cells and leukocytes in the rabbit aorta after balloon injury. Circulation 88: 1788–1803.

Thomas, K. A. and Gimenez-Gallego, G. (1986). Fibroblast growth factors: broad spectrum mitogens with potent angiogenic activity. Trends Pharmacol. Sci. 11: 81–84.

Thompson, W. D., Harvey, J. A., Kazmi, M. A. and Stout, A. J. (1991). Fibrinolysis and angiogenesis in wound healing. J. Pathol. 165: 311–318.

Thompson, M. M., Jones, L., Nasim, A., Sayers, R. D., and Bell, P. R. (1996). Angiogenesis in abdominal aortic aneurysms. Eur. J. Vasc. Endovasc. Surg. 11: 464–469.

van der Wal, A. C., Das, P. K., Bentz van de Berg, D., van der Loos, C. M., and Becker, A. E. (1989). Atherosclerotic lesions in humans. In situ immunophenotypic analysis suggesting an immune mediated response. Lab. Invest. 61: 166–170.

Williams, J. K., Armstrong, M. L., and Heistad, D. D. (1988). Vasa vasorum in atherosclerotic coronary arteries: responses to vasoactive stimuli and regression of atherosclerosis. Circ. Res. 62: 515–523.

Winternitz, M. C., Thomas, R. M., and LeCompte, P. M. (1938). The Biology of Arteriosclerosis. Charles C. Thomas, Springfield, IL.

Wolinsky, H. and Glagov, S. (1967). Nature of species differences in the medial distribution of aortic vasa vasorum in mammals. Circ. Res. 20: 409–421.

Yamada, K. M. (1983). Cell surface interactions with extracellular materials. Annu. Rev. Biochem. 52: 761–799.

Yamagishi, M., Miyatake, K., Tamai, J., Nakatani, S., Koyama, J., and Nissen, S. E. (1994). Intravascular ultrasound detection of atherosclerosis at the site of focal vasospasm in angiographically normal or minimally narrowed coronary segments. J. Am. Coll. Cardiol. 23: 352–357.

Zamir, M. and Silver, M. D. (1985). Vasculature in the walls of human coronary arteries. Arch. Pathol. Lab. Med. 109: 659–662.

Zemplenyi, T., Crawford, D. W., and Cole, M. A. (1989). Adaptation of arterial wall hypoxia demonstrated in vivo with oxygen microcathodes. Atherosclerosis 76: 173–179.

Zhang, Y., Cliff, W. J., Schoefl, G. I., and Higgins, G. (1993). Immunohistochemical study of intimal microvessels in coronary atherosclerosis. Am. J. Pathol. 143: 164–172.

8

Collateral Circulation of the Heart

WOLFGANG SCHAPER, JAN J. PIEK,
RAMON MUNOZ-CHAPULI,
CLAUDIA WOLF, AND WULF ITO

The purpose of this chapter is to describe the process of cardiac angiogenesis and neoarteriogenesis in response to coronary artery disease and to discuss the role of growth factors, extracellular matrix proteins, and circulating angiogenic cells. It is clearly desirable to understand the extent of spontaneous collateral development to appreciate changes induced by exogenous growth factor application or gene therapy. Thus this chapter will build on presentation of animal models discussed in Chapter 10 and will lay the foundation for subsequent discussions of therapeutic angiogenesis in Chapters 13 and 14.

TWO TYPES OF COLLATERAL CIRCULATION

Occlusions of one or more coronary arteries can occur unnoticed and may develop without overt myocardial infarction or result in only minor scar formation because of the timely development of a collateral circulation. Many such cases have been described postmortem in patients dying of noncardiac causes who had been completely unaware of the presence of coronary artery disease (Fig. 8.1.A and B). Other patients with symptomatic ischemic heart disease have had occlusions of all three major coronary arteries or even of the left main coronary artery but did not suffer from infarction. These infrequent patients had apparently profited from slowly progressing disease that allowed for sufficient time to develop extensive collateral circulation.

Collateral vessels, especially the epicardial collaterals that have well developed tunica media, are derived from preexisting arterioles (Baroldi, 1967 and 1974). New vessels sprouting from capillaries and postcapillary

A

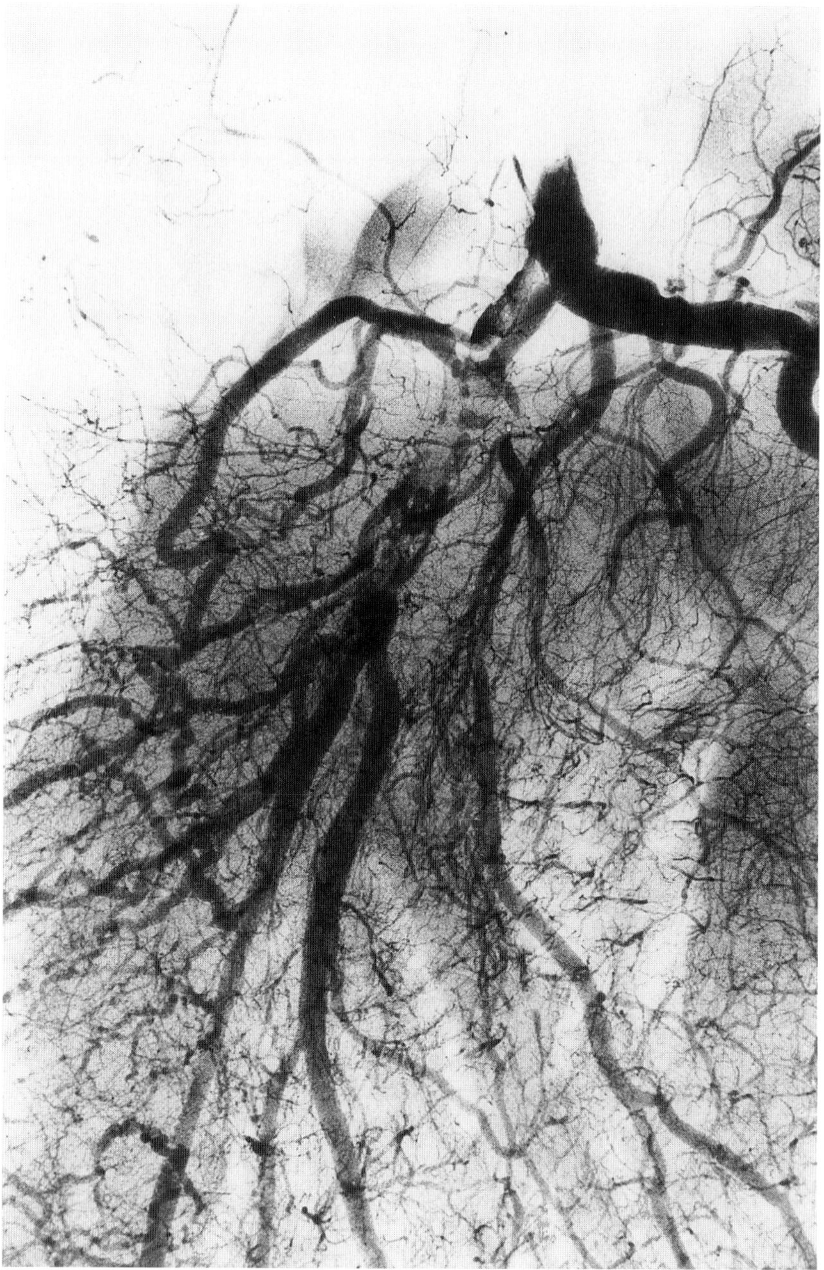

Figure 8.1. A. Postmortem coronary angiogram of a patient with symptomatic diffuse coronary artery disease with multiple lesions in all three coronary arteries and diffuse narrowing of the left anterior descending coronary artery (LAD).

B

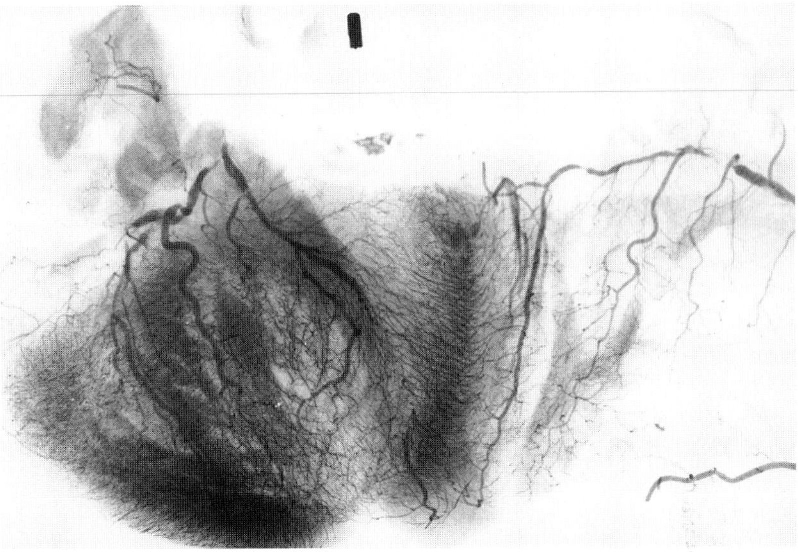

Figure 8.1. (continued) B. Numerous collateral vessels traverse the interventricular septum that originate from the LAD to supply the perfusion region of the recipient right coronary artery (RCA), which exhibits one occlusion and one tight stenosis. The heart was "unrolled" to obtain a quasi two-dimensional image.

venules, a process called angiogenesis, is a second form of neovascularization found in these patients, that leads to formation of thousands of small vessels throughout the compromised areas of the myocardium. Both angiogenesis and collateral vessel development can occur in the same heart as compensatory processes in ischemic heart disease, but collaterals are by far the more physiologically important ones since only arterial vessels deliver the large amounts of blood necessary to maintain structure and function of substantial parts of the left ventricle, or of an entire limb in case of obstruction of femoral or iliac arteries. In contrast, it is not clear if the sprouting of capillaries in the presence of epicardial coronary obstruction is sufficient to supply a large tissue mass.

The following calculations further illustrate the functional advantage of large vessel over small vessel neovascularization. A coronary artery with an internal diameter of 3 mm can be efficiently (but not completely) replaced by three or four smaller collateral arteries. In contrast, over a million new capillaries would be needed to replace the lumenal area of such an artery while, according to Poisoeuille's law, about 25 million capillaries would be needed to compensate for the increase in resistance. The wall thickness area of these vessels would exceed by a factor of 1,000 that of the native vessel and the new tissue needed for the walls would be several thousand times in excess of the material that has to be replaced (i.e., the wall of the defunct artery). Furthermore, although new capillaries can reduce the minimal resistance of the region at risk, they will require substantial new space. Thus, either myocytes are replaced by a growing capillary network or the capillaries remain in a collapsed state (Görge et al., 1989). Thus, collateral artery growth is a much more effective adaptational process when the blood supply to a large tissue mass is compromised.

The most common term used to describe vascular growth in response to developmental and physiological stimuli and to adaptational responses in pathological situations, is angiogenesis. In a strict sense angiogenesis refers to the sprouting of new capillaries from preexisting capillaries or venules (Dumont et al., 1995). The term *vasculogenesis* is reserved for the fetal development of the large blood vessels by angioblasts in situ (Risau and Flamme, 1995). Collateral vessel growth in adult tissues is neither angiogenesis nor vasculogenesis, because the substrate of collateral growth is neither a sprouting capillary nor immature precursor cells but the preexisting interconnecting arteriole. It is certainly unsatisfactory that a most important adaptational vascular growth process has not been named properly. We therefore propose to refer to collateral growth as *neoarteriogenesis* (Fig. 8.2). In this chapter, we will use the term angiogenesis in its re-

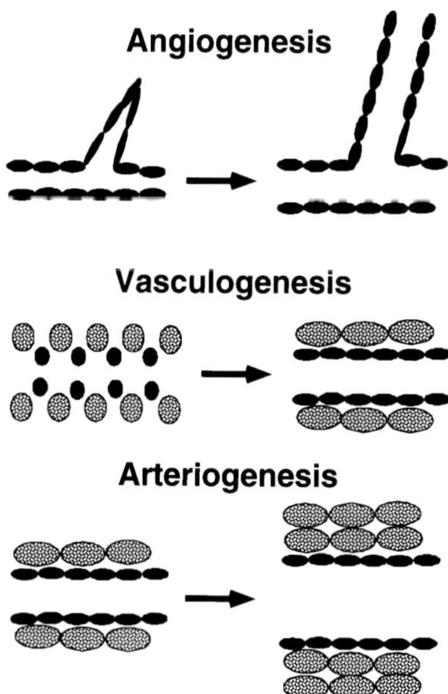

Figure 8.2. Methods of vascular growth. Vascular growth proceeds via three distinct mechanisms: *Angiogenesis*, the sprouting of capillaries; *vasculogenesis*, the in situ development of large vessels from precursor cells (hemangioblasts); and *arteriogenesis*, the in situ growth of arteries from preexisting arteriolar anastomoses.

stricted sense when it is clear that the vessels so named are capillaries that have derived by sprouting from preexisting capillaries. We call the process of development of muscular arterial vessel, the actual collateral vessels, neoarteriogenesis, and we will not use the term vasculogenesis.

Interspecies Diversity in Collateral Networks

Collateral vessels develop from preexisting interconnecting arterioles, but not all species are endowed with a sufficient number of the latter to react rapidly to the development of a critical coronary stenosis. As a way of illustrating this point, consider that acute coronary artery occlusion leads rapidly to transmural myocardial infarction in rats, rabbits, and pigs, and to subendocardial-to-midmyocardial infarction in dogs and cats, but produces no infarction at all in the guinea pig (Fig. 8.3.). Morphological studies of the coronary vessels in these species show that rats, rabbits, and pigs have anatomical end-arteries with no arteriolar connections, dogs and cats are well endowed with these vessels, and guinea pig hearts exhibit a truly abundant arteriolar network (Schaper, 1984). The normal human heart has interconnecting arterioles but fewer than the dog heart (Baroldi, 1967 and 1974). These differences between species are of a genetic nature, and within a given species, they can be enhanced or repressed by selective breeding. The molecular mechanisms of the differences between species must be sought in the fetal development of the coronary vascular system. We hypothesize that they are caused by the degree of differentiation, in that in well-collateralized hearts the differentiation program is

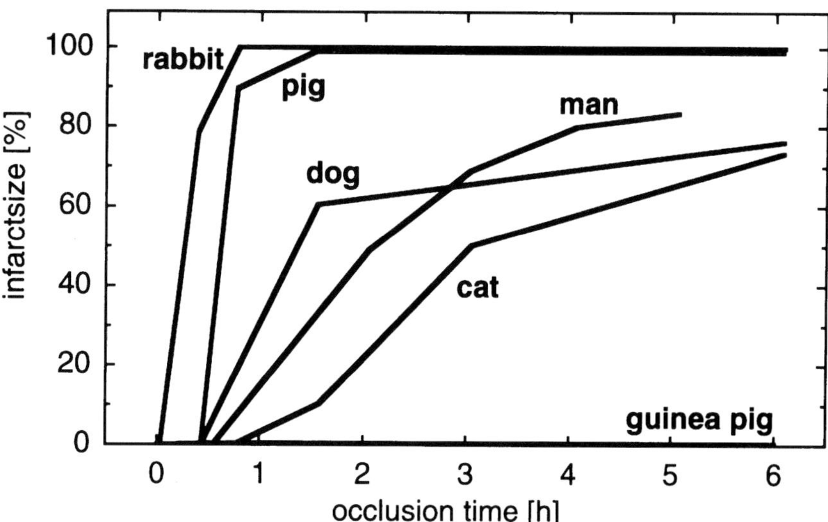

Figure 8.3. Infarct size as a function of occlusion time.

prematurely stopped and retains some features of the fetal system, while the fully differentiated phenotype is the "no-network" anatomical end-artery.

Fetal Development of Collateral Vessels

The first evidence of developing cardiac vessels in the vertebrate heart is the differentiation of a primary capillary plexus that closely follows the epicardial invasion of the myocardial wall. The capillary plexus originates from the coalescence of blood-island-like structures and vasculogenic cells that form a network of vascular channels in the space between the primitive epicardium and the myocardium, especially in the areas where this space is wider, such as around the intercameral grooves. (For a review see Tomanek, 1996.) The sites of origin of the precursors of the primary vascular elements are not well known, but cell lineage experiments (Mikawa and Fischman, 1992) have shown that they are of extracardiac origin and that they arrive to the heart during formation of the primitive epicardium.

After their differentiation, vessels of the subepicardial plexus grow all over the heart and establish intramyocardial links with the intertrabecular sinusoids of the ventricle. This contact allows for an early circulation of blood through the developing compact layer of the myocardium. The importance of these early endocardial–capillary connections has been shown experimentally; the failure to establish the primary plexus induced by genetic manipulations results in embryonic death from pericardial hemorrhage (Kwee et al., 1995). These endocardial–capillary connections seem to be rare in human embryos, however (Hutchins et al., 1988). From the connection of the vascular plexus with the sinus venosus lumen, through the prospective coronary sinus, a directed blood flow presumably originating from the intertrabecular sinusoids to intramyocardial capillaries, subepicardial vascular plexus, and sinus venosus is established (Waldo et al., 1990).

In a later stage of development, the peritruncal network of capillaries establishes a number of connections with the lumen of the aorta at the level of the aortic sinuses (sinuses of Valsalva). Some of these contacts become the definitive orifices of the coronary arteries (Bogers et al., 1989; Poelmann et al., 1993; Waldo et al., 1990). The connection of the vascular plexus with the systemic circulation causes drastic changes in blood pressure and flow inside of the capillary plexus. These changes in conjunction with two concomitant processes, regression of the primary capillary plexus and the progressive arterialization of specific branches, result in formation of the definitive coronary arterial tree.

The regression of the primary capillary plexus of the heart involves disappearance of many subepicardial vessels, as happens in the case of other primitive vascular beds (Risau, 1995). Some of the surviving capillaries are transformed into coronary arteries, some into cardiac veins, and the rest remains as capillaries. The remodeling of the capillary plexus affects also their connections with the intertrabecular sinusoids. Only a few of them, including Thebesian veins, are left open.

The pattern of blood flow seems to determine developmentally programmed vascular regression, although the molecular mechanisms regulating this process in the embryonic capillary beds are not known (Risau, 1995). A recent model proposes a two-step mechanism (Lang and Bishop, 1993; Lang et al., 1994; Meeson et al., 1996). The first event is macrophage-mediated local apoptosis that reduces or blocks the blood flow through the capillary. Lack of flow causes the synchronous apoptosis of endothelial cells within a capillary segment, perhaps from the loss of survival factors present in the plasma.

The increase in blood pressure that follows the opening of the coronary orifices seems to launch the process of arterialization of specific parts of the cardiac vascular plexus. Arterialization involves recruiting of smooth muscle cell (SMC) precursors to form the tunica media, which is followed by expression of smooth muscle α-action. The expression of this specific SMC marker proceeds in an orderly and continuous fashion from the proximal to the distal part of the developing coronary arteries, and from subendothelial to adventitial layers (Hood and Rosenquist, 1992). The initiation of SMC α-action expression is paralleled by development of the vagal parasympathetic plexus. This observation, as well as other experimental findings, suggests that the cardiac neural crest is involved in the patterning of the coronary vascular system (Waldo et al., 1994).

Both remodeling of the primary plexus through vascular regression and arterialization of specific branches are responsible for formation of the definitive arterial tree of the adult heart. Vascular regression eliminates many connecting branches between the primary vessels. Arterialization, however, seems to play a stabilizing role, since the arterialized branches will probably be conserved during subsequent development and become unresponsive to angiogenic stimuli.

The variation observed between species in the number of connecting arterioles between the main coronary arteries might be related to the differential coupling of the two antagonistic processes, vascular regression and arterialization. When the arterialization of the main coronary vessels occurs after the elimination of all connecting branches, the coronary arteries will conform to an end-artery pattern. It is tempting to speculate that a premature arterialization of the capillary network before the conclusion of the process of vascular regression will keep a significant number of connecting arterioles between the main coronary arteries. In fact, postnatal development of transverse arterioles from capillaries connecting terminal arterioles has been demonstrated in the skeletal muscle of the rat (Price et al., 1994). Thus, we can conjecture that the existence and abundance of connecting arterioles in any-one species will depend upon a complex set of factors, including blood flow and blood pressure patterns inside the primary cardiac capillary plexus, the relative cycles of regression and arterialization of this plexus, and possibly the pattern of parasympathetic innervation of the heart.

VESSEL GROWTH AS A RESPONSE TO VESSEL OCCLUSION

Relationship Between Pressure and Flow in the Collateral Circulation

The capacity of a vascular segment to conduct blood flow is best examined by the relationship between pressure and flow. This is usually studied in experimental animals by pump perfusion during maximal vasodilation by varying the flow and determining the corresponding pressure. Endogenous or exogenous growth-factor-stimulated angiogenesis and neoarteriogenesis will shift the pressure–flow relationship curve to the left, i.e., toward higher flows at the same pressure. Indeed, the shift in the pressure flow relationship curve to higher flows at the same pressure (at maximal vasodilation) is the incontrovertible proof of new vascular growth (Schaper et al., 1976a).

Immediately following acute coronary occlusion, the pressure–flow relationship curve shifts to the right and, due to the low flow, the slope becomes flattened. As the collateral circulation develops, the slope of pressure–flow relationship becomes steeper and the curve shifts to the left but does not reach normal values. Typically, only about one-third of the conductance of the normal vasculature that existed before occlusion is replaced by neoarteriogenesis (Schaper et al., 1976a). If the peripheral coronary pressure (PCP) is assumed to be the true perfusion pressure of the collateral-dependent vasculature, the plot of PCP versus collateral blood flow (which equals flow through the dependent vasculature) has the same slope as does the relationship of normal coronary blood flow to aortic perfusion pressure, thus implying that the collateral-dependent microvasculature has not changed in the canine model, with only the epicardial collaterals responding to coronary occlusion. This is different in the pig, in which normal tissue perfusion is obtained at much lower PCPs. The plot of PCP versus collateral flow is thus much steeper, strongly suggesting that, in addition to neoarteriogenesis, a microvascular growth process in the collateral-dependent region occurs (Schaper et al., 1992; White et al., 1981).

If, as occurs under most clinical conditions, collateral flow cannot be measured, it is important to realize that the PCP is only a rough measure of changes in collateral perfusion. This is because PCP is dependent on three variables: (1) the vascular resistance of the collateral-supplied tissue (PCP decreases with increase in flow): (2) the perfusion pressure at the entrance of the collateral vessels (therefore PCP is usually expressed as the ratio of PCP and perfusion pressure)? and (3) the tone (conductance) of the proper collaterals (any fall in the tone will increase PCP and vice versa). A drug that reduces the tone of the collateral vessels and increases collateral blood flow may not change PCP, because the effects may cancel each other; the fall in PCP due to increased flow may be counteracted by the fall in collateral resistance. A high PCP relative to aortic pressure in patients with one-vessel disease is a relatively good indicator that compensation occurred from the development of large-caliber muscular collateral vessels. When collateral development occurs predominantly via small microvessels (as is the case in the pig and in many human hearts), however, the PCP even in well-adapted cases remains low because of the large energy losses that occur in the microcirculation. In this case the PCP is not a useful indicator of the extent of collateral development.

Neovascularization in Animal Models

The canine ameroid model is characterized by the development of large muscular collateral arteries predominantly with only limited new capillary growth, and is hence the ideal model for the study of neoarteriogenesis (Schaper, 1971). The early stages of neoarteriogenesis are characterized by thin-walled vessels that look rather like veins on histologic examinations. Plasma proteins that had seeped through the vessel are all found in the periarterial space and in the adventitia; monocytes are observed adhering to the endothelium and invading the subintimal space. Almost 10% of all endothelial and smooth muscle cells are preparing for, or are in the process of, cell division. At later stages the wall-to-lumen ratio is normalized and a subintimal layer of smooth muscle cells has formed and becomes arranged along the long axis of the vessel. An internal elastic lamina no longer separates tunica media from tunica intima. Remnants of the old internal elastic lamina are found displaced toward the adventitia. At a later time a new internal elastic lamina is formed by the smooth muscle cells of the neointima (Schaper et al., 1976a, b; Schaper and Schaper, 1993).

The magnitude of the growth process is impressive: The radius of the interconnecting arteriole increases by a factor of 20 while the final tissue mass of the vascular wall increases nearly 50-fold. In spite of these impressive numbers, only about 30% of the ability to conduct flow at maximal vasodilation in the compromised territory is restored, as shown below. It is not clear why the adaptation remains incomplete, but there is apparently enough range for further improvement, as has been shown in studies of therapeutic angiogenesis.

In contrast to the canine model, neovascularization that develops in response to ischemia in the ameroid pig model consists mainly of small vessels about the size or somewhat larger than capillaries that lack an arterial coat. These vessels develop preferentially around areas of focal necrosis (Schaper and Schaper, 1993) although they can be found throughout the ischemic territory of the heart. Similar neovascularization in pigs can also be induced by microembolization with 15μm microspheres. This has the advantage of a more predictable time course of angiogenesis, a prerequisite for the investigation of growth factor expression. The fact that pig collaterals originate from capillary-like structures explains the low peripheral coronary pressure in the distal stump of the occluded artery. The low pressure in the collateral system is perhaps one of the reasons why these vessels remain thin-walled but do not leak. Another explanation could be that porcine myocardium does not have an efficient smooth-muscle-recruiting mechanism such as the angiopoietin–tie-2 system (Folkman and D'Amore, 1996).

The Human Collateral Circulation

Autopsy experience demonstrates variable and sometimes impressive evidence of collateral development in the human heart including the autopsy cases described earlier. The true frequency and extent of protection extended by developing collateral vessels is not precisely known. An early attempt to quantify protection by collaterals divided coronary angiograms into one-, two-, and three-vessel disease with or without demonstrable collaterals. About 30% of patients with one-vessel disease had no collaterals, but not a single patient in a sizable population of patients with three-vessel disease had no collaterals, probably because their absence was not compatible with survival (Gottwik et al., 1984). Thus, important questions in the study of the human collateral circulation include (1) what type of collateral vessel is formed (e.g., dog-like muscular vessels or pig-like small ones), (2) how fast do human collaterals develop, and (3) how good are mature human collaterals?

A number of studies have suggested that mature human collaterals are predominantly muscular and are the product of neoarteriogenesis. The arguments in favor of this concept include observations that the peripheral coronary pressure in patients with angiographically documented collaterals can be as high as that seen in the canine model (see below). Since high PCPs can only be reached with large-caliber connections and since typical "small vessel" neovascularization produces low PCPs, these findings argue in favor of the presence of large-caliber muscular vessels. In addition to earlier histological studies that confirmed the muscular nature of human collaterals, recent clinical studies produced functional evidence supporting their presence. Administration of smooth muscle vasodilators (nitroglycerine and adenosine) demonstrates no consistent fall in PCP despite increases in coronary blood flow, thus implying a decrease in collateral resistance that is consistent with the presence of newly developed muscular conduits. Near doubling of collateral flow observed in patients with an extensive collateral network under the influence of vasodilators is in the range of flows found in mature collateral circulation in the dog model. While strongly implying the presence of "conduit"-type collaterals, however, these data do not exclude the development of additional "small vessel type" (capillaries and venules) vasculature.

There is limited information regarding factors influencing collateral vascular growth in humans. Extensive collateral vascular development in severe obstructive coronary artery disease of longstanding duration has been documented (Fulton, 1964, 1965; Zoll et al., 1951). These observations suggest that severity of a coronary lesion and duration of symptoms are contributing factors for stimulation of collateral vessel growth. The angiographic studies confirm the data obtained from these investigations, although the results are not uniform. Several studies have suggested that the duration of symptomatic disease is a predominant factor, while other investigations indicated that the severity of coronary lesions is a major determinant of collateral vessel growth (Cohen et al., 1989; Fujita et al., 1987; Muller et al., 1989). These conflicting results may be related to differences in study design, patient selection, or documentation of recruitability of collateral vessels, but they also indicate that factors influencing collateral vessel growth in humans are not well established.

Coronary angioplasty can serve as a useful model for studies of human collateral circulation during coronary occlusion. We evaluated factors influencing collateral vascular development in a homogeneous group of these patients by relating clinical, electrocardiographic, and angiographic parameters to the presence of collateral vessels during coronary occlusion. Of 103 consecutive patients with single-vessel coronary disease referred for coronary angioplasty, 42 demonstrated the presence of recruitable collaterals during balloon inflation. The ability to recruit collaterals correlated with the duration of angina (with patients with symptoms of angina less than 3 months' duration having markedly less collateral vessel development than did patients with a duration of angina for more than 3 months) and coronary lesion severity (Fig. 8.4.). In addition, electrocardiographic signs of ischemia during coronary occlusion were reduced in the presence of collateral vessels (ST shift 0.38 ± 0.33 mV versus 0.14 ± 0.19 mV, $p<0.0001$) (Piek et al., 1997b).

The time span necessary for collateral vascular growth in humans is uncertain. In a recent prospective study, Rentrop et al. showed that there is a marked increase in angiographic appearance of collateral vessels 10 to 14 days after persistent coronary occlusion in postthrombolytic patients (Rentrop et al., 1989). These findings are in accordance with experimental data demonstrating restoration of flow to normal values by collateral vessels within 2 weeks after total coronary occlusion (Schaper et al., 1975).

The relationship between collateral vascular growth and coronary lesion severity is in keeping with experimental and clinical studies demonstrating a threshold of coronary narrowing beyond which there is an increase in collateral flow or angiographic appearance of collateral vessels (Gregg, 1974). Moreover, experimental work has demonstrated that the development of the collateral circulation is accelerated when a coronary artery becomes progressively narrowed (Schaper, 1979). Thus, the minimal time period for collateral development in subtotal occlusions is likely at least two weeks and perhaps longer in less severe coronary obstructions.

Our current understanding of the dynamics of the collateral circulation

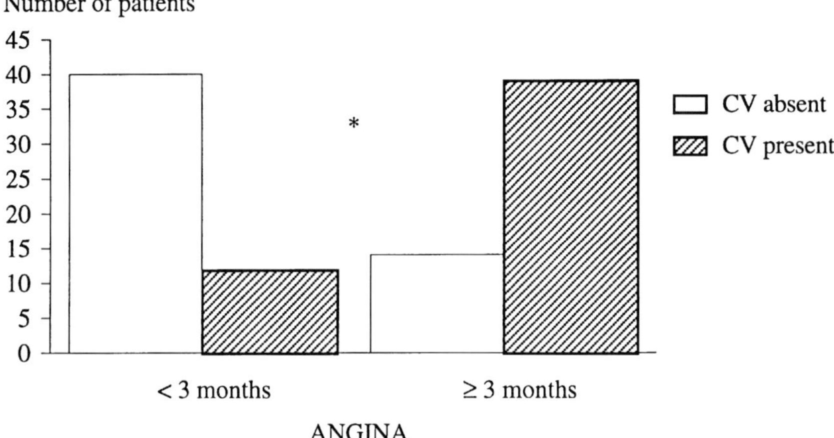

Figure 8.4. Ability to recruit collateral arteries in correlation to severity of angina.

in the clinical setting is limited because of the dependence upon coronary angiography. Only a few clinical studies have attempted to describe the development of the collateral vascular bed in terms of flow or resistance (Feldman and Pepine, 1984; Goldstein et al., 1974). Analysis of blood flow velocity in the donor coronary artery during transient coronary occlusion of the recipient artery allows assessment of collateral flow between the two vascular beds (Fujita et al., 1988). An example of this approach is shown in Figure 8.5. for a patient with subtotal occlusion of right coronary artery and recruitable LAD to RCA collaterals. Recruitability of collateral vessels is associated with a transient increase of blood flow velocity in the donor artery in conjunction with collateral flow in the recipient artery that is not seen in the absence of recruitability (Piek et al., 1997c).

The assessment of coronary flow changes in the contralateral donor coronary artery can be used to calculate the collateral vascular resistance (*Rcoll*), in relation to the resistance of the contralateral peripheral vascular bed (*Rcoll/R3*, see appendix and Figure 8.6.).

$$\mathrm{Rcoll/R3} = \frac{\mathrm{Pao} - \mathrm{Pw}}{\mathrm{Pao}} \cdot \frac{\mathrm{dMPVdef}}{\mathrm{dMPVinf} - \mathrm{dMPVdef}}$$

Figure 8.5. Blood flow velocity analysis of the donor LAD before, during, and after balloon coronary occlusion (BCO) of the RCA showing a 30% increase in maximal diastolic blood flow velocity during coronary occlusion. These alterations in blood flow velocity of the donor coronary artery coincide with collateral flow in the recipient coronary artery. The blood flow velocity signal in the recipient coronary artery was retrograde (below zero-line), but is displayed antegrade (above zero-line) demonstrating a predominant systolic flow velocity signal and a complete diastolic flow velocity signal.

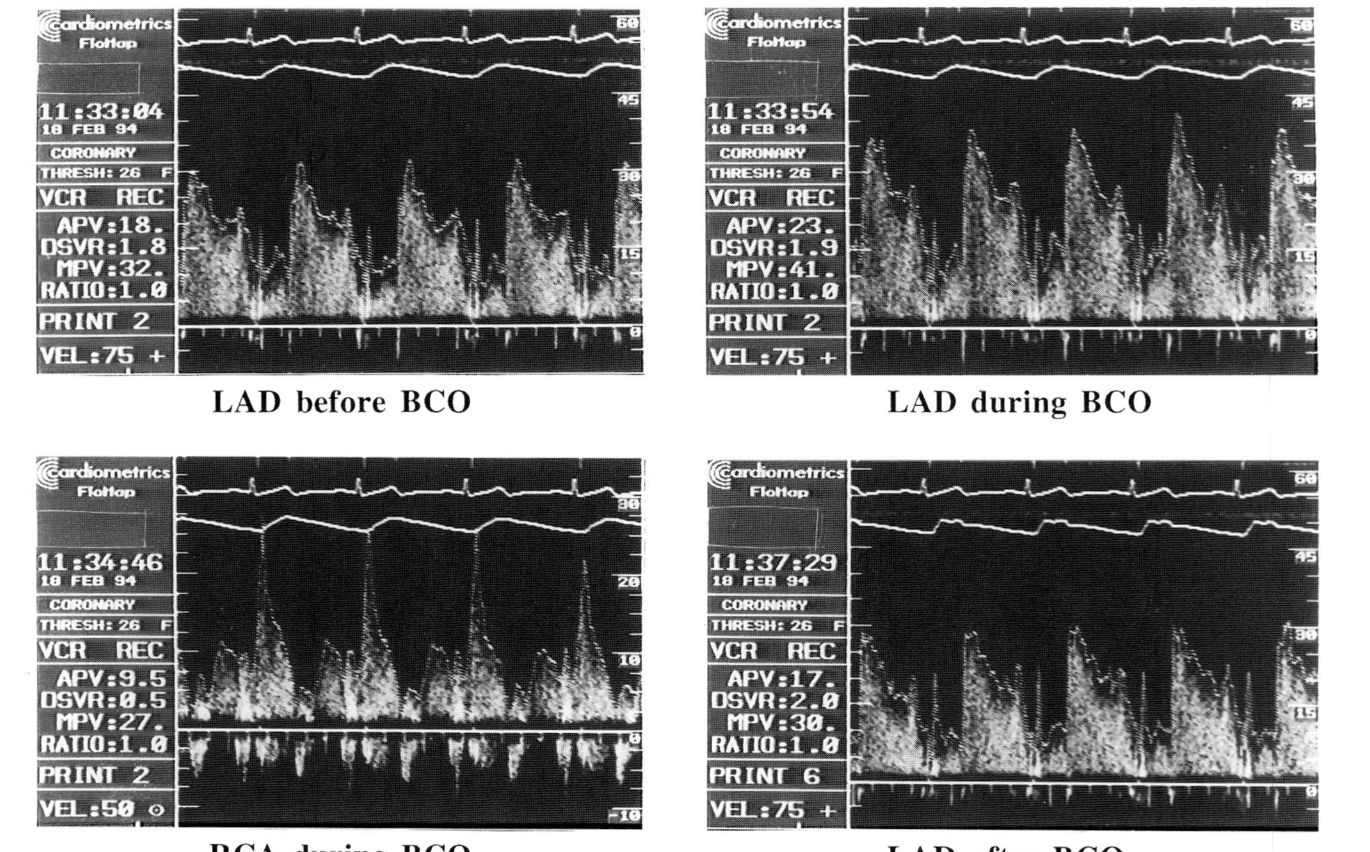

LAD before BCO

LAD during BCO

RCA during BCO

LAD after BCO

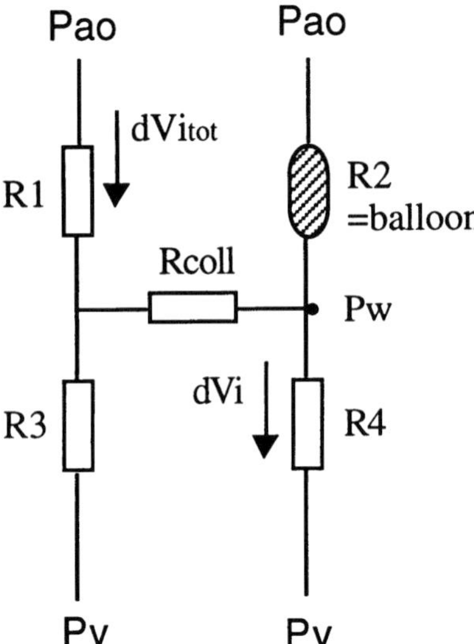

Figure 8.6. The coronary arterial circulation schematically represented as an electrical analog model.

Another approach to evaluation of collateral vascular resistance is to relate the antegrade or retrograde collateral blood flow velocity during balloon inflation in the recipient coronary artery to the pressure gradient upon the collateral vascular bed (see appendix): $Rcoll = Pao - Pw/\ dVi$ (mmHg/cm/sec). The first approach provides information on the interpatient variability of the collateral vascular resistance. The application of the latter approach is limited to serial studies in the same patient such as alterations of the collateral vascular resistance after subsequent balloon inflations or following pharmacological modulation. In addition, the coronary wedge/aortic pressure ratio provides information regarding the relationship between the peripheral vascular resistance of the recipient coronary (*R4*) and the collateral vascular resistance (see appendix): $Pw/Pao = R4/Rcoll + R4$.

The application of this technique to the evaluation of the pharmacologic responsiveness of the coronary collateral vascular resistance and peripheral vascular resistance of the recipient coronary artery is illustrated in Figure 8.7.C. There is limited information in the literature regarding the responsiveness of the collateral circulation in humans. Studies measuring great cardiac vein flow have been performed during coronary angioplasty, but the accuracy of this technique for collateral flow assessment has been questioned.

A noninvasive study using perfusion scintigraphy in patients with chronic coronary occlusion reported an improvement of flow to collateral-dependent vascular regions after intravenous administration of nitroglycerine (Aoki et al., 1991). Similar findings were reported after intravenous administration of dipyridamole evaluated by positron emission tomography in similar patients (McFalls et al., 1993; Vanoverschelde et al., 1993). The ratio of hyperemic versus baseline myocardial blood flow to the collateral-dependent areas varied in these studies between 1.4 ± 0.6 and 1.9 ± 1.0, respectively. The observed improvement in myocardial perfusion after the administration of vasodilators may have been the result of alterations in preload or afterload as well as a direct vasodilating effect on collateral vessels, although these influences can be somewhat minimized by intracoronary administration.

Our current experience with the illustrated protocol (see Fig. 8.7C) indicates that the administration of adenosine or nitroglycerine to patients with recruitable collateral vessels does not induce a change in the collateral blood flow velocity integral or the coronary wedge/aortic pressure ratio. In contrast, in patients with one-vessel disease and spontaneously visible collateral vessels, the diastolic collateral blood flow velocity integral increased from 8.0 ± 4.5 to 10.8 ± 8.0 cm/sec ($p=0.01$) after adenosine and from 7.4 ± 4.5 to 10.3 ± 6.9 cm/sec ($p=0.003$) after nitroglycerine while the overall coronary wedge/aortic pressure ratio remained unchanged after adenosine and nitroglycerine (Piek et al., 1997a).

During coronary angioplasty, the angiographic development of collateral vessels is directly related with the coronary wedge/aortic pressure ratio, presumably related to a reduction in collateral vascular resistance (Meier et al., 1987; Mizuno et al., 1988; Rentrop et al., 1988). In patients with one-vessel disease and spontaneously visible collateral vessels, collateral vascular resistance decreased from 10.3 ± 9.5 to 8.6 ± 8.5 mmHg/cm ($p=0.01$) after adenosine and from 11.6 ± 10.4 to 8.3 ± 8.9 mmHg/cm ($p<0.001$) after nitroglycerine. At the same time, the peripheral resistance of the recipient coronary artery decreased from 7.7 ± 5.5 to 5.9

Figure 8.7. (On Next Two Pages) A and B Angiography of a 59-year-old male with angina pectoris, functional class I according to the Canadian Cardiovascular Society Classification following an non-Q anteroseptal myocardial infarction. Angiography of the left coronary artery revealed a coronary narrowing (65% diameter stenosis) of the left anterior descending coronary artery and spontaneously visible collateral vessels originating from the right coronary artery. Fig. 8.7C. Coronary blood flow velocity during balloon coronary occlusion of the left anterior descending coronary artery (recipient artery) showed a 2.7-fold increase after the administration of a bolus of 12 mg adenosine in the right donor coronary artery. The administration of a bolus of 0.2 mg nitroglycerine during a subsequent balloon coronary occlusion resulted in a 2.2-fold increase of blood flow velocity in the recipient coronary artery. Coronary wedge pressure was measured through the fluid-filled lumen during subsequent balloon inflations after withdrawal of the guide wire. The coronary wedge/aortic pressure ratio remained decreased 0.56 to 0.47, unchanged after the administration of adenosine, and increased from 0.44 to 0.49 after the administration of nitroglycerine.

A

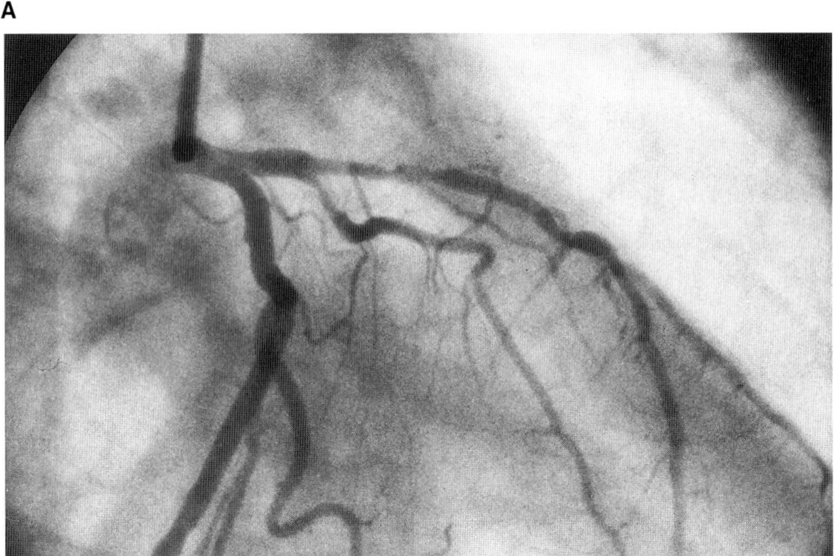

B

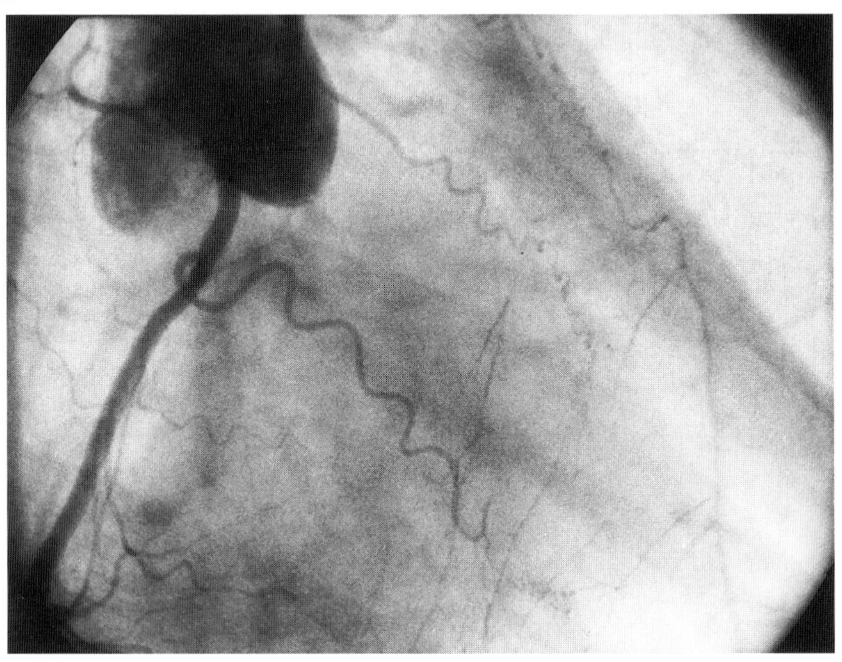

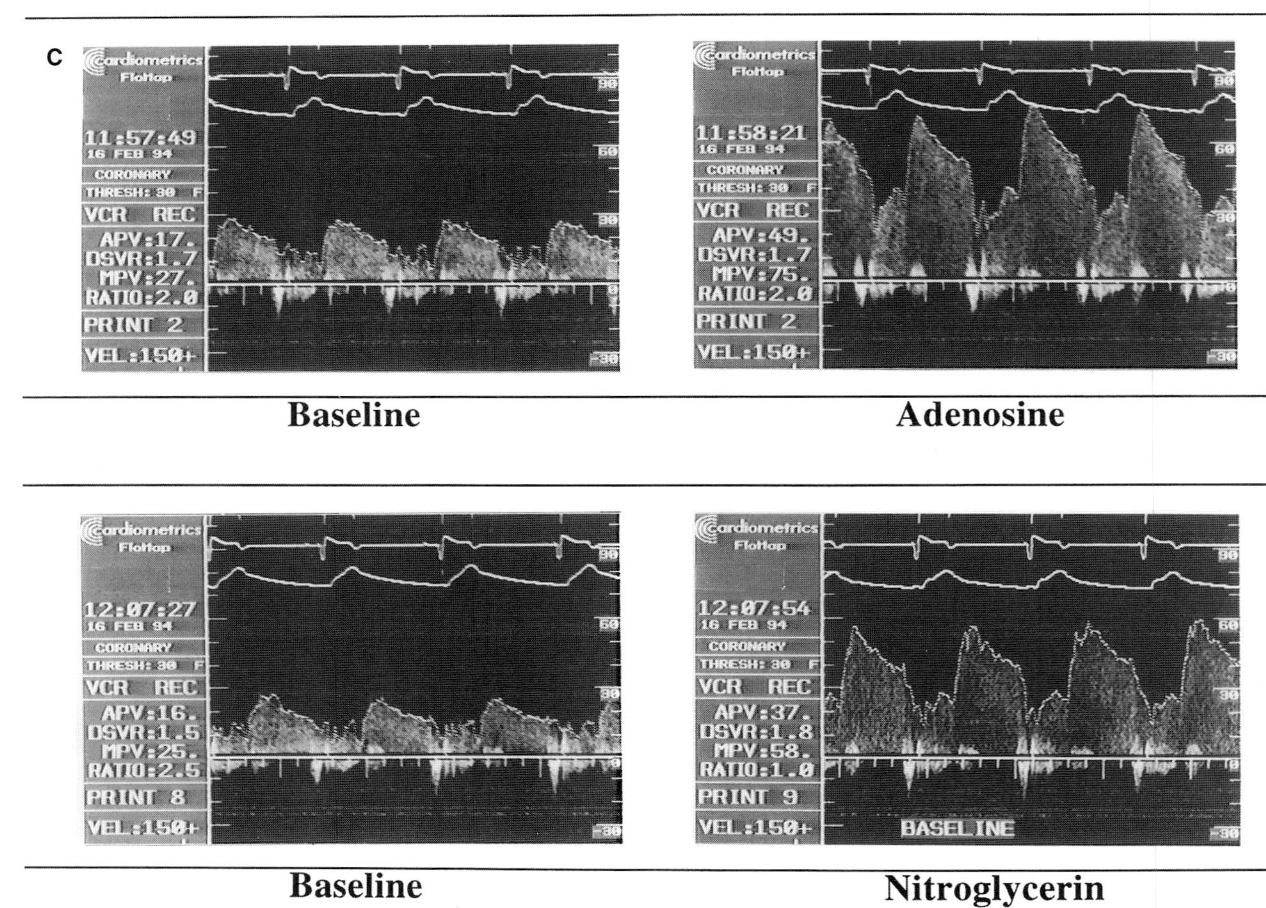

C
Cardiometrics
FloMap
11:57:49
16 FEB 94
CORONARY
THRESH: 30 F
VCR REC
APV:17.
DSVR:1.7
MPV:27.
RATIO:2.0
PRINT 2
VEL:150+
90
60
30
0
-30
Baseline
Cardiometrics
FloMap
11:58:21
16 FEB 94
CORONARY
THRESH: 30 F
VCR REC
APV:49.
DSVR:1.7
MPV:75.
RATIO:2.0
PRINT 2
VEL:150+
90
60
30
0
-30
Adenosine
Cardiometrics
FloMap
12:07:27
16 FEB 94
CORONARY
THRESH: 30 F
VCR REC
APV:16.
DSVR:1.5
MPV:25.
RATIO:2.5
PRINT 8
VEL:150+
90
60
30
0
-30
Baseline
Cardiometrics
FloMap
12:07:54
16 FEB 94
CORONARY
THRESH: 30 F
VCR REC
APV:37.
DSVR:1.8
MPV:58.
RATIO:1.0
PRINT 9
VEL:150+
BASELINE
90
60
30
0
-30
Nitroglycerin

± 5.1 mmHg/cm ($p<0.001$) after adenosine and from 8.4 ± 6.6 to 7.1 ± 7.2 mmHg/cm ($p=0.01$) after nitroglycerine (Piek et al., 1997a).

Thus, coronary collateral blood flow can be increased by adenosine and nitroglycerine in patients with one-vessel disease and spontaneously visible collateral vessels, in contrast to the case with patients with recruitable collateral vessels. This effect is the result of a reduction of the collateral vascular resistance and the peripheral vascular resistance of the recipient coronary artery. The increase of the collateral blood flow velocity after the administration of adenosine or nitroglycerine is the result of a reduction of both the collateral vascular resistance itself and the microvascular resistance of the recipient bed.

The Coronary Collateral Circulation in Relation to Clinical Outcome and Prognosis

Initial angiographic studies demonstrated that collateral vessels are only visualized in the presence of subtotal or total obstructive coronary lesions. Nonetheless, the angiographic manifestation of collaterals has been related to the clinical outcome of various coronary syndromes (Cohen, 1985). The angioplasty studies mentioned above documented a marked discrepancy in angiographic appearance of collateral vessels depending on the pressure gradient exerted on the vascular bed. The majority of symptomatic patients with one-vessel disease exhibited recruitment of collateral vessels that were not seen in previous angiographic studies.

Recruitment of collateral vessels can also be documented by hemodynamic measurements. The initial report by Rentrop was followed by several other studies that showed that spontaneously visible and recruitable collateral vessels in one-vessel disease are related to the coronary wedge pressure, which can also be used for documentation of collateral vessels during coronary occlusion (Meier et al., 1987; Rentrop et al., 1988). These investigations demonstrated that a coronary wedge pressure of more than 30 mmHg is indicative of angiographic appearance of collateral vessels during coronary occlusion.

Presence of collateral vessels during brief coronary occlusion, documented by angiography or coronary wedge pressure measurements, results in reduction of electrocardiographic signs of ischemia and left ventricular dysfunction (Cohen and Rentrop, 1986; Dervan et al., 1987; Hill et al., 1985; Macdonald et al., 1986; Mizuno et al., 1988). The functional importance of the presence of collateral vessels during coronary occlusion was not further evaluated in these studies by assessment of the size of the myocardium at risk. In addition, a reduction of myocardial ischemia by pharmacologic modulation of the collateral vascular resistance was evaluated only indirectly by coronary sinus measurements (Feldman et al., 1986, 1987; Feldman and Pepine, 1984; Kern et al., 1990); the accuracy of this technique for assessment of collateral flow has been subject to criticism (Cohen et al., 1988).

A recent study extended these observations by relating the collateral vascular growth assessed by the coronary wedge/aortic pressure ratio to the clinical outcome during a mean follow-up period of 16 months. Coronary ischemic events occurred mostly in patients with insufficiently developed collateral vessels, assessed during the previous coronary angioplasty, indicating that physiologic estimates of collateral vascular resistance may yield prognostic information (Pijls et al., 1995). These studies suggest a beneficial effect of collateral vessels during brief coronary occlusion; however, these reports do not permit conclusions regarding the relevance of collateral vascular supply during prolonged ischemia, such as in acute myocardial infarction.

Coronary arteriography during the acute phase of myocardial infarction for the evaluation of thrombolytic therapy provides information on the time span necessary for collateral vascular development. Collateral vessels, initially absent, became angiographically apparent within 10–14 days after sustained coronary occlusion (Nitzberg et al., 1985; Rentrop et al., 1989; Schwartz et al., 1984). Several clinical studies have claimed a protective effect of collateral vessels in acute myocardial infarction. Conclusions drawn from these retrospective studies, however, are limited, as coronary angiography was only performed several days to weeks after the acute coronary event (Fuster et al., 1979; Hamby et al., 1976; Williams et al., 1976). In contrast, coronary arteriography performed during the acute phase of myocardial infarction for the evaluation of thrombolytic therapy yields relevant information on the functional significance of collateral vessels. The angiographic appearance of collateral vessels, combined with thrombolytic therapy, exerts a beneficial effect on left ventricular function as manifested by restoration of global and regional ejection fraction at follow-up (Blanke et al., 1985; Nohara et al., 1983; Saito et al., 1985; Schwartz et al., 1985; Sheehan et al., 1987). Moreover, the presence of collateral flow to the jeopardized myocardium during acute myocardial infarction may explain the beneficial effect of late thrombolytic therapy (more than 7 hours after onset of complaints) or nitroglycerine therapy and explain reduction in aneurysm formation (Rogers et al., 1984; Hirai et al., 1987; Lamas et al., 1991; Rentrop et al., 1989).

A report from the thrombolysis in myocardial infarction (TIMI)-1 trial convincingly supports the functional importance of collateral vessels in acute myocardial infarction (Habib et al., 1991). In this study patients were included only if coronary arteriography revealed absence of reperfusion 90 minutes after the onset of thrombolytic therapy, thereby reducing interference of antegrade flow on limitation of myocardial damage. Under these conditions, collateral vascular supply reduced myocardial infarct size by 35% as assessed by enzymatic means an global ejection fraction by 12% at follow-up. In a prospective study of myocardial viability in the vascular territory of an occluded coronary artery following myocardial infarction, the improvement of myocardial function following successful reperfusion was associated with the size of the collateral-dependent vascular bed as assessed with myocardial contrast echocardiography (Sabia et al., 1992). Adequate perfusion to collateral-dependent vascular areas, assessed with positron emission tomography, is important for preservation of myocardial contractile function and, hence, clinical outcome (Vanoverschelde et al., 1993).

In summary, clinical studies performed in the setting of coronary angioplasty and acute myocardial infarction underscore the functional significance of collateral circulation during acute coronary occlusion and its relevance to prognosis following myocardial infarction.

MECHANISMS OF COLLATERAL VESSEL GROWTH

Role of Tissue Ischemia

Many believe that tissue ischemia governs the development of collateral vessels, although this view has recently been challenged (Ito et al., 1997a; Paskins-Hurlburt and Hollenberg, 1992; Schaper and Ito, 1996). The ischemia hypothesis is attractive because it is undeniable that coronary occlusion, even the slowly progressing variety, will cause ischemia eventually. Furthermore, ischemia upregulates expression of a number of angiogenic molecules including VEGF and FGFs (Fischer et al., 1995; Ikeda et al., 1995; Ladoux and Frelin, 1993). Nevertheless, there are important discrepancies between the presence of tissue ischemia and vascular growth. First, muscular collateral arteries, especially the *stem* and *midzone* segments, are surrounded by myocardium that is not ischemic because it is situated outside the region at risk for infarction. Even in cases in which the midzone segments lie within the region at risk, the myocardium in the vicinity of the growing vascular segment does not become ischemic. This can be demonstrated by injecting radioactive tracer microspheres during an acute but transient occlusion of a coronary artery into a dog at the time of implantation of an ameroid constrictor. Evaluation of coronary flow six weeks later, when collateral vessels have formed in response to chronic ameroid occlusion, finds no evidence of underperfusion of myocardial tissue in the direct vicinity of now-enlarged collaterals. There is also evidence of severe perfusion deficit during acute occlusion in the subendocardium, but no collateral growth occurs there (Schaper, 1971a; Schaper and Schaper, 1993). Thus, the site of ischemia can be dissociated from the site of collateral formation.

Second, collateral growth continues after cessation of ischemia, i.e., there is a temporal dissociation between tissue ischemia and collateral vessel growth. This point has been demonstrated in an experiment (Franklin et al., 1985) in which the left circumflex coronary artery was briefly occluded with a chronically implanted device for 30 seconds every 2 minutes. Between 80 and 200 occlusions were necessary to avoid the con-

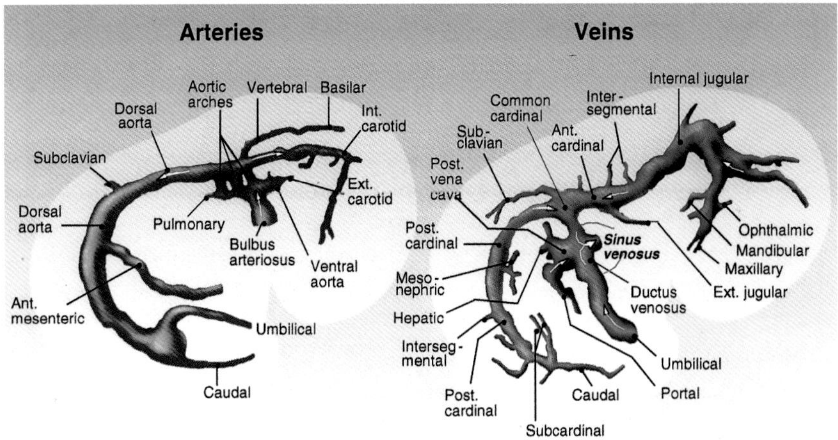

Plate 1. Drawing of mouse vasculature at embryonic day 11 (the midday of the vaginal plug is defined as day 0.5; birth at day 21). Only the major arteries and veins are shown. The direction of blood flow is indicated by white arrows.

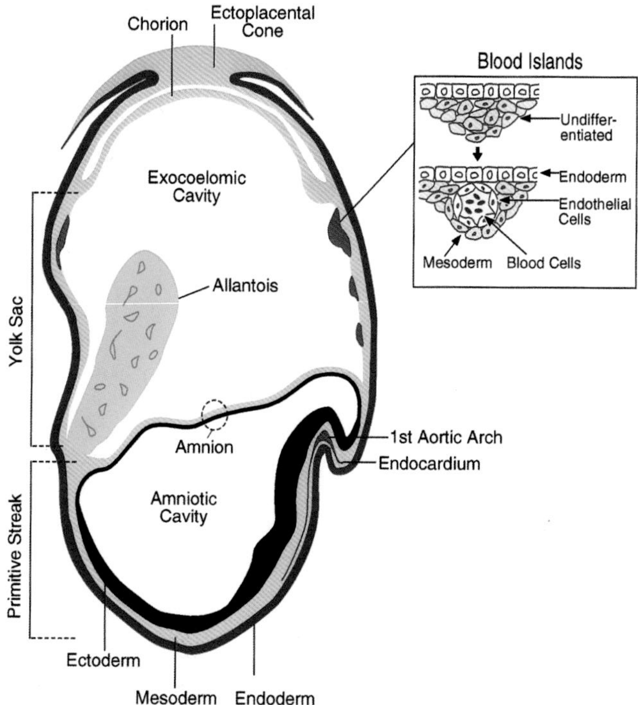

Plate 2. Schematic drawing of a sagittal section of a mouse embryo around day 7.8 of development. Blood islands begin to form in the extraembryonic mesoderm of the yolk sac (right upper corner insert). Intraembryonic vascular development also starts with the assembly of the endocardial tubes in the proximal lateral mesoderm. In parallel, vascular cords form inside the allantois.

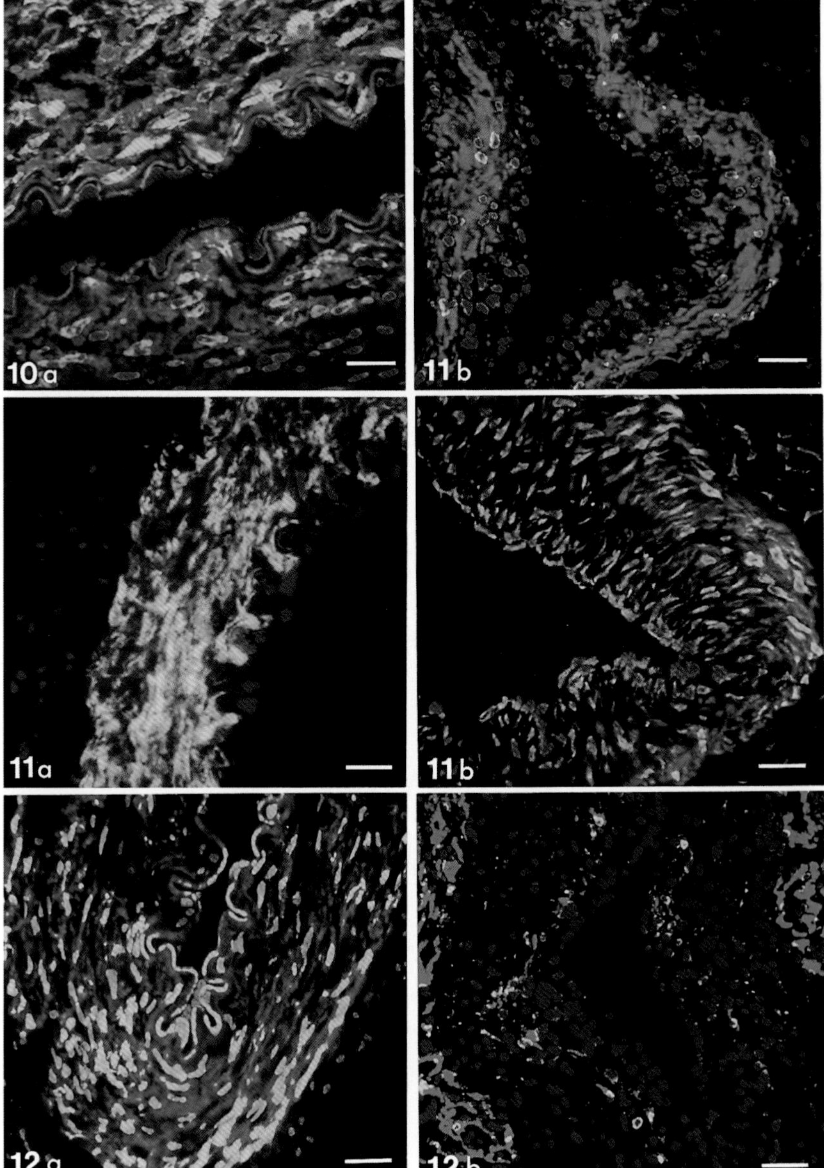

Plate 3. In normal vessels α-smooth muscle actin is present in the media (10A) while in collateral vessels the α-smooth muscle actin is reduced particularly in the smooth muscle cells of the neointima (10B).

Plate 4. Localization of calponin in the media of a normal coronary artery (11A) and in the collateral vessel (11B)—note weak expression in neointima.

Plate 5. In normal vessels desmin is distributed in the entire media (12A) while in growing collateral vessels only small amounts of desmin are detectable in the media and is nearly absent in the neointima (12B).

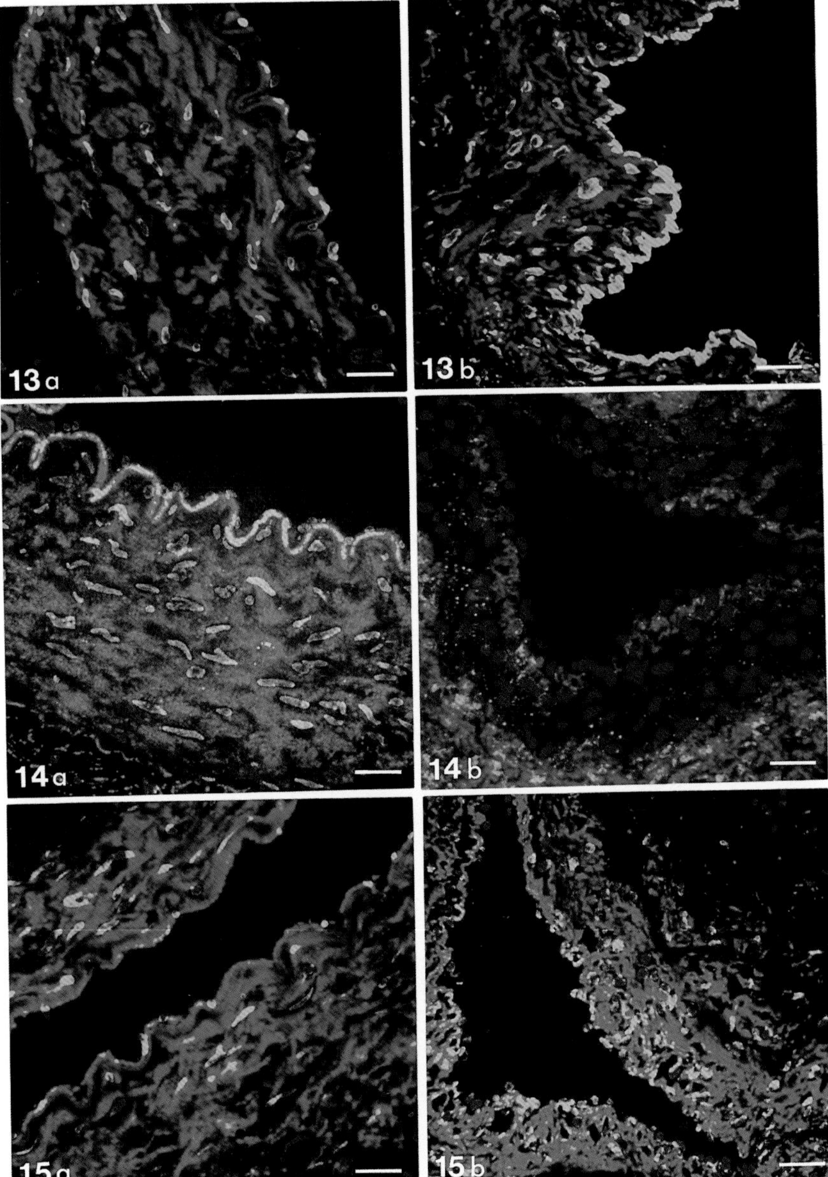

Plate 6. Vimentin is stained evenly in normal coronary arteries (13A) while in growing collateral arteries vimentin is increased mainly in the endothelium and the neointima (13B).

Plate 7. Chondroitin sulfate expression is increased in growing collateral vessels (14A) while the inner elastic membrane is missing or only present in fragmental remnants (14B).

Plate 8. Fibronectin is present in the vessel wall of normal coronary arteries (15A). Increase of fibronectin in the neointima and the media of collateral vessels is evident (15B).

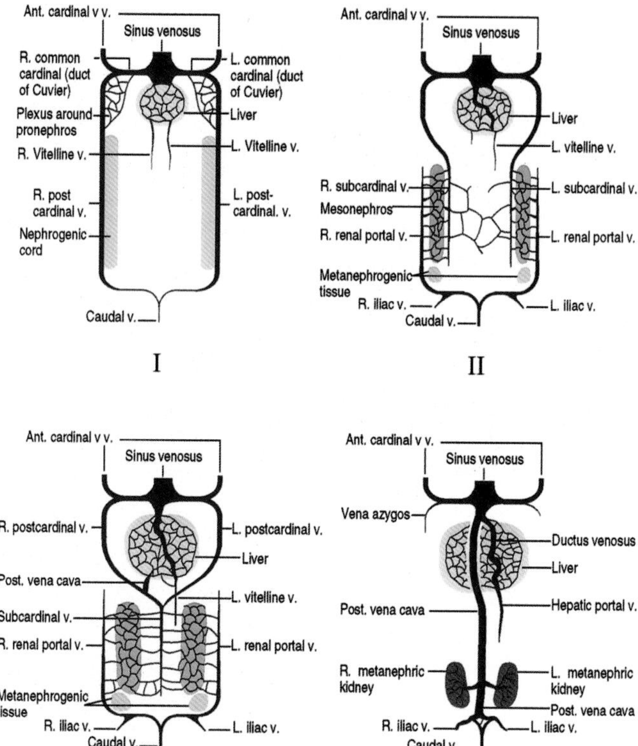

Plate 9. Transformation of posterior veins during embryonic development in vertebrates.

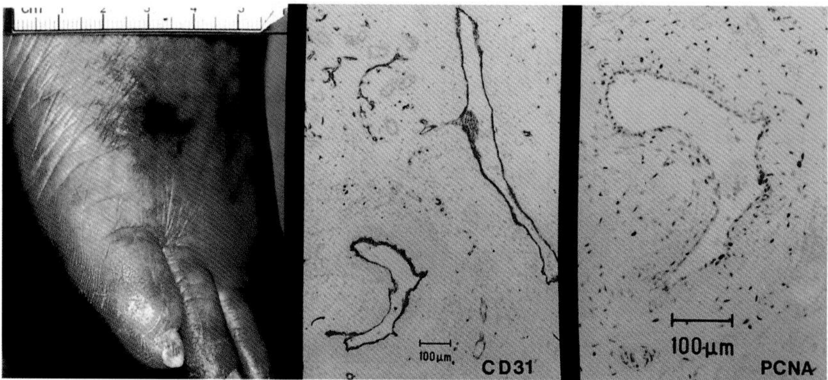

Plate 10. One spider angiomata that developed approximately 1 week post gene therapy in distal portion of ischemic limb. Photomicrographs of tissue sections immunostained with antibody to endothelial antigen CD31 indicate vascularity of lesion, while immunostain of adjacent section for proliferating cell nuclear antigen (PCNA) indicates extent of proliferative activity among endothelial cells in lesion. [Reproduced from Isner et al (1996) with permission.]

tractile dysfunction caused by blood flow deprivation, by developing a collateral circulation. A reactive hyperemia was also no longer visible. Although at first glance this experiment can be interpreted as support for the ischemia hypothesis, a more detailed analysis reveals that dogs with good collateral blood flow from the start needed fewer occlusions to reach the desired results—that is, those with less ischemia had a faster-progressing collateral development. This observation argues strongly against the role of ischemia. Our group repeated these experiments in the pig heart and needed about 600 occlusions to obtain some evidence of vascular growth. However, this type of vascular growth was not distinguishable from that of inflammatory adhesions that had formed between the epicardium, the lungs, and the chest wall in response to the chronic implants. Thus, in this experiment we showed that a very high number of intensely ischemic episodes did not produce a relevant collateral circulation, thus suggesting that ischemia did not play a decisive role and that inflammatory mechanisms were more closely related. A capillary collateral circulation appears to require some focal necrosis as a stimulus for angiogenesis (Schaper and Schaper, 1993).

Thus, the association between tissue ischemia and neoarteriogenesis appears to be somewhat circumstantial. Growth of muscular collateral arteries is almost always associated with ischemia, but this association has nothing to do with the cellular and molecular mechanisms. These mechanisms are strictly local and involve the actions of shear forces and the invasion of circulating cells that are attracted to regions of high shear stress, such as those that occur in preformed network arterioles when a large artery becomes stenosed.

Role of Monocytes, Cytokines, and Growth Factors

One model of collateral growth favors strictly local changes near the interconnecting arteriole that alter its endothelium and attract circulating cells capable of production of growth factors, or possibly stem cells that can then actively participate in new vessel formation. These local changes may include chronic increase in shear stress in response to coronary stenosis and enhanced adhesive properties of the endothelium that may promote attachment of circulating cells.

This model is supported by the finding that monocytes invade into the subintimal space of growing collaterals (Schaper et al., 1976a). These monocytes become activated and produce a number of growth factors including tumor necrosis factor alpha (TNF-α) and acidic and basic fibroblast growth factors (FGF-1 and FGF-2) (Arras et al., 1996; Arras et al. 1998). These growth factors can then initiate endothelial and smooth muscle migration and proliferation as well as vessel wall remodeling, which includes the controlled destruction of the old internal elastic lamina and removal of a significant proportion of the preexisting smooth muscle cells by apoptosis. The result of this process in dogs is a 20-fold increase in the collateral vessel diameter and a 50-fold increase in collateral tissue mass.

Similar observations have been made in growing collateral arteries of the rabbit hindlimb (Ito et al., 1997a). Already 3 days after femoral artery occlusion monocytes adhere and migrate into collateral arteries, accompanied by a massive proliferation of endothelial and smooth muscle cells. As in the heart of microembolized pigs these monocytes are the main source of FGFs and TNF-α. An increased accumulation and activation of monocytes at the site of collateral growth either induced by a single lipopolysaccharide injection or locally by a continuous infusion of the monocyte-specific chemoattractant protein (MCP-1) lead to an increase of the collateral conductance by up to 250% and to a marked increase in the density of collateral arteries (Ito et al., 1997b). In contrast to the dog heart, the preexisting arteriolar connections are not visible angiographically. A pressure waveform in the periphery of an acutely occluded hindlimb suggests that preexisting arteriolar connections are present. Collateral arteries are already visible 3 days after occlusion, demonstrating a massive proliferation of endothelial as well as smooth muscle cells over a distance of up to 5 cm. The magnitude of this response makes it unlikely that the source of these collateral arteries is sprouting capillaries. These findings furthermore suggest that neoarteriogenesis is a very rapid adaptive response to vessel occlusions, with the main increase in collateral conductance occurring within the first week after femoral artery occlusion.

Similar to neoarteriogenesis, angiogenesis is also associated with accumulation and activation of monocytes/macrophages. In the microembolization-pig-heart model, morphologic evidence of angiogenesis is observed around the 3rd day in areas of focal necrosis (Bernotat-Danielowski et al., 1993; Schaper and Schaper, 1993). Monocyte-macrophage accumulation and strong FGF-1 expression occur in these foci at the same time (Bernotat-Danielowski et al., 1993). In the rabbit hindlimb, histological and hemodynamic evidence of angiogenesis is observed in the calf muscle one week after occlusion and it is also associated with accumulation of FGF-producing monocytes/macrophages (Ito et al., 1997a). Thus, both neoarteriogenesis and angiogenesis, in the heart and in the periphery, are associated with the accumulation and activation of monocytes-macrophages which, in the case of neoarteriogenesis, are the main source of FGF.

Another circulating cell that can promote angiogenesis and that has also been associated with collateral growth is the basophilic lymphocyte, which matures into a mast cell once it has invaded the vessel wall. These mast cells, in turn, produce large amounts of heparin, which is essential for the action of growth factors such as FGF and VEGF (Meininger and Zetter, 1992) as well as growth factors themselves.

Recently, endothelial stem cells have been isolated from circulating human blood that possesses the angioblast-like marker antigens CD-34 and flk-1 (Asahara et al., 1997). These cells develop into tube-like structures in culture and adhere, after injection, to places of angiogenesis in adult mice and rabbits following femoral artery excision. The finding of circulating cells that became incorporated in a new vessel changes the paradigm of angiogenesis, which, in its classical and restricted definition, describes the sprouting of capillaries from preexisting capillaries.

Growth Factors

A number of growth factors are involved in the development of coronary collaterals. FGF-2 is expressed in the neointima of canine collateral vessels, where its expression correlates with mitotic activity. In a model of myocardial angiogenesis following microsphere embolization, FGF-1 expression is increased severalfold but parallels, rather than precedes, capillary sprouting (Schaper and Schaper, 1993). FGF-1 expression remains elevated for about 2 weeks, i.e., long after angiogenesis has stopped, thus suggesting that FGF-1 may have functions other than that of mitogen. VEGF is very rapidly overexpressed in porcine myocardium following brief, but not repeated, episodes of ischemia, although increased expression is also found in chronically ischemic myocardium. PDGF-AA is expressed in the neointima of canine collaterals, a place of intense cellular migration. Myocytes in the vicinity of sprouting capillaries in the pig heart produce IGF-1-mRNA and the class IV neurofilament nestin (Kluge et al., 1995).

Initially, VEGF appeared to be an ideal candidate for the link between tissue ischemia and collateral vessel growth; VEGF-mRNA expression is upregulated by a decrease in oxygenation due to the presence of hypoxia-inducible-factor (HIF-1)-sensitive elements in the VEGF promoter that leads to increase in transcription (Ikeda et al., 1995). Furthermore, a significant part of the steady-state increase in VEGF-mRNA expression is caused by enhanced message stability, brought about by expression of a protein that binds to several AUUA-rich untranslated regions at the 3' end of the mRNA and thereby increases its half-life (Ikeda et al., 1995). As already mentioned, although VEGF expression is very sensitive to even brief periods of ischemia/reperfusion (Sharma et al., 1992; Hashimoto et al., 1994), this increase is not necessarily followed by an angiogenic response. In other settings such as acute pulmonary pressure overload, VEGF expression is upregulated as fast as expression of nuclear protooncogenes c-fos and c-jun, again producing an angiogenic response (Kuki et al., 1997). For instance, a rapid increase in VEGF expression is noted in a rat heart subjected to a sudden increase in left ventricular end-diastolic pressure, (unpublished observation) but without angiogenesis. Thus, VEGF may have functions other than angiogenesis, such as maintaining survival of stressed endothelium.

The increase in VEGF message stability caused by hypoxia/ischemia may be mediated via the adenosine receptor (Fischer et al., 1997). This is an appealing mechanism since myocardial hypoxia leads to increased adenosine production via breakdown of ATP, and adenosine is known to be angiogenic. The decline of VEGF expression following repeated exposures to hypoxia (Levy et al., 1995; Fischer et al., 1997) might be explained by the well-known "exhaustion" of the adenosine system. Only the first two brief coronary occlusions produce adenosine, and the recovery of the response requires more than 24 hours.

Regulation of Collateral Growth by Receptors and Inhibitors

Many angiogenic growth factors such as VEGF are constitutively expressed in the normal heart without causing vessel proliferation. While this may reflect either the absence of receptors or the sequestration of the growth factors in the extracellular matrix, it is also possible that negative regulators present in normal tissues inhibit both angiogenesis and neoarteriogenesis. One such inhibitor recently isolated from normal bovine heart shows homology to the B-cell translocation gene btg-1 (Westernacher and Schaper, 1995). Thus, vessel growth in the adult heart might not only require upregulation of growth factors and their receptors but also inhibitors.

Is Embryonic Vasculogenesis Recapitulated in Neoarteriogenesis?

Significant progress in the understanding of angiogenesis has been made using murine and avian embryos as well as cells in culture. Until recently very little was known about the step following angiogenesis in the embryo—namely, the "arterialization" of the capillary sprouts and their growth in diameter, which is a process that most closely resembles collateral growth. It now appears, however, that the tie-2/angiopoietin system that is critical for the recruitment of smooth muscle cells and the formation of arterial vessels may play an important role in this process (Davis et al., 1996; Suri et al., 1996). By analogy with this embryonic process, a proposed scheme for the orderly assembly of the venous system (Folkman and D'Amore, 1996) may be, in our opinion, even better suited to explain the arterialization of the capillary plexus of the coronary vasculature. Thus, following VEGF-dependent invasion of the myocardium by capillaries, "arterialization" of the plexus and the regression of the network commences under the influence of angiopoietin/tie-2 signaling, inducing PDGF expression in endothelial cells, which is in turn chemoattractive and mitogenic for smooth muscle cells. The process is then completed by induction of TGF-β expression.

It, however, remains to be determined whether "arterialization" of capillary sprouts occurs in adult tissues and whether, in addition to a possible role in embryonic development, the above described sequence is recapitulated in collateral vessel growth, or neoarteriogenesis, which starts with thinning and dedifferentiation of the preexisting interconnecting arteriole and then, after several rounds of endothelial and smooth muscle cell mitosis, develops an arterial coat and a new muscular intima.

Dedifferentiation of Smooth Muscle Cells in Growing Collateral Arteries

Most of the cells in the neointima show characteristics of smooth muscle cells. They are spindle-like in shape and most show expression of smooth muscle marker proteins such as α-SM actin (Plate 3A). In vascular smooth muscle cells, α-actin forms thin filaments consisting of two helical strands of actin monomers. These filaments insert at cytoplasmic dense bodies and have a function in smooth muscle cells similar to that of the Z-bands in striated muscle cells; α-smooth muscle actin is able to bind tropomyosin, caldesmon, calponin, and myosin, thereby participating in regulation of smooth muscle contraction (Jiang and Stephens, 1994). Unlike mature quiescent smooth muscle cells, proliferating smooth muscle cells present in the neointima following balloon angioplasty express reduced amounts α-SM actin. The same change in α-SM actin is observed after a few days in culture (Orlandi et al., 1994).

This change in smooth muscle cell phenotype, from normal contractile to ''synthetic,'' is accompanied by an increase in the number of mitochondria and the size of the Golgi apparatus. The same phenotypic changes have been observed by electron microscopy in growing collateral vessels (Schaper, 1971a). Cells in the neointima of developing collateral vessels express α-SM actin, but the staining is irregular while the cells close to the lumen of the vessel show no α-SM actin expression at all (Plate 3B). These observations suggest that smooth muscle cells in growing collateral vessels are dedifferentiated and immature.

Calponin, another protein responsible for cell contraction, inhibits actin-mediated activation of the Mg^{2+}-ATPase by the myosin heads. Like smooth muscle actin, calponin is present in differentiated, contractile smooth muscle cells. Cultured smooth muscle cells lose their ability to express calponin in a time-dependent fashion and reduced calponin expression in smooth muscle cells correlates with an increase in their migration ability (Birukov et al., 1991; Takahashi et al., 1993). In normal coronary arteries, calponin is present in the smooth muscle cells of the media, with all cells appearing equally stained with an anticalponin antibody, while no calponin expression is found in the intima or adventitia. Growing collaterals show a reduction in calponin expression in the neointima, whereas calponin is regularly observed in the cells of the underlying media, thus again suggesting that smooth muscle cells in the neointima are in the dedifferentiated state (Plate 4).

Changes in the expression of cytoskeletal proteins that are responsible for cell shape and stability also point toward a recapitulation of embryonic patterns of vessel growth. The expression of desmin, a muscle-specific intermediate filament, switches to expression of vimentin in smooth muscle cells of growing collateral arteries (Plates 5 and 6). The reverse happens during embryonic development where vimentin is replaced by desmin in some tissues (Vincent et al., 1991). For this reason vimentin has been named an *embryonic filament.* The desmin-vinculin switch has also been observed when the formation of neointima was stimulated by angioplasty (Gabbiani et al., 1982). Similar changes are observed in expression of another cytoskeletal protein, meta-vinculin, which decreases in smooth muscle cells of neointima (Belkin et al., 1988; North et al., 1993).

Another important extracellular matrix constituent involved in vessel remodeling is chondroitin sulfate, which is produced by both endothelial cells and smooth muscle cells (Wight et al., 1986). Chondroitin sulfates are found on the cell surface and in the extracellular matrix, where they form spot-like structures (Avnur and Geiger, 1984); in vivo, chondroitin sulfates localize to the extracellular matrix of the media and the adventitia, but not intima, of normal vessels (Lark et al., 1988). Proliferating smooth muscle cells increase chondroitin sulfate expression (Wight et al., 1989). Higher than normal expression is also seen in the neointima of atherosclerotic vessels (Li et al., 1993), in vessels following balloon angioplasty (Galis and Alavi, 1993), and in the neointima of growing collateral vessels. In addition, while chondroitin sulfate expression in the media of collaterals is similar to that seen in normal vessels, collaterals display a very intense labeling in the adventitia, nearly as strong as that in the neointima.

The presence of chondroitin sulfate reduces the adhesive ability of other matrix proteins, including fibronectin and collagen (Knox and Wells, 1979), and promotes smooth cell migration (Morriss-Kay and Tuckett, 1989). In addition, chondroitin sulfate promotes SMC migration by inhibiting elastin-dependent formation of the internal elastic lamina, the natural barrier between intima and media. The effect on elastic lamina formation is observed in fetal ductus arteriosus. Under conditions with increased chondroitin sulfate expression the formation of the inner elastic membrane is disturbed (Hinek et al., 1992). It is interesting to note that, in growing collateral vessels, the internal elastic membrane is either missing or present only in fragmentary remnants, a feature that may facilitate migration of the SMCs from the media into the neointima (Plate 7).

The neointima of proliferating collateral arteries also shows increased expression of collagen VI, which can be detected intracellularly in some of the neointimal cells, thus suggesting a high degree of synthesis while other parts of the vessel wall show normal collagen VI expression. While the exact role of collagen VI is unclear, it is thought to promote cell adhesion in the neointima and thus provide stability for the developing vessel. This is accomplished in part by association with collagens I and III via collagen I binding sites (Bonaldo et al., 1990) and with integrins via the RGD domains.

Another extracellular matrix protein, laminin, is found in basement membranes where it forms close connections with collagen IV and it seems to participate in early embryogenesis, since it can be detected in two-cell mice embryos (Kleinman et al., 1993). In normal vessels, laminin is found in the extracellular matrix around the smooth muscle cells of the media, while no laminin is detectable beneath the endothelium in the intima. In the adventitia moderate laminin expression can be seen in the connective tissue. Growing collateral vessels express an increased amount of laminin in the extracellular space in the media and in the neointima. Endothelial cells plated on laminin substrates form tube-like structures similar to capillaries, while cells plated on plastic dishes develop single-layer cultures (Vernon et al., 1992), thus suggesting that the extracellular matrix is able to influence the phenotype and the differentiation state of endothelial cells. Laminin expression in the course of angiogenesis is an indication of vascular maturation (Risau and Lemmon, 1988).

Fibronectin, yet another extracellular matrix protein, promotes cytokinesis, and may influence cell migration in the ductus arteriosus; antibodies against fibronectin inhibit smooth muscle cell migration in collagen networks (Boudreau et al., 1991). Fibronectin is present in the developing ventricular outflow tract, where smooth muscle cells that are migrating to the neointima to attach to the matrix (Burke et al., 1994). In developing coronary collateral vessels, fibronectin is highly expressed, particularly in vessels in which the neointima proliferates to such an extent that the lumen decreases instead of widening (Plate 8). Actually, in most collateral arterioles that initially participate in the growth process eventually regress again in favor of a few that mature into small arteries, a process called "pruning" in analogy to the vascular regression that leads to avascular areas in the embryo.

Altered expression of intracellular marker proteins of smooth muscle cells leading to a dedifferentiated phenotype and increased expression of certain matrix proteins is a pattern that is not unique to collateral vessel formation but is rather typical for vascular remodeling. The trigger for the master switch that activates and inhibits this battery of genes is unknown. Growth factors are most probably involved in these changes in gene expression. Studies exploring the expression of these genes during embryonic arteriogenesis and the study of the tie-2/angiopoietin system during neoarteriogenesis may promote our understanding of the recapitulation of embryonic patterns of development in collateral growth.

Regression of Collaterals

When studying the collateral circulation in the dog heart, we observed that only a limited number of the originally formed collateral vessels survived. In most collateral arteries, an exuberant proliferation of smooth muscle cells and an increase of extracellular matrix formation without a concomitant enlargement of the lumen finally leads to the obliteration of these vessels. This phenomenon most likely reflects the competition for flow. Provided that growth of collateral vessels is dependent upon blood flow velocity, larger vessels initially have a growth advantage. As they enlarge, these vessels conduct an increasingly larger proportion of the total blood flow, thereby reducing shear stress forces within smaller vessels. Reduction of shear forces within smaller vessels that are already mitotically stimulated reduces the remodeling influence and leads to intimal proliferation and increased fibronectin expression without the adequate enlargement of the vessel. The exuberant intimal proliferation and increased fibronectin expression may be caused by increased PDGF production, as suggested by studies in prosthetic arteries (Geary et al., 1994) and by the fact that increased shear stress decreases PDGF expression.

The model presented here for the regression of collateral arteries is also supported by clinical findings. Since the advent of bypass grafting cardiac surgeons have observed that only those bypass grafts that carry large flows to the otherwise-underperfused territories will remain patent. On the other hand, the presence of collateral arteries is a risk factor for early closure of coronary artery lesions undergoing percentaneous transluminal coronary angioplasty (PTCA) (Pijls and Bracke, 1995; Probst et al., 1991). Following successful PTCA, enlarged collaterals regress because the stenotic pressure difference does not exist anymore. If that balloon-dilated artery now develops restenosis, no new collaterals are present because, as explained in the paragraph on fetal development, only a limited number of preformed, preexisting arteriolar collateral vessels exists. The majority of the new collaterals perish by "pruning" during the first wave of adaptive collateral growth. Only a few large ones that are functional remain. If these regress when the diseased artery becomes recanalized no other arteriolar structures will be present if restenosis occurs.

The Limits of Growth

Neoarteriogenesis is a powerful adaptive response to arterial occlusion but it has limitations. One limitation is the time requirement for vascular growth; another is the incomplete nature of adaptation. The latter is particularly significant since, even under the best circumstances, collateral development usually remains incomplete; only about 30% of the maximal blood flow capacity is restored, and collateral artery growth stops for unknown reasons. Whereas normal coronary flow reserve is about five times the normal resting flow, maximal collateral flow reserve is about twofold. Thus, the shear forces in the greatly enlarged vessels are substantially decreased and the receptors for growth factors are probably downregulated. Thus, it is possible that the exogenous application of growth factors at this stage might be without effect.

The tortuosity of collateral vessels is another factor that limits optimal adaptation because of the energy losses that occur at higher flow rates. Stimulated growth may also increase tortuosity which may curtail the beneficial effect.

Also, the progression of coronary artery disease can occlude the "stem" artery of the collateral vessels. When this occurs as slowly as the first occlusion, another set of anastomoses could form and the previous vessels assume the status of a secondary network because the blood flow has to overcome the resistance of two collateral systems in series before it can perfuse capillaries. The effect is the same as if the primary network has to carry a chronically increased flow. If only one coronary artery remains patent and total coronary flow and muscle mass are preserved, the patent artery has now to conduct about triple the normal flow on a long term basis. This should increase the size and the capacity to conduct flow of the arterial tree as well as that of the primary network of collaterals, if shear stress is indeed a critical factor.

The "in-series" configuration of collateral resistance reduces the effective perfusion pressure for the last recipient bed. The stenosis of another stem artery may lead to the well-known observation of "infarction-at-a-distance" (Fig. 8.8.). The reduction of perfusion pressure as illustrated in the figure is even more pronounced when the diastolic pressure in the left ventricle is elevated, as is often the case in advanced coronary disease. Diastolic pressure must then be subtracted from the secondary PCP, and the resulting effective perfusion pressure may come close to (or actually

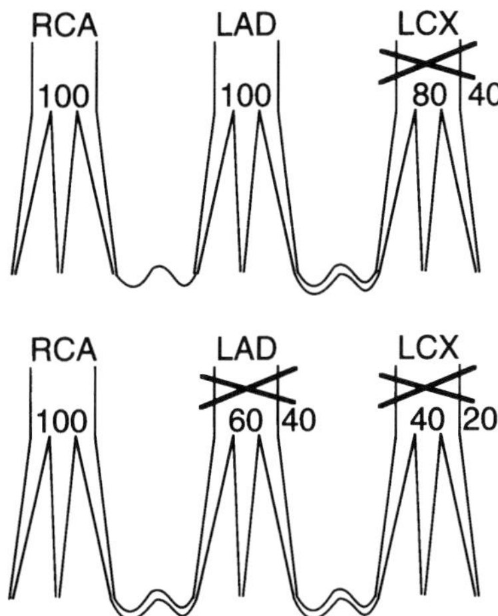

Figure 8.8. Schematic and simplified version of the development of secondary collateral networks when the feeder artery proper (LAD) becomes itself occluded. The RCA is now the only source of blood flow. Energy losses lead to pressure gradients with isolated LCX occlusion. These become amplified with vasodilation and pressure falls to 40 mmHg with additional LAD occlusion so that the perfusion pressure for the LCX territory falls to 40 under normal conditions and further to 20 with vasodilation; i.e., the LCX tissue becomes actually underperfused. Left ventricular end diastolic pressure may rise due to LCX ischemia thereby further reducing subendocardial LCX flow.

reach) critical closing pressure or P at zero flow (P_{zf}) with myocardial ischemia as the consequence, which occurs, of course, already above P_{zf}.

Outlook

That complete occlusion of one or more coronary arteries may lead to symptomless adaptation and normalization of coronary blood flow should encourage us to repeat this experiment of nature in those cases where nature obviously failed. Reasons for such failures include the fact that sudden occlusions do not respect the time requirements of arterial growth, insufficient endogenous growth factor may be produced, or insufficient numbers of growth factor receptors may be present on target cells. A lack of growth factor production can be corrected by exogenous supplementation with either growth factor proteins or by gene therapy.

REFERENCES

Aoki, M., Sakai, K., Koyanagi, S., Takeshita, A., and Nakamura, M. (1991). Effect of nitroglycerin on coronary collateral function during exercise evaluated by quantitative analysis of thallium-201 single photon emission computed tomography. Am. Heart J. 121: 1361–1366.

Arras, M., Mohri, M., Sack, S., Schwarz, E. R., Schaper, J., and Schaper, W. (1992). Macrophages accumulate and release tumor necrosis factor-alpha in the ischemic porcine myocardium. Circulation 86 (Suppl. I): 0129 (abstr.).

Arras, M., Ito, W. D., Scholz, D., Winkler, B., Schaper, J. and Schaper, W. (1998). Monocyte activation in angiogenesis and collateral growth in the rabbit hindlimb capillary sprouting in a rabbit model of hindlimb ischemia J. Clin. Invest. 101: 40–50.

Asahara, T., Murohara, T., Sullivan, A., Silver, M., van der Zee, R., Li, T., Witzenbichler, B., Schatteman, G., and Isner, J. M. (1997). Isolation of putative progenitor endothelial cells for angiogenesis. Science 275: 964–967.

Avnur, Z. and Geiger, B. (1984). Immunocytochemical localization of native chondroitin-sulfate in tissues and cultured cells using specific monoclonal antibody. Cell 38: 811–811.

Baroldi, G. and Scomazzoni, G. (1967). Coronary Circulation in the Normal and the Pathologic Heart. Office of the Surgeon General, Department of the Army, Washington.

Baroldi, G., Radice, F., Schmid, G., and Leone, A. (1974). Morphology of acute myocardial infarction in relation to coronary thrombosis. Am. Heart J. 87: 65–75.

Belkin, A. M., Ornatsky, O. I., Glukhova, M. A., and Koteliansky, V. E. (1988). Immunolocalization of meta-vinculin in human smooth and cardiac muscles. J. Cell Biol. 107: 545–553.

Bernotat-Danielowski, S., Sharma, H. S., Schott, R. J., and Schaper, W. (1993). Generation and localisation of monoclonal antibodies against fibroblast growth factors in ischaemic collateralised porcine myocardium. Cardiovasc. Res. 27: 1220–1228.

Birukov, K. G., Stepanova, O. V., Namaev, A. K. and Shirinsky, V. P. (1991) Expression of calponin in rabbit and human aortic smooth muscle cells. Cell. Tissue Res. 266: 579–584.

Blanke, H., Cohen, M., Karsch, K. R., Fagerstrom, R., and Rentrop, K. P. (1985). Prevalence and significance of residual flow to the infarct zone during the acute phase of myocardial infarction. J. Am. Coll. Cardiol. 5: 827–831.

Bogers, A. J. J. C., Gittenberger-de Groot, A. C., Poelmann, R. E., Peault, B. M., and Huysmans, H. A. (1989). Development of the origin of the coronary arteries, a matter of ingrowth or outgrowth? Anat. Embryol. 180: 437–441.

Bonaldo, P., Russo, V., Bucciotti, F., Doliana, R., and Colombatti, A. (1990). Structural and functional features of the alpha 3 chain indicate a bridging role for chicken collagen VI in connective tissues. Biochemistry 29: 1245–1254.

Boudreau, N., Turley, E., and Rabinovitch, M. (1991). Fibronectin, hyaluronan, and hyaluronan binding protein contribute to increased ductus arteriosus smooth muscle cell migration. Dev. Biol. 143: 235–247.

Burke, R. D., Wang, D., and Jones, V. M. (1994). Ontogeny of vessel wall components in the outflow tract of the chick. Anat. Embryol. 189: 447–456.

Cohen, M. and Rentrop, K. P. (1986). Limitation of myocardial ischemia by collateral circulation during sudden controlled coronary artery occlusion in human subjects: a prospective study. Circulation 74: 469–476.

Cohen, M. V., Matsuki, T., and Downey, J. M. (1988). Pressure-flow characteristics and nutritional capacity of coronary veins in dogs. Am. J. Physiol. 255: H834–H846.

Cohen, M., Sherman, W., Rentrop, K. P., and Gorlin, R. (1989). Determinants of collateral filling observed during sudden controlled coronary-artery occlusion in human-subjects. J. Am. Coll. Cardiol. 13: 297–303.

Davis, S., Aldrich, T. H., Jones, P. F., Acheson, A., Compton, D. L., Jain, V., Ryan, T. E., Bruno, J., Radziejewski, C., Maisonpierre, P. C., and Yancopoulos, G. D. (1996). Isolation of angiopoietin-1, a ligand for the TIE2 receptor, by secretion-trap expression cloning. Cell 87: 1161–1169.

Dervan, J. P., McKay, R. G., and Baim, D. S. (1987). Assessment of the relationship between distal occluded pressure and angiographically evident collateral flow during coronary angioplasty. Am. Heart J. 114: 491–497.

Dumont, D. J., Fong, G. H., Puri, M. C., Gradwohl, G., Alitalo, K., and Breitman, M. L. (1995). Vascularization of the mouse embryo: a study of flk-1, tek, tie, and vascular endothelial growth factor expression during development. Dev. Dyn. 203: 80–92.

Feldman, R. L. and Pepine, C. J. (1984). Evaluation of coronary collateral circulation in conscious humans. Am. J. Cardiol. 53: 1233–1238.

Feldman, R. L., Macdonald, R. G., Hill, J. A., Limacher, M. C., Conti, C. R., and Pepine, C. J. (1986). Effect of propranolol on myocardial ischemia occurring during acute coronary occlusion. Circulation 73: 727–733.

Feldman, R. L., Macdonald, R. G., Hill, J. A., and Pepine, C. J. (1987). Effect of nicardipine on determinants of myocardial ischemia occurring during acute coronary occlusion produced by percutaneous transluminal coronary angioplasty. Am. J. Cardiol. 60: 267–270.

Fischer, S., Sharma, H. S., Karliczek, G. F., and Schaper, W. (1995). Expression of vascular permeability factor/vascular endothelial growth factor in pig cerebral microvascular endothelial cells and its upregulation by adenosine. Mol. Brain Res. 28: 141–148.

Fischer, S., Knöll, R., Renz, D., Karliczek, G. F., and Schaper, W. (1997). Role of adenosine in the hypoxic induction of vascular endothelial growth factor in porcine brain derived microvascular endothelial. Endothelium 5: 155–165.

Folkman, J. and D'Amore, A. (1996). Blood vessel formation: what is its molecular basis? Cell 87: 1153–1155.

Fujita, M., McKnown, D. P., and McKnown, M.D. Franklin, D. (1990). Coronary collateral regression in conscious dogs. Angiology 41: 621–630.

Fujita, M., Sasayama, S., Ohno, A., Nakajima, H., and Asanoi, H. (1987). Importance of angina for development of collateral circulation. Br. Heart J. 57: 139–143.

Fujita, M., McKnown, D. P., McKnown, M.D., and Franklin, D. (1988). Electrocardiographic evaluation of collateral development in conscious dogs. J. Electrocardiol. 21: 55–63.

Fulton, W. F. M. (1964). The time factor in the enlargement of anastomoses in coronary artery disease. Scot. Med. J. 9: 18–23.

Fulton, W. F. M. (1965). Arterial anastomoses in the coronary circulation. In "The Coronary Arteries. Arteriography, Microanatomy, and Pathogenesis of Obliterative Coronary Artery Disease" (W. F. M. Fulton, ed.) pp. 72–128. Thomas, C. C., Springfield, IL.

Fuster, V., Frye, R. L., Kennedy, M. A., Connolly, D. C., and Mankin, H. T. (1979). The role of collateral circulation in various coronary syndromes. Circulation 59: 1137–1144.

Gabbiani, G., Rungger-Brandle, E., de Chastonay, C., and Franke, W. W. (1982). Vimentin-containing smooth muscle cells in aortic intimal thickening after endothelial injury. Lab. Invest. 47: 265–269.

Galis, Z. S. and Alavi, M. Z. (1993). Co-localization of aortic apoliprotein B chondroitin sulfate in an injury model of atherosclerosis. Am. J. Pathol. 142: 1432–1438.

Geary, R. L., Kohler, T. R., Vergel, S., Kirkman, T. R., and Clowes, A. W. (1994). Time course of flow induced smooth muscle cell proliferation and intimal thickening in endothelialized baboon vascular grafts. Circ. Res. 74: 14–23.

Goldstein, R. E., Stinson, E. B., Scherer, J. L., Senigen, R. P., Grehl, R. M., and Epstein, S. E. (1974). Intraoperative coronary collateral function in patients with coronary occlusive disease. Nitroglycerine responsiveness and angiographic correlations. Circulation 49: 298–308.

Görge, G., Schmidt, T., Ito, B. R., Pantely, G. A., and Schaper, W. (1989). Microvascular and collateral adaptation in swine hearts following progressive coronary artery stenosis. Basic Res. Cardiol. 84: 524–535.

Gottwik, M., Stämmler, G., Schaper, W., and Schlepper, M. (1984). Collateral development and function in jeopardized human myocardium [abstract]. Circulation 70 Suppl. II: 94.

Gregg, D. E. (1974). The natural history of coronary collateral development. Circ. Res. 35: 335–344.

Habib, G. B., Heibig, J., Forman, S. A., Brown, B. G., Roberts, R., Terrin, M. L., Bolli, R., (1991). Influence of coronary collateral vessels on myocardial infarct size in humans. Results of Phase I thrombolysis in myocardial infarction (TIMI) trial. Circulation 83: 739–746.

Hamby, R. I., Aintablian, A., and Schwartz, A. (1976). Reappraisal of the functional significance of the coronary collateral circulation. Am. J. Cardiol. 38: 305–309.

Hashimoto, E., Ogita, T., Nakaoka, T., Matsuoka, R., Takao, A., and Kirka, Y.

(1994). Rapid induction of vascular endothelial growth factor expression by transient ischemia in rat heart. Am. J. Physiol. 267: H1948–H1954.

Hill, J. A., Feldman, R. L., Macdonald, R. G., and Pepine, C. J. (1985). Coronary artery collateral visualization during acute coronary occlusion. Am. J. Cardiol. 55: 1216–1218.

Hinek, A., Boyle, J., and Rabinovitch, M. (1992). Vascular smooth msucle cell detachment from elastin and migration through elastic laminae is promoted by chondroitin sulfate-induced "shedding" of the 67-kDa cell surface elastin binding protein. Exp. Cell Res. 203: 344–353.

Hirai, T., Fujita, M., Sasayama, S., Ohno, A., Yamanishi, K., Nakajima, H., and Asanoi, H. (1987). Importance of coronary collateral circulation for kinetics of serum creatine kinase in acute myocardial infarction. Am. J. Cardiol. 60: 446–450.

Hood, L. and Rosenquist, T. H. (1992). Coronary artery development in the chick: origin and development of smooth muscle cells, and the effects of neural crest ablation. Anat. Rec. 234: 291–300.

Hutchins, G. M., Kessler-Hanna, A., and Moore, G. W. (1988). Development of the coronary arteries in the embryonic human heart. Circulation 77: 1250–1257.

Ikeda, E., Achen, M. G., Breier, G., and Risau, W. (1995). Hypoxia-induced transcriptional activation and increased mRNA stability of vascular endothelial growth factor in C6 glioma cells. J. Biol. Chem. 270: 19761–19766.

Ito, W. D., Arras, M., Winkler, B., Scholz, D., Htun, P., and Schaper, W. (1997a). Angiogenesis but not collateral growth is associated with ischemia after femoral artery occlusion. Am. J. Physiol., 273: H1255–H1265.

Ito, W. D., Arras, M., Winkler, B., Scholz, D., Schaper, J., and Schaper, W. (1997b). Monocyte chemotactic protein-1 increases collateral and peripheral conductance after femoral artery occlusion. Circ. Res. 80: 829–837.

Jiang, H. and Stephens, N. L. (1994). Calcium and smooth muscle contraction. Mol. Cell Biochem. 135: 1–9.

Kern, M. J., Deligonal, U., and Labovitz, A. J. (1990). Effects of diltiazem and nifedipine on systemic and coronary hemodynamics and ischemic responses during transient coronary artery occlusion. Am. Heart J. 119: 47–54.

Kleinman, H. K., Weeks, B. S., Schnaper, H. W., Kibbey, M. C., Yamamura, K., and Grant, D. S. (1993). The laminins: a family of basement membrane glycoproteins important in cell differentiation and tumor metastases. Vitam. Horm. 47: 161–186.

Kluge, A., Zimmermann, R., Münkel, B., Mohri, M., Schaper, J., and Schaper, W. (1995). Insulin-like growth factor I is involved in inflammation linked angiogenic processes after microembolization in porcine heart. Cardiovasc. Res. 29: 407–415.

Knox, P. and Wells, P. (1979). Cell adhesion and proteoglycans. I. The effect of exogenous proteoglycans on the attachment of chick embryo fibroblasts to tissue culture plastic and collagen. J. Cell Sci. 40: 77–88.

Kuki, S., Bauer, E. P., Arras, M., Zimmermann, R., and Schaper, W. (1997). Pulmonary artery banding upregulates vascular endothelial growth factor and its flk-1 receptor in pig hearts. J. Am. Coll. Cardiol. 29: 41141.

Kwee, L., Baldwin, H. S., Shen, H. M., Stewart, C. L., Buck, C., Buck, C. A., and Labow, M. A. (1995). Defective development of the embryonic and extraembryonic circulatory system in vascular cell adhesion molecule (VCAM-1) deficient mice. Development 121: 489–503.

Ladoux, A. and Frelin, C. (1993). Hypoxia is a strong inducer of vascular endothelial growth factor mRNA expression in the heart. Biochem. Biophys. Res. Commun. 195: 1005–1010.

Lamas, G. A., Pfeffer, M. A., and Braunwald, E. (1991). Patency of the infarct-related coronary artery and ventricular geometry. J. Am. Coll. Cardiol. 68: 41D–51D.

Lang, R. A. and Bishop, J. M. (1993). Macrophages are required for cell death and tissue remodeling in the developing mouse eye. Cell 74: 453–462.

Lang, R. A., Lustig, M., Francois, F., Sellinger, M., and Plesken, H. (1994). Apoptosis during macrophage-dependent tissue remodeling. Development 12: 3395–3403.

Lark, M. W., Yeo, T. K., Lara, S., Hellstrom, I., Hellstrom, K. E., and Wight, T. N. (1988). Arterial chondroitin sulfate proteoglycan: localization with a monoclonal antibody. J. Histochem. Cytochem. 36: 1211–1221.

Lazarous, D. F., Shou, M., Scheinowitz, M., Hodge, E., Thirumurti, V., Kitsiou, A. N., Stiber, J. A., Lobo, A. D., Hunsberger, S., Guetta, E., Epstein, S. E., and Unger, E. F. (1996). Comparative effects of basic fibroblast growth factor and vascular endothelial growth factor on coronary collateral development and the arterial response to injury. Circulation 94: 1074–1082.

Levy, A. P., Levy, N. S., Loscalzo, J., Calderone, A., Takahashi, N., Yeo, K. T., Koren, D., Colucci, W. S., and Goldberg, M. A. (1995). Regulation of vascular endothelial growth factor in cardiac myocytes. Circ. Res. 76: 758–766.

Li, Z., Alavi, M. Z., Wasty, F., Galis, Z., and Moore, S. (1993). Proteoglycan synthesis by the neointimal smooth muscle cells cultured from rabbit aortic explants following de-endothelialization. Pathobiology 61: 89–94.

Macdonald, R. G., Hill, J. A., and Feldman, R. L. (1986). ST segment response to acute coronary occlusion: coronary hemodynamic and angiographic determinants of direction of ST segment shift. Circulation 74: 973–979.

McFalls, E. O., Araujo, K. I., Lammertsma, A., Rhodes, C. G., Bloomfield, P., Pupita, G., Jones, T., and Maseri, A. (1993). Vasodilator reserve in collateral-dependent myocardium as measured by positron emission tomography. Eur. Heart J. 14: 336–343.

Meeson, A., Palmer, M., Calfon, M., and Lang, R. (1996). A relationship between apoptosis and blood flow during programmed capillary regression is revealed by vital analysis. Development 122: 3929–3938.

Meier, B., Luethy, P., Finci, L., Steffenino, G. D., and Rutishauser, W. (1987). Coronary wedge pressure in relation to spontaneously visible and recruitable collaterals. Circulation 75: 906–913.

Meininger, C. J. and Zetter, B. R. (1992). Mast cells and angiogenesis. Semin. Cancer Biol. 3: 73–79.

Mikawa, T. and Fischman, D. A. (1992). Retroviral analysis of cardiac morphogenesis: discontinuous formation of coronary vessels. Proc. Natl. Acad. Sci. USA 89: 9504–9508.

Mizuno, K., Horiuchi, K., Matui, H., Miyamoto, A., Arakawa, K., Shibuya, T., Kurita, A., and Nakamura, H. (1988). Role of coronary collateral vessels during transient coronary occlusion during angioplasty assessed by hemodynamic, electrocardiographic and metabolic changes. J. Am. Coll. Cardiol. 12: 624–628.

Morriss-Kay, G. and Tuckett, F. (1989). Immunohistochemical localization of chondroitin sulphate proteoglycans, and the effects of chondroitinase ABC in 9-to 11-day rat embryos. Development 106: 787–798.

Muller, D. W. M., Topol, E. J., Califf, R. M., Sigmon, K. N., Gorman, L., George, B. S., Kereiakes, D. J., Lee, K. L., Ellis, S. G., (1989). Relationship between antecedent angina pectoris and short-term prognosis after thrombolytic therapy for acute myocardial infarction. Am. Heart J. 13: 297–303.

Nitzberg, W. D., Nath, H. P., and Rogers, W. J. (1985). Collateral flow in patients with acute myocardial infarction. Am. J. Cardiol. 56: 729–736.

Nohara, R., Kambara, H., Murakami, T., Kadota, K., Tamaki, S., and Kawai, C. (1983). Collateral function in early acute myocardial infarction. Am. J. Cardiol. 52: 955–959.

North, A. J., Galazkiewicz, B., Byers, T. J., Glenney, J. R., and Small, J. V. (1993). Complementary distribution of vinculin and dystrophin define two distinct sarcolemma domains in smooth muscle. J. Cell Biol. 120: 1159–1167.

Orlandi, A., Ehrlich, H. P., Ropraz, P., Spagnoli, G., and Gabbiani, G. (1994). Rat aortic smooth muscle cells isolated from different layers and at different times after endothelial denudation show distinct biological features in vitro. Arterioscler. Thromb. 14: 982–989.

Paskins-Hurlburt, A. and Hollenberg, N. K. (1992). "Tissue need" and limb collateral arterial growth. Skeletal contractile power and perfusion during collateral development in the rat. Circ. Res. 70: 546–553.

Piek, J. J., Koolen, J. J., Metting van Rijn, A. C., Bot, H., Hoedemaker, G., David, G. K., Dunning, A. J., Spaan, J. A. E., and Visser, C. A. (1993). Spectral analysis of flow velocity in the contralateral artery during coronary angioplasty: a new method for assessing collateral flow. J. Am. Coll. Cardiol. 21: 1574–1582.

Piek, J. J., van Liebergen, R. A. M., Koch, K. T., deWinter, R. J., Peters, R. J. G., and David, G. K. (1997a). Pharmacologic modulation of the human collateral vascular resistance in acute and chronic coronary occlusion assessed by intracoronary blood flow velocity analysis in an angioplasty model. Circulation 96: 106–115.

Piek, J. J., van Liebergen, R. A. M., Koch, K. T., Peters, R. J. G., and David, G. K. (1997b). Clinical, angiographical and hemodynamic predictors of recruitable collateral flow assessed during balloon angioplasty coronary occlusion. J. Am. Coll. Cardiol. 29: 275–282.

Piek, J. J., van Liebergen, R. A. M., Koch, K. T., Peters, R. J. G., and David, G. K. (1997c). Comparison of collateral vascular responses in the donor and recipient coronary artery during transient coronary occlusion assessed by intracoronary blood flow velocity analysis in patients. Am. Coll. Cardiol. 29: 1528–1535.

Pijls, N. H. and Bracke, F. A. (1995). Damage to the collateral circulation by PTCA of an occluded artery. Cathet. Cardiovasc. Diagn. 34: 61–64.

Pijls, N. H. J., Bech, G. J. W., El Gamal, M. I. H., Bonnier, H. J. R. M., De Bryne, B., Van Gelder, B., Michels, H. R., and Koolen, J. J. (1995). Quantification of recruitable coronary collateral blood flow in conscious humans and its potential to predict future ischemic events. J. Am. Coll. Cardiol. 25: 1522–1528.

Poelmann, R. E., Gittenberger-de Groot, A. C., Mentink, M. M. T., Bökenkamp, R., and Hogers, B. (1993). Development of the cardiac coronary vascular endothelium, studied with antiendothelial antibodies, in chicken-quail chimeras. Circ. Res. 73: 559–568.

Price, R. J., Owens, G. K., and Skalak, T. C. (1994). Immunohistochemical identification of arteriolar development using markers of smooth muscle differentiation. Evidence that capillary arterialization proceeds from terminal arterioles. Circ. Res. 75: 520–527.

Probst, P., Baumgartner, C., and Gottsauner-Wolf, M. (1991). The influence of the presence of collaterals on restenoses after PTCA. Clin. Cardiol. 14: 803–807.

Rentrop, K. P., Thornton, J. C., Feit, F., and Van Buskirk, M. (1988). Determinants and protective potential of coronary arterial collaterals as assessed by an angioplasty model. Am. J. Cardiol. 61: 677–684.

Rentrop, K. P., Feit, F., Sherman, W., Stecy, P., Hosat, S., Cohen, M., Rey, M., Ambrose, J., Nachamie, M., and Schwartz, W. (1989). Late thrombolytic therapy preserves left ventricular function in patients with collateralized total coronary occlusion: primary end-point findings of the 2nd Mount-Sinai New York University Reperfusion Trial. J. Am. Coll. Cardiol. 14: 58–64.

Risau, W. (1995). Differentiation of endothelium. FASEB J. 9: 926–933.

Risau, W. and Flamme, I. (1995). Vasculogenesis. Annu. Rev. Cell Dev. Biol. 11: 73–91.

Risau, W. and Lemmon, V. (1988). Changes in the vascular extracellular matrix during embryonic vasculogenesis and angiogenesis. Dev. Biol. 125: 441–450.

Rogers, W. J., Hodd, W. P., Jr., Mantle, J. A., Baxley, W. A., Kirklin, J. K., Zorn, G. L., and Nath, H. P. (1984). Return of left ventricular function after reperfusion in patients with myocardial infarction: importance of subtotal stenoses or intact collaterals. Circulation 69: 338–349.

Sabia, P. J., Powers, E. R., Ragosta, M., Sarembock, I. J., Burwell, L. R., and Kaul, S. (1992). An association between collateral blood flow and myocardial viability in patients with recent myocardial infarction. N. Engl. J. Med. 327: 1825–1831.

Saito, Y., Yasuno, M., Ishida, M., Suzuki, K., Matoba, Y., Emura, M., and Takahashi M., (1985). Importance of coronary collaterals for restoration of left ventricular function after intracoronary thrombolysis. Am. J. Cardiol. 55: 1259–1263.

Schaper, W. (1971). The Collateral Circulation of the Heart. Elsevier North Holland, Amsterdam.

Schaper, W. (1979). The Pathophysiology of Myocardial Perfusion. Elsevier/North-Holland Biomedical Press, Amsterdam.

Schaper, W. (1984). Experimental infarcts and the microcirculation. In "Therapeutic Approaches to Myocardial Infarct Size Limitation" (D. J. Hearse and D. M. Yellon, eds.) pp. 79–90. Raven Press, New York.

Schaper, W. and Ito, W. (1996). Molecular mechanisms of coronary collateral vessel growth. Circ. Res. 79: 911–919.

Schaper, W. and Schaper, J. (1993). Collateral Circulation—Heart, Brain, Kidney, Limbs. Kluwer Academic, Boston.

Schaper, W. and Winkler, B. (1978). Determinants of peripheral coronary pressure in coronary occlusion. In "Primary and Secondary Angina Pectoris" (A. Maseri, M. Lesch, and G. A. Klassen, eds.) pp. 351–361. Grune and Stratton, New York.

Schaper, W., Wüsten, B., Flameng, W., Scholtholt, J., Winkler, B., and Pasyk, S. (1975). Local dilatory reserve in chronic experimental coronary occlusion without infarction. Quantitation of collateral development. Basic Res. Cardiol. 70: 159–173.

Schaper, W., Flameng, W., Winkler, B., Wuesten, B., Türschmann, W., Neugebauer, G., Carl, M., and Pasyk, S. (1976a). Quantification of collateral resistance in acute and chronic experimental coronary occlusion in the dog. Circ. Res. 39: 371–377.

Schaper, W., Koenig, R., Franz, D., and Schaper, J. (1976b) Scanning electron microscopy of developing coronary arterial blood vessels. Tal Intern. Publ. Comp. Israel 2: 438–440.

Schaper, W., Bernotat-Danielowski, S., Nienaber, C., and Schaper, J. (1992). Collateral circulation. In "The Heart and Cardiovascular System" (H. Fozzard, E. Haber, R. Jennings, A. Katz, and H. Morgan, eds.) Volume Two, pp. 1427–1464. Raven Press, New York.

Schwartz, H., Leiboff, R. H., Bren, G. B., Wasserman, A. G., Katz, R. J., Varghese, P. J., Sokil, A. B., and Ross, A. M. (1984). Temporal evolution of the human coronary collateral circulation after myocardial infarction. J. Am. Coll. Cardiol. 4: 1088–1093.

Schwartz, H., Leiboff, R. L., Katz, R. J., Wasserman, A. G., Bren, G. B., Varghese, P. J., and Ross, A. M. (1985). Arteriographic predictors of spontaneous improvement in left ventricular function after myocardial infarction. Circulation 71: 466–472.

Sharma, H. S., Sassen, L., Knöll, R., and Verdouw, P. D. (1992). Myocardial expression of vascular endothelial growth factor: enhanced transcription during ischemia and reperfusion [abstract]. Circulation 86 Suppl. I: 1168.

Sheehan, F. H., Braunwald, E., Canner, P., Dodge, H. T., Gore, J., Van Natte, P., Passamani, E. R., Williams, D. O., and Zaret, B. (1987). The effect of intravenous thrombolytic therapy on left ventricular function: a report on tissue-type plasminogen activator and streptokinase from the Thrombolysis in Myocardial Infarction (TIMI Phase I) trial. Circulation 75: 817–829.

Suri, C., Jones, P. F., Patan, S., Bartunkova, S., Maisonpierre, P. C., Davis, S., Sato, T. N., and Yancopoulos, G. D. (1996). Requisite role of angiopoietin-1, a ligand for the TIE2 receptor, during embryonic angiogenesis. Cell 87: 1171–1180.

Takahashi, K., Takagi, M., Ohgami, K., Nakai, M., Kojima, A., Nadal-Ginard, B., and Shibata, N. (1993). Inhibition of smooth muscle cell migration and proliferation caused by transfection of the human calponin gene is associated with enhanced cell-matrix adhesion and reduced PDGF responsiveness. Circulation 88: 174.

Tomanek, R. J. (1996). Formation of the coronary vasculature: a brief review. Cardiovasc. Res. 31: E46–E51.

Vanoverschelde, J. L., Wijns, W., Depré, C., Essamri, B., Heyndrickx, G. R., Borgers, M., Bol, A., and Melin, J. A. (1993). Mechanisms of chronic regional postischemic dysfunction in humans: new insights from the study of noninfarcted collateral-dependent myocardium. Circulation 87: 1513–1523.

Vernon, R. B., Angello, J. C., Iruela-Arispe, M. L., Lane, T. F., and Sage, E. H. (1992). Reorganization of basement membrane matrices by vellular traction promotes the formation of cellular networks in vitro. Lab. Invest. 66: 536–547.

Vincent, M., Levasseur, S., Currie, R. W., and Rogers, P. A. (1991). Persistence of an embryonic intermediate filament-associated protein in the smooth muscle cells of elastic arteries and in Purkinje fibres. J. Mol. Cell. Cardiol. 23: 873–882.

Waldo, K., Willner, W., and Kirby, M. L. (1990). Origin of the proximal coronary artery stems and a review of ventricular vascularization in the chick embryo. Am. J. Anat. 188: 109–120.

Waldo, K. L., Kumski, D. H., and Kirby, M. L. (1994). Association of the cardiac neural crest with development of the coronary arteries in the chick embryo. Anat. Rec. 239: 315–331.

Westernacher, D. and Schaper, W. (1995). A novel heart derived inhibitor of vascular cell proliferation. Purification and biological activity. J. Mol. Cell. Cardiol. 27: 1535–1543.

White, F. C. and Bloor, C. M. (1981). Coronary collateral circulation in the pig: correlation of collateral flow with coronary bed size. Basic Res. Cardiol. 76: 189–196.

Wight, T. N., Kinsella, M. G., Lark, M. W., and Potter-Perigo, S. (1986). Vascular cell proteoglycans: evidence for metabolic modulation. Ciba Found. Symp. 124: 241–259.

Wight, T. N., Potter-Pergio, S., and Aulinskas, T. (1989). Proteoglycans and vascular cell proliferation. Am. Rev. Respir. Dis. 140: 1132–1135.

Williams, D. O., Amsterdam, E. A., Miller, R. R., and Mason, D. T. (1976). Functional significance of coronary collateral vessels in patients with acute myocardial infarction: relation to pump performance, cardiogenic shock and survival. Am. J. Cardiol. 37: 345–351.

Zoll, P. M., Wessler, S., and Schlesinger, M. J. (1951). Interarterial coronary anastomoses in the human heart, with particular reference to anemia and relative cardiac anoxia. Circulation 4: 797–819.

APPENDIX. EVALUATION OF COLLATERAL CIRCULATION

The coronary arterial circulation can be schematically represented as an electrical analog model (see Fig. 8.6):

Pao = mean aortic pressure

Pv = central venous pressure

P = mean coronary wedge pressure

*R*1 = resistance of the epicardial donor coronary artery

*R*2 = resistance of the epicardial recipient coronary artery

*R*3 = resistance of the peripheral vascular bed of the donor coronary artery

Rcoll = resistance of the collateral vascular bed

*R*4 = resistance of the peripheral vascular bed of the recipient coronary artery

dVi = diastolic collateral blood flow velocity integral of the recipient coronary artery

dVitot = diastolic coronary blood flow velocity of the donor coronary artery during balloon occlusion of the recipient coronary artery

$dMPV_{def}$ = maximal diastolic blood flow velocity of the donor coronary artery during balloon deflation

$dMPV_{inf}$ = maximal diastolic blood flow velocity of the donor coronary artery during balloon inflation

Calculation of the Collateral Vascular Resistance by Coronary Blood Flow Velocity Analysis of the Donor Coronary Artery

The assessment of coronary flow changes in the donor coronary artery can be used to calculate the collateral vascular resistance (*Rcoll*) in relation to the resistance of the donor (*Rcoll/R3*) (Piek et al., 1993). In this calculation *Rcoll* and *R3* are considered to remain constant, i.e., independent of flow and pressure, *R1* is considered negligible compared to all other resistances in patients with one-vessel disease, and the central venous pressure is considered to be zero in patients with a normal left ventricular function. Assuming that the diameter of the donor coronary artery before and during balloon inflation remains constant:

$$\text{coronary blood flow} = k \cdot dMPV \tag{1}$$

where k is a constant

Application of Ohm's law to blood flow provides the following equations:

$$\text{Balloon deflated: } k \cdot dMPV_{def} = \frac{Pao}{R3} \tag{2}$$

$$\text{Balloon inflated: } k \cdot dMPV_{inf} = \frac{Pao}{R3} + \frac{Pao - Pw}{Rcoll} \tag{3}$$

The relative resistance of the collateral vascular bed (Rcoll/R3) can be calculated from Eq. 2 and Eq. 3:

$$Rcoll/R3 = \frac{Pao - Pw}{Pao} \cdot \frac{dMPV_{def}}{dMPV_{inf} - dMPV\ def} \tag{4}$$

Calculation of the Collateral Vascular Resistance by Coronary Blood Flow Velocity Analysis of the Recipient Coronary Artery

The coronary vasculature is represented as resistors exhibiting ideal current–voltage behavior: $V = I^{*}R$. The voltage (V) is expressed as the pressure gradient and the current (I) as the diastolic blood flow velocity integral.

$$Pao = dVI_{tot} * (R1 + R3//(Rcoll + R4) \tag{5}$$

$$\text{where } R3 \mathbin{//} (Rcoll + R4) = \frac{R3 * (Rcoll + R4)}{R3 + Rcoll + R4}$$

Pao can also be expressed according to the following equation:

$$Pao = dVI_{tot} * R1 + dVI\ (Rcoll + R4) Pw = dVi * R4 \tag{6}$$

The coronary wedge/aortic pressure ratio can be expressed by eliminating the dVi and dVi_{tot} from the Eqs. 1, 2, and 3, which provides the following equation (Schaper and Winkler, 1978):

$$\frac{Pw}{Pao} = \frac{R3 + R4}{(Rcoll + R4) + (R3 + R1) + R1 * R3} \tag{8}$$

$$\frac{Pw}{Pao} = \frac{R4}{Rcoll + R4} \tag{9}$$

The collateral vascular resistance (*Rcoll*) and the peripheral vascular resistance of the recipient coronary artery (*R*4) can be expressed according to the following equations:

$$Rcoll = \frac{Pao - Pw}{dVI} \tag{10}$$

$$R4 = \frac{Pw}{dVI} \tag{11}$$

9

Angiogenesis in Nonischemic Myocardium

ROBERT J. TOMANEK

The high oxygen consumption of the myocardium necessitates abundant perfusion, which is facilitated by a rich vascular supply. Capillary density (number of capillaries/per mm^2) is about 2,000 to >4,000, depending on the species and method of processing the tissue for microscopic analysis. Figure 9.1, a micrograph of the myocardium, illustrates the extensiveness of the capillary bed. Most capillaries are arranged parallel to the long axes of cardiac myocytes, but anastomotic channels and obliquely oriented segments occur. The latter are due to branching.

Coronary angiogenesis during normal growth and development is a well-recognized event. This phenomenon also occurs in cardiac hypertrophy and other conditions that require adaptive growth of the coronary bed in order to meet requirements for enhanced perfusion, such as exercise stress. This chapter documents conditions in which coronary angiogenesis is activated and addresses the potential mechanisms that may be responsible for neovascularization of the nonischemic postnatal myocardium.

EXPANSION OF THE CAPILLARY BED BY ANGIOGENESIS

As heart mass increases during postnatal growth, or in response to increased work in the adult, adequate angiogenesis must occur to assure a normal coronary reserve and to preserve normal intercapillary distances. As myocytes grow in diameter and length, the surrounding capillary channels must also increase in length. This necessitates the elongation of both longitudinally and laterally oriented capillaries (A and B, respectively in Fig. 9.2). To maintain a consistent numerical or length density, new cap-

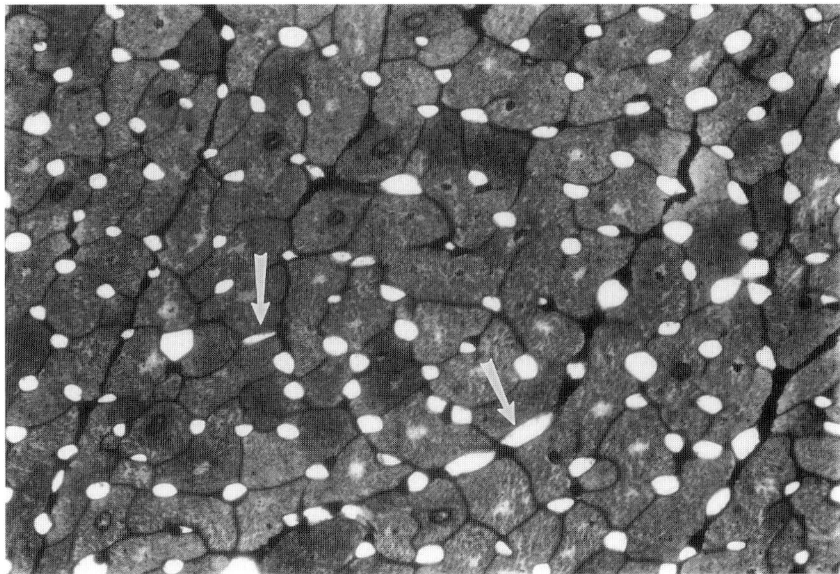

Figure 9.1. Cardiac myocyte and capillary profiles (translucent in this micrograph) from an adult rat heart that has been fixed by vascular perfusion under physiological pressure. The section, cut perpendicular to the long axis of myocytes, shows that most capillary profiles are aligned parallel to the myocytes, with some passing obliquely or nearly transversely (arrows).

illary channels need to be formed, since the only other way that normal numerical and length density could be maintained is by extensive elongation of capillaries, causing them to become more tortuous. The latter has not been demonstrated. The formation of new capillaries can occur by either sprouting (C in Fig. 9.2), as commonly described, or splitting, i.e., partitioning a capillary to form two daughter capillaries (D in Fig. 9.2), as proposed by Van Groningen and colleagues (1991). Therefore, capillary angiogenesis can occur by three methods: (1) elongation via addition of endothelial cells within a capillary unit, (2) sprouting, and (3) partitioning. All of these forms of growth necessitate endothelial cell proliferation and migration. Formation of new arterioles is also necessary during cardiac growth if maximal myocardial flow per unit mass is to be maintained. These vessels are formed by an expansion of capillaries and the addition of smooth muscle cells to form tunica media.

ANGIOGENESIS IN THE HYPERTROPIC HEART

It is well documented that coronary vascular growth is marked during the prenatal period and during early postnatal life. Coronary angiogenesis in the adult, however, is generally thought to be very limited. The belief that

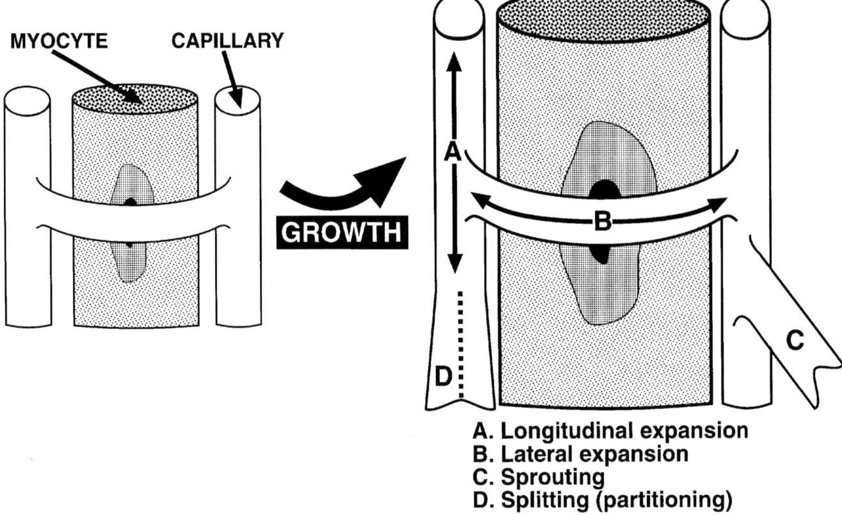

Figure 9.2. Comparison of the three ways that coronary capillaries can grow. A capillary can increase its length by endothelial cell proliferation along its course to produce longitudinal (A) or lateral (B) expansion of the capillary bed. New capillary channels can be formed by either sprouting (C) or splitting of an existing capillary channel to form two daughter channels (as proposed by van Groningen et al., 1991). See text for details.

cardiac hypertrophy associated with pressure overload in adults is not accompanied by growth of the coronary vasculature was based on human postmortem studies, which revealed that capillary numerical density (number of capillaries/mm^2) was lower in such enlarged hearts (reviewed in Rakusan, 1987). Moreover, in patients with long-term left ventricular hypertrophy associated with hypertension (Marcus et al., 1982) or aortic stenosis (Strauer, 1979), coronary reserve is usually markedly depressed. Thus, it is evident that major resistance vessels, as well as capillaries, are compromised in pressure-overload-induced hypertrophy of the heart. That growth of the coronary vasculature is severely limited in adults is suggested by an investigation that found that hearts with congenital aortic valve stenosis had normal capillary densities, whereas those with acquired aortic valve stenosis had markedly reduced capillary densities (Rakusan et al., 1994). Although such data on the surface appear to support the idea that in the adult heart vascular growth does not accompany ventricular enlargement, a more accurate conclusion is that coronary growth does not parallel myocardial growth. An examination of the literature indicates that capillary growth during or after cardiac hypertrophy in response to pressure overload is variable. Much of this variability can be attributed to differences in models of enhanced afterload, duration and magnitude of pressure overload, age, and species (reviewed in Tomanek, 1990).

In two models of pressure overload, we found that with time microvascular growth can match, or nearly match, the magnitude of ventricular enlargement. In the spontaneously hypertensive rat with moderate cardiac hypertrophy, neither capillary growth nor that of the major resistance vessels parallels the growth of the myocardium during the first 4 months of life in this species (Tomanek et al., 1982; Wangler et al., 1982). Upon the cessation of the increase in hypertrophy, however, vascular growth is sufficient to normalize capillary numerical and volume densities and maximal myocardial perfusion. The latter, when adjusted for perfusion pressure, is an index of the cross-sectional area of the coronary bed. Similarly, in long-term, "one-kidney, one-clip" hypertension in dogs, maximal myocardial perfusion is normalized and a substantial growth of the capillary bed nearly parallels the increase in ventricular mass (Tomanek et al., 1989; 1991). It should be emphasized that this compensatory growth is dependent upon the model of hypertension and perhaps other factors as well. When cardiac hypertrophy occurs in response to thyroxine, volume overload, or exercise training, a fully compensatory angiogenesis is not unusual (Tomanek and Torry, 1994, Chen et al., 1994; Tomanek et al., 1998; Tomanek, 1990, 1994).

ANGIOGENESIS AS A COMPONENT OF POSTNATAL GROWTH

Early postnatal growth is characterized by a high rate of capillary angiogenesis which far exceeds myocardial growth (Fig. 9.3). In the rat, left ventricular volume increases 12-fold, while absolute capillary length increases 21-fold during the first 11 days of postnatal life (Olivetti et al., 1980). This angiogenesis reduces mean intercapillary distance from 30 μm at day 1 to 17.5 μm at day 11. Capillary growth continues into adult life as overall capillary length increases between 5 and 52 weeks in this species (Mattfeld and Mall, 1987). Ventricular volume grows more, however, thus increasing mean intercapillary distance. Postnatal growth is also characterized by a maturation process involving biochemical changes and a remodeling process that adjusts orientation and increases homogeneity of spacing of capillaries (Rakusan et al., 1994).

Heart weight and cardiac myocyte size in mammals increase over the life span while capillary density tends to decrease slightly (Rakusan et al., 1994). The finding that arteriolar density decreases sharply during senescence suggests that angiogenesis is limited by factors associated with aging. This view is further supported by the observation of a marked decline in vascularity and maximal perfusion when cardiac hypertrophy develops in senescent rats as a consequence of late-onset hypertension (Tomanek et al., 1990, 1993). Data from senescent rats with hypertrophy induced by a 2-month treatment with thyroxine indicate that a significant coronary angiogenesis can occur, however, and that maximal myocardial perfusion can be maintained despite the development of cardiac hypertrophy (To-

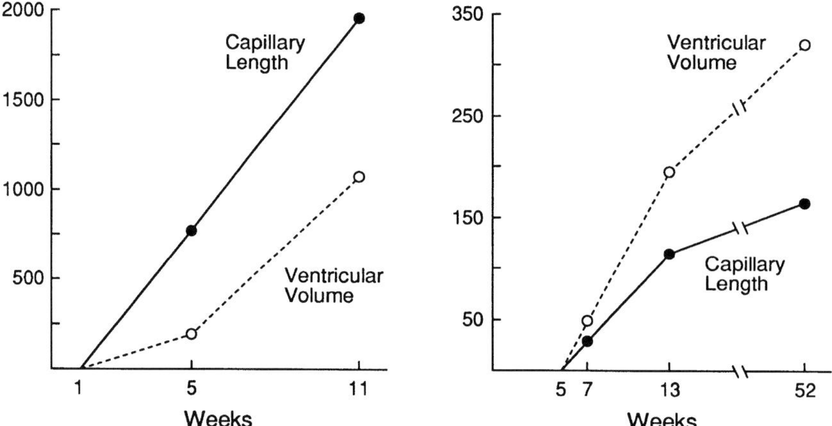

Figure 9.3. Capillary postnatal growth (capillary length) in relationship to ventricular growth (volume) for the rat. (Left) During the first 5 weeks capillary length increases more rapidly than than ventricular volume, but between weeks 5 and 11 capillary and ventricular growth are nearly parallel. (Right) In contrast, after the 13th week of postnatal life growth of the myocardium exceeds that of the capillary bed. Data on the Left are from Olivetti et al. (1980); data on the right are from Mattfeldt and Mall (1987).

manek et al., 1995). These findings suggest that the model of hypertrophy is a critical factor in determining the angiogenic response. In conclusion, age is a factor in coronary angiogenesis, but is not a major limiting factor when the appropriate stimulus for vascular growth is present.

PRESSURE AND VOLUME OVERLOAD

Ventricular hypertrophy in response to pressure or volume overload is commonly encountered in the clinical setting. Hypertension and vascular coarctation are common causes of pressure overload, while valvular disease is a major cause of volume overload. As noted earlier in this review, coronary angiogenesis occurs when an appropriate stimulus is present. Since pressure overload in adults is usually associated with inadequate growth of the coronary vasculature, one assumes that the stimulus for growth is inadequate. Despite the evidence from animal studies on long-term hypertension and hypertrophy that suggest that coronary vascular growth over time may compensate for the increased ventricular mass, data in humans indicate that long-term aortic stenosis or hypertension severely impairs coronary reserve (Harrison et al., 1991). This impairment may not be due entirely to the increase in ventricular mass, however, since vasoreactivity is affected by the presence of hypertension (Harrison et al., 1991). When cardiac hypertrophy occurs in response to a volume overload, such as is seen following experimentally induced aortocaval shunts, capillary and arteriolar growth have often been found to parallel the magnitude of hypertrophy in experimental volume overload (Tomanek and Torry, 1994). The arteriolar growth in the hypertrophic ventricle maintains the characteristic hierarchy of this segment of the vascular tree. Moreover, maximal coronary perfusion is normal in volume-overloaded hearts, a finding that indicates that capillary and precapillary growth are compensatory. These findings again support the concept that the stimulus for cardiac hypertrophy is an important determinant for coronary angiogenesis in the enlarged heart.

EXERCISE TRAINING, HYPOBARIC HYPOXIA, AND ANGIOGENESIS

The degree to which coronary angiogenesis occurs in response to exercise training has been controversial. The variable results reported in the literature (Laughlin and McAllister, 1992; Tomanek, 1994) can be explained by differences in experimental protocols regarding age, species, and type and intensity of training. It is clear that capillary proliferation is commonly observed in young, growing animals. The severity of the aerobic training is another important determinant of microvascular growth, with moderate training apparently being more conducive to capillary proliferation than strenuous training. Capillary density may be normal in hearts from trained animals with cardiac hypertrophy, a finding that indicates that a capillary growth proportional to the increase in ventricular mass occurred. At the same time, angiogenesis is apparently not dependent upon the presence of cardiac hypertrophy, since capillary density may increase even though heart weight is unchanged. Exercise training stimulates capillary growth in hearts of young, but not adult, hypertensive rats. This finding further supports the conclusion that capillary growth is more likely to occur in the young than in the adult. Arteriolar proliferation and an increase in diameter have also been documented in exercise-trained humans, monkeys, pigs, dogs, and rats.

Exposure to chronic hypobaric hypoxia for 2 weeks or longer, i.e., during actual or simulated high altitude, triggers cardiovascular adaptations, including ventricular hypertrophy. Most studies have found that capillary growth is stimulated under this condition (reviewed in Lund and Tomanek, 1980; and Turek et al., 1985). A common finding is that the degree of angiogenesis is proportional to the magnitude of right or left ventricular enlargement. In young guinea pigs exposed to hypobaric hypoxia, however, capillary density and capillary/fiber ratio were higher in both ventricles than in controls, even though only the right ventricle was significantly enlarged in the hypoxic group. Thus, capillary growth was not limited to hypertrophic myocardium. That vascular growth under hypobaric conditions is not linked to the development of cardiac hypertrophy is further supported by evidence that chronic exposure to hypobaria in rats with previously developed hypertrophy triggers angiogenesis without further cardiac enlargement (Lund and Tomanek, 1980). The degree of hypoxia at the tissue level is probably minimal during hypobaric exposure, since the hematocrit is increased. Thus, hypoxia is probably not a direct stimulus for endothelial cell proliferation, at least under these conditions.

THYROID HORMONE-INDUCED CARDIAC HYPERTROPHY AND ANGIOGENESIS

Most studies have found that cardiac hypertrophy in response to thyroid hormones is accompanied by a coronary angiogenesis that is clearly more marked than in other models, so that angiogenesis exceeds the magnitude of hypertrophy (Tomanek et al., 1995). Growth of both capillaries and resistance vessels occurs in this model, which is characterized by an enhanced coronary flow in response to a high metabolic rate and a volume overload of the ventricles (reviewed in Tomanek et al., 1995). The angiogenic response to thyroxine is rapid since endothelial cells of myocardial capillaries show an increase in DNA synthesis within 24 hours of a single thyroxine injection (Tomanek et al., 1998). Fibroblast growth factor-2 (basic FGF) mRNA is also upregulated in this model. Although the growth response is most marked in young rats, growth of capillary and precapillary vessels during cardiac hypertrophy in senescent rats is of sufficient magnitude to compensate for the additional myocardial mass. Thus, maximal coronary perfusion not compromised. These data indicate that age does not markedly affect coronary angiogenesis when the stimulus for growth is thyroxine. Such a finding stands in contrast to other models of cardiac hypertrophy, most notably pressure overload. As noted earlier, when experimental hypertension (''one-kidney, figure 8 renal wrap model'') was induced in senescent rats, capillary growth not only failed to occur, but an absolute reduction of capillaries was documented. Hypertension, however, has direct effects on the vasculature that may limit expansion of the microvascular bed. In addition, various models of hypertension differ with respect to endocrine and other humoral factors that may alter vessels independently of elevated arterial pressure. In sharp contrast to late-onset hypertension and hypertrophy, angiogenic factors regulating vascular growth in thyroxine-induced hypertrophy are not negated in senescence. These findings indicate that coronary angiogenesis can occur during cardiac hypertrophy in the aged if the appropriate stimulus is available. Recent evidence suggests that the thyroxine analog, diiodothyropropionic acid (DITPA) may serve as a useful therapeutic agent in the hypertrophic myocardium surviving infarction (Tomanek et al., 1998). Ten days of DITPA treatment in rats beginning 1 day after infarction induced capillary growth, which was most pronounced in the border region undergoing the most marked hypertrophy.

FACILITATION OF CORONARY ANGIOGENESIS BY AN INCREASED DIASTOLIC INTERVAL

Hudlicka and colleagues (1995) have demonstrated that long-term bradycardia induced by electrical pacing in rabbits and pigs and by the bradycardia drug alinidine in rats is associated with capillary growth. Although blood flow is not enhanced during bradycardiac pacing, the prolongation of the diastolic interval increases the duration of higher wall tension, since wall tension is higher in diastole than in systole. Accordingly, the authors propose that stretch of the capillary's basement membrane, which results from the increased wall tension, may trigger angiogenesis in this model. Whether this mechanical stimulus triggers appropriate growth factors has not been established; however, an increase in mRNA for transforming growth factor-β was noted in paced hearts. In agreement with these findings are data from growing rabbits, either with or without experimentally elevated blood pressure, that show that prolonged diastole due to hypothyroidism is associated with greater capillary growth than that documented in euthyroid rabbits (Tomanek and Torry, 1994).

MECHANISMS OF CORONARY ANGIOGENESIS

Angiogenesis is commonly believed to be triggered by primary stimuli that can be are categorized as (1) mechanical (Hudlicka et al., 1992), (2) energy imbalance due to hypoxia (Adair et al., 1990), or (3) inflammatory processes (Schaper 1993). Although these factors are not mutually exclusive (Rakusan, 1995), the first two are the most likely candidates in the nonischemic heart. While these primary stimuli may initiate a cascade of events that culminate in angiogenesis, there are, of course, many regulatory factors that must be activated. These include growth factors and various components of the extracellular matrix. Pericytes also play a regulatory role in angiogenesis (Tilton, 1991).

Increased Blood Flow as a Mechanical Stimulus for Angiogenesis

Increases in blood flow are accompanied by enhanced shear stress and wall tension, which have been long regarded as stimuli for vascular sprouting (Hudlicka et al., 1992, 1995). Endothelial cells are mechanoreceptors for shear stress and stretch; DNA synthesis in these cells occurs in response to cell flattening as well as by increases in flow or turbulence (Tomanek and Torry, 1994). Endothelial cells are, therefore, subjected to such physical forces in several models of cardiac hypertrophy since substantial blood flow elevations occur in the hyperthyroid state, during exercise, and, to a lesser degree, in altitude hypoxia. As noted earlier, capillary growth occurs under all three of these conditions. Moreover, if flow is elevated by chronic administration of dipyridamole, adenosine, xanthine derivatives, or alcohol, myocardial capillary proliferation is stimulated. Thus, chronic or intermittent elevations in flow are associated with coronary vascular growth. Since enhanced capillary flow results in increased wall shear stress, because capillary diameter is not altered (Hudlicka, 1994), a mechanical stimulus is available for capillary endothelial cell proliferation. In addition, adenosine production may underlie coronary angiogenesis in both the ischemic and nonischemic heart due to direct stimulation of endothelial cell proliferation by adenosine (Granger et al., 1994).

Finally, nitric oxide (NO) may provide a stimulus for angiogenesis related to increased flow (Granger et al., 1994) (see Chapters 2 and 13 for details).

Angiogenesis in Response to Mechanical Stimuli in the Absence of Increased Blood Flow

Coronary angiogenesis may also occur in the nonischemic heart during normal blood flow, as is the case with bradycardia and volume overload. As a consequence of the prolonged diastolic interval, capillary wall tension is higher for a longer period of the cardiac cycle, thus lengthening the time of the mechanical signal for angiogenesis (Hudlicka and Brown (1996)). One can also view the prolonged diastolic interval as enhancing the time that capillary diameter is in its relatively "dilated" state, since diastolic capillary diameter is greater than its systolic diameter (Tomanek and Torry, 1994). Thus, bradycardia prolongs the time that a capillary spends in a relatively elongated or stretched state. Volume overload is not characterized by either a significant increase in coronary perfusion or a protracted diastole. In this model, however, end diastolic ventricular dimensions are larger than hearts with a normal volume load and therefore capillaries must necessarily be subjected to a longitudinal stretch, since they are aligned with myocytes. This stretch occurs in both the transverse and longitudinal axes of the ventricle. Figure 9.4 summarizes the types of mechanical forces discussed in the various models of cardiac hypertrophy.

Molecular Signals for Angiogenesis

While mechanical factors may provide the initial impetus for angiogenesis in the heart, the cascade of events (e.g., cell proliferation and migration, extracellular matrix changes, and tube formation) that constitute angiogenesis require precise signaling mechanisms. These signals must facilitate all of the events in the angiogenic cascade, thus involving not only the endothelial cell, but also its basement membrane and other components of the extracellular matrix. One important effect of stretch on endothelial cells is the activation of Ca^{2+} channels, leading to increased intracellular concentration of this divalent ion, which enables cell proliferation. In this regard, vasodilation may be an important event facilitating angiogenesis. Vasodilation of venules prior to capillary sprouting

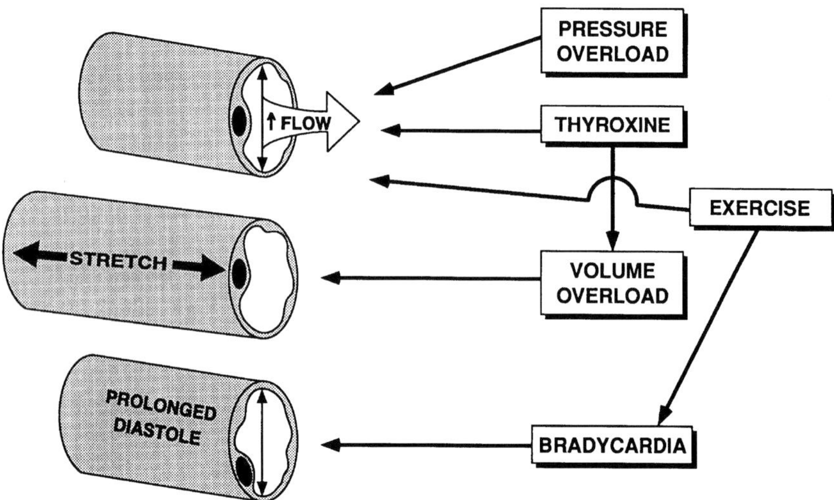

Figure 9.4. A summary of mechanical factors in several models of cardiac hypertrophy. A marked increase in flow occurs with elevated thyroxine levels or during exercise and may provide for enhanced shear stress and wall tension. Angiogenesis over time during pressure overload may also be stimulated by a modest increased flow/capillary as a consequence of increased myocyte mass. Increased diastolic filling, characteristic of volume overload as well as thyroxine, stretches capillaries longitudinally as diastolic cardiac dimensions are enhanced (compared to normal diastolic filling). Volume overload characterizes thyroxine treatment, as well as A-V fistulae. Finally, prolonged diastole during bradycardia enables capillary wall tension to remain elevated for a longer duration of the cardiac cycle, and in addition may provide a longitudinal stretch due to increased diastolic filling. Exercise training, in addition to enhancing flow acutely, facilitates a resting bradycardia.

from these vessels has been noted and may be an important step in the process of angiogenesis (Folkman and Shing, 1992). Indeed, endothelial cells may become more responsive to growth factors when they become stretched. The role of growth factors (reviewed by Klagsbrun and D'Amore, 1991; Folkman and Shing, 1992), well documented in other models of angiogenesis (e.g., tumors), has yet to be established in the nonischemic heart. Of the various angiogenic polypeptides, fibroblast growth factor (FGF−2) and vascular endothelial growth factor (VEGF) are good candidates for the regulation of angiogenesis in the myocardium.

There is some evidence supporting the idea that mechanical stress triggers FGF−2 secretion by cardiac myocytes. Beta-adrenergic stimulation of heart rate and force of contraction, which caused increases in the number of reversibly wounded myocytes, was associated with an enhancement in FGF−1 and FGF−2 release from the heart studied ex vivo (Clarke et al., 1995). Another report indicates that increased mechanical activity due to continuous pacing of rat ventricular myocyte in vitro caused a hypertrophic response of these cells, which could be blocked by neutralizing anti-FGF−2 antibodies (Kaye et al., 1996). Moreover, the media from the paced cells contained higher titers of FGF−2. In contrast, neither FGF−1 nor FGF−2 was upregulated in response to banding of the pulmonary artery of swine (Carroll et al., 1995). Thus, while there is evidence for mechanical stimulation of FGF release in the myocardium, there are no data available to support the hypothesis that FGF plays a key role during cardiac hypertrophy.

VEGF has been implicated in angiogenesis in models of ischemia and/or hypoxia (Banai et al., 1994). Moreover, evidence of its upregulation in pressure-overload-induced cardiac hypertrophy in a nonischemic model has also been demonstrated (Carroll et al., 1995). Three to seven hours after banding of the pulmonary artery, a three to fourfold increase in mRNA for VEGF in the right ventricle, as well as increases in urokinase-type plasminogen activator at these time points, was noted. The latter is important in angiogenesis because it facilitates the breakdown of the basement membrane. (See Chapter 2 for details.) Evidence of cell damage and inflammation was documented by histological changes and increases in JE (an early gene which encodes a cytokine chemoattractant) and intercellular adhesion molecule (which plays a role in extravasation of monocytes). Whether some degree of hypoxia occurs in the myocytes of the right ventricle in this model during the early phase of pressure overload has not been determined. Accordingly, the stimulus for upregulation of VEGF during the acute phase of cardiac hypertrophy due to sudden and marked increase in ventricular pressure cannot be ascertained; however, muscle cell injury appears to be one explanation. Recent experimental evidence supports stretch as a mechanical trigger for VEGF. Li and colleagues (1997) demonstrated that stretch stimulated an upregulation of VEGF message in rat hearts subjected to an end-diastolic overload of 35 mmHg for 30 minutes. This increase was mediated by TGF-β since inhibition of this growth factor prevented VEGF mRNA upregulation. These data support the hypothesis that stretch is an important signal for VEGF and, therefore, angiogenesis.

Some increase in transforming growth factor-β (TGF-β) in bradycardiac paced hearts which undergo capillary proliferation has been reported (Hudlicka and Brown, 1996). This growth factor has not been shown to be a mitogen for coronary endothelial cells, but plays a role in extracellular matrix formation. Two other angiogenic molecules have been found in hearts after long-term bradycardiac pacing: (1) a low molecular weight angiogenic factor previously identified in hearts with myocardial infarction and (2) endothelial cell stimulating angiogenic factor, which has been identified in many other tissues (Hudlicka and Brown, 1996). We have recently documented an increase in both VEGF mRNA and protein in hearts of rats with bradycardia induced by the drug alinidine (Zheng and Tomanek, 1998). In this model, VEGF mRNA was elevated after 1 week of pacing, prior to an increase in capillary length density. The latter was enhanced by 40% after 3 weeks of pacing.

SUMMARY AND CONCLUSIONS

Angiogenesis in the nonischemic myocardium occurs during normal postnatal growth and to a variable degree during cardiac hypertrophy. Although age plays a role in most models of cardiac enlargement, angiogenesis occurs if an appropriate stimulus is provided, e.g., thyroxine. The extent of angiogenesis in the hypertrophic heart is dependent upon the stimulus evoking the hypertrophy. Data from animals with experimentally induced cardiac hypertrophy suggest that the presence of mechanical factors that place endothelial cells in a relatively stretched position favor angiogenesis. Thus, a substantial microvascular growth has been documented in models in which increases occur in (1) coronary flow, (2) diastolic interval, or (3) ventricular filling. Stretch of endothelial cells is a likely mechanical factor that is available in all three model types. The link between the mechanical factors and the molecular signals for angiogenesis is not established in the nonischemic myocardium. The extracellular matrix and growth factors and their receptors are almost undoubtedly involved. FGF−2 and VEGF are two growth factors implicated in this process, as both have been shown to be effective in facilitating neovascularization of the nonischemic myocardium. Nevertheless, the synergistic actions of these and other growth factors in angiogenesis during postnatal growth and in adaptive growth in the adult are not understood.

REFERENCES

Adair, T. H., Gay, W. J., and Montani, J. P. (1990). Growth regulation of the vascular system: evidence for a metabolic hypothesis. Am. J. Physiol. 259: R393–R404.

Banai, S., Jaklitsch, M. T., Shou, M., Lazarous, D. F., Scheinowitz, M., Biro, S., Epstein, S. E., and Unger, E. F. (1994). Angiogenic-induced enhancement of collateral blood flow to ischemic myocardium by vascular endothelial growth factor in dogs. Circulation 89: 2183–2189.

Carroll, S. M., Nimmo, L. E., Knoepfler, P. S., White, F. C. and Bloor, C. M. (1995). Gene expression in a swine model of right ventricular hypertrophy: intercellular adhesion molecule, vascular endothelial growth factor and plasminogen activators are upregulated during pressure overload. J. Mol. Cell. Cardiol. 27: 1427–1441.

Chen, Y., Torry, R. J., Baumbach, G. L., and Tomanek, R. J. Proportional arteriolar growth accompanies cardiac hypertrophy induced by volume overload. (1994). Am. J. Physiol. 267: H2132–H2137.

Clarke, M. S., Caldwell, R. W., Chiao, H., Miyake, K., and McNeil, P. L. (1995). Contraction-induced cell wounding and release of fibroblast growth factor in heart. Circ. Res. 76: 927–934.

Folkman, J. and Shing, Y. (1992). Angiogenesis. J. Biol. Chem. 16: 10931–10934.

Granger, H. J., Ziche, M., Hawker, J. R., Meininger, C. J., Czisny, L. E., and Zawieja, D. C. (1994). Molecular and cellular basis of myocardial angiogenesis. Cell. Mol. Biol. 40: 81–85.

Harrison, D. G., Marcus, M. L., Dellsperger, K. C., Lamping, K. G., and Tomanek, R. J. (1991). Pathophysiology of myocardial perfusion in hypertension. Circulation 83 Suppl. III: III–14–III–18.

Hudlicka, O. (1994). Mechanical factors involved in the growth of the heart and its blood vessels. Cell. Mol. Biol. Res. 40: 143–152.

Hudlicka, O. and Brown, M.D. (1996). Postnatal growth of the heart and its blood vessels. J. Vasc. Res. 33(4): 266–287.

Hudlicka, O., Brown, M.D., and Egginton, S. (1992). Angiogenesis in skeletal and cardiac muscle. Physiol. Rev. 72: 369–417.

Hudlicka, O., Brown, M.D., Walter, H., Weiss, J. B., and Bate, A. (1995). Factors involved in capillary growth in the heart. Mol. Cell. Biochem. 147: 57–68.

Kaye, D., Pimental, D., Prasad, S., Maki, T., Berger, H. J., McNeil, P. L., Smith, T. W., and Kelly, R. A. (1996). Role of transiently altered sarcolemmal membrane permeability and basic fibroblast growth factor release in the hypertrophic response of adult rat ventricular myocytes to increased mechanical activity in vitro. J. Clin. Invest. 97: 281–291.

Klagsbrun, M. and D'Amore, P. A.. (1991) Regulators of angiogenesis. Annu. Rev. Physiol. 53: 217–239.

Laughlin, M. H. and McAllister, R. M. (1992). Exercise training-induced coronary vascular adaptation. J. Appl. Physiol. 73: 2209–2225.

Lund, D. D. and Tomanek, R. J. (1980). The effects of chronic hypoxia on the myocardial cell of normotensive and hypertensive rats. Anat. Rec. 196: 421–430.

Marcus, M. L., Doty, D. B., Hiratzka, L. F., Wright, C. B. and Eastham, C. L. (1982) Decreased coronary reserve mechanism for angina pectoris in patients with aortic stenosis and normal coronary arteries. N. Engl J. Med. 307: 1362–1367.

Mattfeldt, T. and Mall, G. (1987). Growth of capillaries and myocardial cells in normal rat heart. J. Mol. Cell. Cardiol. 19: 1237–1246.

Olivetti, G., Anversa, P., and Loud, A. V. (1980). Morphometric study of early postnatal development in the left and right ventricular myocardium of the rat. II. Tissue composition, capillary growth, and sarcoplasmic alterations. Circ. Res. 46: 503–512.

Rakusan, K. (1987). Microcirculation in the stressed heart. In "The Stressed Heart" (M. J. Legato, ed.) pp 107–123. Nijhoff, Boston.

Rakusan, K. (1995). Coronary angiogenesis—from morphometry to molecular biology and back. Ann. N.Y. Acad. Sci. 752: 257–266.

Rakusan, K., Cicutti, N., and Flanagan, M. F. (1994). Changes in the microvascular network during cardiac growth, development, and aging. Cell. Mol. Biol. Res. 40: 117–122.

Schaper, W. (1993). New paradigms for collateral vessel growth [editorial]. Basic Res. Cardiol. 88(3): 193–198.

Strauer, B. E. (1979). Ventricular function and coronary hemodynamics in hypertensive heart disease. Am. J. Cardiol. 44: 999–1007.

Tilton, R. G. (1991). Capillary pericytes: perspectives and future trends. J. Electron Microsc. Tech. 19: 327–344.

Tomanek, R. J. (1990) Response of the coronary vasculature to myocardial hypertrophy. J. Am. Coll. Cardiol. 15: 528–533.

Tomanek, R. J. (1994). Exercise induced coronary angiogenesis. Med. Sci. Sports Exerc. 26: 1245–1251.

Tomanek, R. J. and Torry, R. J. (1994) Growth of the coronary vasculature in hypertrophy; mechanisms and model dependence. Cell. Mol. Biol. Res. 40: 129–136.

Tomanek, R. J., Searls, J. C., and Lachenbruch, P. A. (1982). Quantitative changes in the capillary bed during developing peak and stabilized cardiac hypertrophy in the spontaneously hypertensive rat. Circ. Res. 51: 295–304.

Tomanek, R. J., Schalk, K. A., Marcus, M. L., and Harrison, D. G. (1989). Coronary angiogenesis during long-term hypertension and left ventricular hypertrophy in dogs. Circ. Res. 65: 352–359.

Tomanek, R. J., Aydelotte, M. R., and Butters, C. A. (1990). Late-onset renal hypertension in old rats alters myocardial microvessels. Am. J. Physiol. 259: H1681–H1687.

Tomanek, R. J., Wessel, T. J. and Harrison, D. G. (1991). Capillary growth and geometry during long-term hypertension and myocardial hypertrophy in dogs. Am. J. Physiol. 261: H1011–H1018.

Tomanek, R. J., Aydelotte, M. R., Anderson, K. E., and Torry, R. J. (1993). Coronary blood flow in senescent rats with late-onset hypertension. Am. J. Physiol. 264: H1854–H1860.

Tomanek, R. J., Connell, P. M., Butters, C. A., and Torry, R. J. (1995). Compensated coronary microvascular growth in senescent rats with thyroxine-induced cardiac hypertrophy. Am. J. Physiol. 268: H419–H425.

Tomanek, R. J., Doty, M. K., and Sandra, A. (1998). Early coronary angiogenesis in response to thyroxine: growth characteristics and upregulation of basic fibroblast growth factor. Circ. Res. 82: 587–593.

Tomanek, R. J., Zimmerman, Suvarna, P. R., Morkin E., Pennock, G. D. and Goldman, S. (1998). A thyroid hormone analog stimulates angiogenesis in the postinfarcted rat heart. J. Molec. Cell Cardiol., 30: 923–932.

Turek, Z., Hoofd, L. J. C., Ringnalda, B. E., and Rakusan, K. (1985). Myocardial capillarity of rats exposed to simulated high altitude. Adv. Exp. Med. Biol. 191: 249–255, 1985.

Van Groningen, J. P., Wenink, A. C. G., and Testers, L. H. M. (1991). Myocardial capillaries: increase in number by splitting of existing vessels. Acta Embryol. 184: 65–70.

Wangler, R. D., Peters, K. G., Marcus, M. L., and Tomanek, R. J. (1982). Effects of duration and severity of arterial hypertension and cardiac hypertrophy on coronary vasodilator reserve. Circ. Res. 51: 10–18.

Zheng, W., and Tomanek, R. J. VEGF is upregulated in bradycardia-induced coronary angiogenesis in rat. FASEB J. 12: A71, 1998.

10

Animal Models of Angiogenesis in Cardiovascular Tissues

J. GARY MESZAROS, LAURENCE L. BRUNTON, AND COLIN M. BLOOR

Assessment of the physiologic triggers of angiogenesis and growth factors with therapeutic potential in myocardial ischemia (described elsewhere in this book) have depended on the use of large animal models of myocardial ischemia and collateral flow. Understanding the rationale behind, and the limitations of, these animal models is important for interpreting the results of interventions that alter angiogenesis. In this chapter, large-animal models of coronary collateral formation and angiogenesis will be described, along with a model of peripheral ischemia.

EFFECTS OF A DECREASE IN VESSEL DIAMETER ON THE RESISTANCE TO BLOOD FLOW

Genesis of new blood vessels in the heart can be studied during embryonic development and in the early postnatal period. After that, the vascularization of the heart may be considered mature but subject to predictable changes with the time. Chief among these are responses to the rise in both diastolic and systolic blood pressure that occurs with age, due mainly to the progressive deposition of atherosclerotic material on vessel walls. This reduction in radius of the arterial vessels greatly increases the resistance to flow. By Poiseuille's equation,

$$\Delta\text{Pressure} = (\text{Flow})\ (\text{Resistance})$$

If flow is to be constant, then, as resistance increases, the pressure gradient across the resistance must increase. This increase may be interpreted as either a requirement for higher pressure to maintain adequate perfusion through progressively smaller vessels or as diminution of flow with constant pressure.

Modest occlusion of vessels has an effect that is larger than one might expect, that is, flow is not proportional to the cross-sectional area of a vessel (πr^2) as intuition might suggest. Rather, flow varies with the fourth power of the radius, due to the contribution of friction. In terms of resistance, Poiseuille's equation states that

$$\text{Resistance} = (\Delta\text{Pressure})/(\text{Flow}) = (8L\nu)/(\pi r^4),$$

where L = length of the blood vessel, ν = viscosity of the blood, and r = radius of the vessel. Thus, resistance varies *inversely* with the fourth power of r. A reduction of r by 10%, to $0.9r$, would increase resistance by $L/(0.9)^4$, which is 1.52. This analysis shows that diminishing vessel radius by 10% can increase resistance by more than 50%. Thus, the physiologic effects of clogging of the arteries are a complex combination of direct and indirect changes in both the cardiovascular system and in all tissues to be perfused. Pressure in the system can rise; tissue perfusion, oxygen delivery, and removal of metabolic products may be reduced. Among the responses to those changes is proliferation in the coronary circulation.

FORMATION OF COLLATERAL VESSELS AS A PHYSIOLOGIC COMPENSATION FOR REDUCED OXYGEN DELIVERY AND INCREASED WORKLOAD

Pumping blood against increased peripheral resistance causes the heart to do more work, and thus to require more oxygen. Among the changes that one notices in a heart that is working substantially harder on a long-term basis are hypertrophy and increased vascularization. These responses can be thought of as physiologic compensations for stress on the heart, or, put another way, as intrinsic mechanisms by which the heart changes so that oxygen supply will meet oxygen demand.

An abrupt reduction in flow and oxygenation of cardiac tissue, such as that produced by ischemia accompanying severe angina or a myocardial infarction, also produces conditions that promote angiogenesis. Repetitive but reversible periods of ischemia that mimic angina in humans also produce an angiogenic response.

STIMULATION OF ANGIOGENESIS BY EXPERIMENTAL ALTERATION OF BLOOD FLOW

There are many experimental paradigms for altering flow, but common mechanisms probably mediate the angiogenic response. By altering blood flow, researchers can experimentally establish conditions in laboratory animals that will cause angiogenic responses in the heart. Although most research has focused on models that induce angiogenesis of coronary collateral vessels in the heart, some studies have been conducted on the peripheral circulation and on other organs, such as the lung. In all of the experimental tissues, the stimuli for angiogenesis probably all upregulate polypeptide growth factors and proteolytic enzymes. By light microscopy, the first response to an angiogenic stimulus is the growth of endothelial cells in capillaries, and to a lesser extent, in small arterioles and venules. Remodeling of capillary-size vessels to small arterioles and venules quickly follows this early response.

FACTORS THAT INFLUENCE THE CHOICE OF LARGE ANIMAL MODELS OF ANGIOGENESIS

In evaluating the utility of any animal model of a human disease, one should consider to what extent the experimental animal system mimics the disease. Such evaluation is frequently superficial, since the biology of the human disease under study (in this case, myocardial ischemia) may not be fully understood. In the case of models of angiogenesis, it is important to consider whether one species is experimentally advantageous over another, whether a model is readily and reproducibly established in the laboratory, whether the data obtained are reproducible, and whether the model produces the desired angiogenic response without obvious and limiting side effects (such as morbidity). Each model has its own strengths and weaknesses; for instance, a model may mimic specific aspects of a human disease but not others. Also, different models may provide cellular material suitable for studying distinct aspects of angiogenesis using different types of analysis; for instance, a model selected to produce tissue for in situ cytochemical staining may differ from one designed to produce a relatively homogeneous population of cells for extraction of mRNA. Thus, the choice of a particular experimental model of angiogenesis may depend on factors as disparate as experimental goals, available expertise and equipment, budget, and intuition.

THE AMEROID CONSTRICTOR MODEL

Slow, progressive coronary artery occlusion can be achieved by use of an ameroid occluder. Ameroid is a modified casein substance that expands as it becomes hydrated. An elder statesman of pathology can recall a time just after World War II when the buttons of raincoats were made of ameroid. This gives rise to a picture—in black and white, of course—of Humphrey Bogart at the end of a long wet day as a gumshoe, trapped in his trench coat, struggling to get his buttons, newly swollen to 30 mm in diameter, through 25-mm button holes.

If a slotted ring of ameroid is put over a vessel, such as a coronary artery, and outward expansion is prevented by an outer ring of an inflexible material (stainless steel), then the expansion of the ameroid as it hydrates will be directed inward. As hydration proceeds, the central hole in the ameroid through which the vessel passes becomes gradually smaller. If the size of the initial hole and the quantity of ameroid are sufficient, the vessel will become occluded. Figure 10.1 shows the details of the positioning of an ameroid occluder and two designs for occluders.

Choosing the type and size of an ameroid occluder is not always straightforward. Fortunately, many studies using these methods have been performed, and it is usually possible find a description of the methods used for a particular animal according to age (size) and vessel that one wishes to occlude in the published literature (Schaper et al., 1969; White et al., 1992; Carroll, 1997). The dimensions shown in Table 10.1 are helpful for planning experiments using laboratory pigs or dogs. Installing the occluder is not a trivial process for either the experimental subject or the experimenter. The occluder must be inserted surgically with a procedure that requires maintenance of surgical anesthesia and a monitored postoperative period (see Schaper et al., 1969; White et al., 1992, for details of anesthesia for dogs and pigs). Generally, ameroid occluders are placed on the left circumflex coronary artery after a sterile left lateral thoracotomy in the fourth intercostal space, opening of the pericardial sac, and isolation of the left circumflex artery. To monitor the progress of constriction and subsequent recovery of blood flow, the experimenter also implants a coronary flow probe and a cuff occluder that is used to obtain zero flow for calibration of the flow probe. Depending on the nature of the study, it may be desirable to implant probes for ventricular pressure development and wall motion and for ECG measurements. After all instruments have been inserted, the pericardium and then the thoracotomy are closed. Animals usually are allowed to recover from surgery for 2 weeks before studies are performed; thus, animal care costs are significant.

Although these methods reliably produce vascular occlusion, the timing of such an occlusion is difficult to control or predict. Figure 10.2 shows the rate at which flow is occluded in a pig using the experimental approach shown in Figure 10.1. The sequence of events as the occluder hydrates includes increased dilation of the blood vessel downstream of the occluder to sustain flow until no more dilation is possible; then, as the occluder continues to expand inward, flow decreases, and finally ceases altogether. No systematic study of how shape and thickness of the ameroid ring affect the rate of occlusion has been reported. Thus, it is not clear whether the rate of occlusion in this model can be varied precisely. Total occlusion occurs about 10–17 days following insertion of the ameroid device (Carroll, 1997). From microsphere and morphometric studies, it is clear is that angiogenesis is well under way by day 14 after implantation

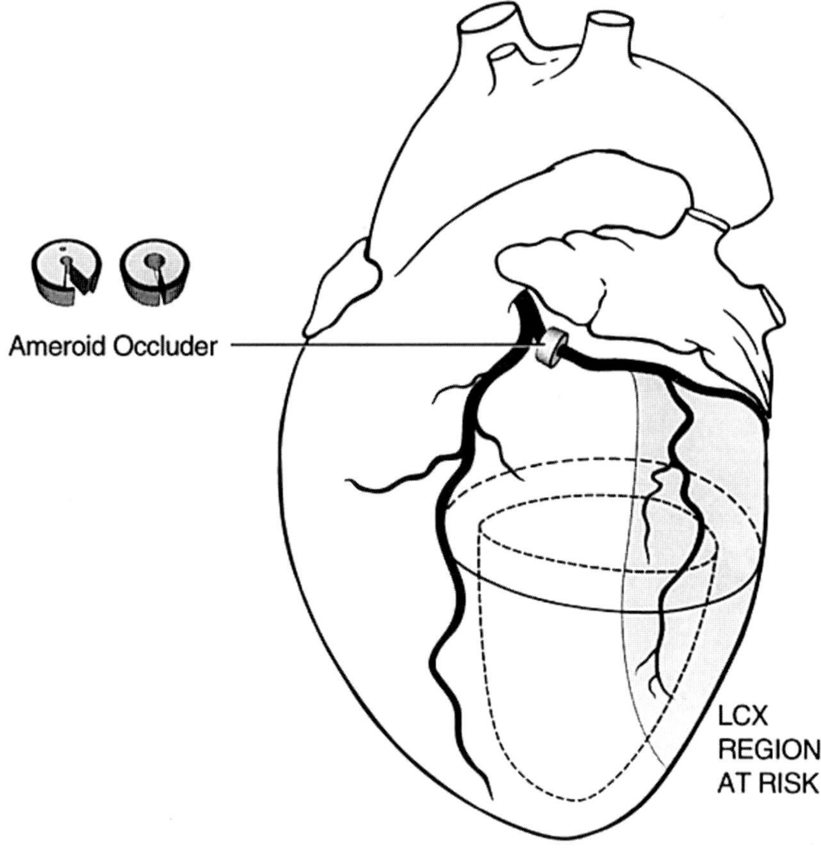

Figure 10.1. Ameroid occlusion of a coronary artery. The ameroid occluder is placed on the left circumflex artery (LCX); then a stainless steel band is placed outside the ameroid to focus the swelling of the material inward. The gray area indicates the vascular bed of the LCX, which is at risk when gradual coronary occlusion occurs as the ameroid device constricts the vessel. The dashed lines indicate the chamber of the left ventricle. Collateral vessels develop from neighboring vessels such as the LAD. Ameroid occluders come in several geometries: the original design (above, left) was a central hole (2.5–3 mm) for the vessel with a slot to the edge for putting the ameroid onto the vessel. Occlusion with this design is not always complete. A more recent design is the example on the right in which the vessel is placed in the wedge-shaped area (3.5–4 mm wide at the maximum radius) and held in place by the outer steel ring. This design presses the vessel shut more reliably and quickly than the old design. In either case, the overall diameter of the device is approximately 9 mm. (Figure taken from Carroll [1997] and used with permission.)

Table 10.1 Coronary Blood Vessel Diameters[a]

HUMAN	
Right coronary artery	1.5–5.5 mm
Left coronary artery	5–10 mm
Left circumflex artery	1.5–5 mm
Interventricular arteries	2–5 mm
INNATE COLLATERALS	
Human	40–500 μm
Dog	40–200 μm
Pig	40–80 μm
CORONARY ARTERIOLES[b]	20–100 μm
CORONARY CAPILLARIES[b]	4–12 μm

[a] Measurements are valid for humans, dogs, and pigs.
[b] Target vessels most used for microembolization.

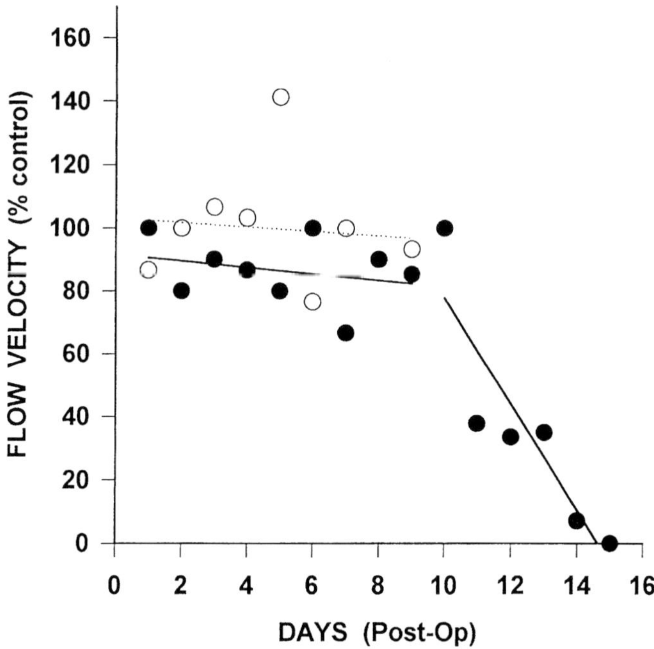

Figure 10.2. Flow measurements in control and ameroid-occluded pigs. Doppler flow velocity measurements were made in a control pig (sham operated; open circles) and a pig in which an ameroid occluder had been placed (closed circles). The data show peak diastolic flow in the LCX (distal to the occluder in the ameroid pig). Flow in the control pig was relatively constant during the entire experiment. In the ameroid-implanted pig, flow was constant for 10 days and then fell over the next 4 to 5 days.

of the occluder (White et al., 1992). The resulting occlusion is relatively reproducible and the variability of the method is within that of most physiologic systems. The time at which the angiogenic response occurs following occlusion varies among experiments and is difficult to predict. Thus, it is essential to assess the time course of flow distribution (using radiolabeled microspheres) and to quantify regional angiogenesis via morphometric analysis and other techniques. These procedures have been well summarized (White et al., 1992). Failure to correlate molecular changes with assessment of the tissue can result in a false impression of the relationship between angiogenesis and molecular events.

Ameroid occlusion has been applied successfully to dogs and pigs. In the dog, evidence of occlusion followed by collateral vessel development is dramatic and reproducible. Measured flow through the left circumflex artery decreases to 5% to 15% of control by 10 to 14 days. By 4 to 6 weeks, flow into the ischemic region has returned to normal levels, indicating that the angiogenic response (collateral vessel development) has fully compensated for the blockade of flow by the ameroid constrictor. After the flow has been restored by the development of collateral or new vessels, pharmacological or physiological vasodilation causes blood flow to increase above resting levels in the region downstream from the ameroid occluder, indicating that a significant coronary collateral reserve is available for recruitment. Thus, the ameroid model induces the development of a large quantity of physiologically and pharmacologically responsive vessels in the dog.

In the pig, ameroid occlusion produces a somewhat different series of events (White et al., 1992). Following insertion of an ameroid device around the left circumflex artery, there is a gradual occlusion of the artery that results in small uniform infarcts with minimal contractile dysfunction. In this model, the ameroid occluder induces pathophysiological responses that resemble those of the chronically ischemic myocardium. Studies using this model suggest that collateral development abruptly ceases early after ameroid placement and that there is a general lack of coronary collateral reserve.

The pig has few innate coronary collaterals. Thus, abrupt occlusion of a coronary artery in a pig results in either death or a large infarct. Gradual occlusion of the pig's left circumflex artery, however, leads to collateral development and preservation of tissue. Unlike the case in some other mammals, the left circumflex artery of the pig delivers blood to only 25% of the left ventricle and there is little collateral circulation in this region (collateral flow is about 60 μl/min/g of ventricle). As a result, a model that features occlusion of the left circumflex artery is attractive to researchers because of the possibility that collateral growth is easy to detect and might be very effective in supplying blood flow to a small region of myocardium following application of an ameroid occluder to the left circumflex artery. In fact, experiments have shown that within 2 weeks of occlusion collateral circulation develops to a level that provides normal coronary blood flow. This flow is still limiting when the pig is subjected to exercise, however; indeed, exercise-induced ischemia persists for as long as 6 months following occlusion of the left circumflex artery. This exercise-induced underperfusion occurs primarily in the endocardium and midmyocardium; the epicardial region shows normal blood flow. Thus, gradual occlusion of the left circumflex artery of the pig induces an angiogenic response, and also provides a stable model of persistent exercise-induced ischemia (White et al., 1992).

The time courses of vessel development and physical appearances of the vessels have been compared in swine and canine models in which ameroid occlusion is used. The rate of development of the medial layer in emerging collaterals during the first month after ameroid placement is similar in dogs and pigs. In subsequent months, however, maturation of the medial wall of the collaterals (seen in microscopic sections as wall thickening, due to accumulation of smooth muscle in the wall) continues in the dog, whereas collateral vessels in the pig show little further development and have distinctly thinner walls than do normal vessels of the same diameter. The total number of collateral vessels increases within 8 weeks of ameroid occlusion in the pig (White et al., 1992). The number of collateral vessels doubled in the "ameroid occluded" animals compared to the control animals. The regional distribution of these new collateral vessels was similar to that of the collaterals seen in control animals. In addition to the increased number of collaterals in the "ameroid occluded" animals, there was also a significant increase in the number of larger collaterals, ranging in diameter from 20 to 60 μm. This morphologic change has functional significance, since flow through these channels is critical in perfusing the ischemic regions of the heart. The time courses of the morphologic changes in the dog are similar to those in the pig model (Schaper, 1971). Additionally, ameroid occlusion of the pig heart may also lead to the development of numerous small vessels (< 20 μm diameter) that, because of their small radii and the consequences of Poiseuille's law, would not be expected to contribute significantly to flow. In contrast to the underdeveloped vessels that are found in swine and humans, the coronary collaterals of the dog are well developed, with a medial wall thickness that approaches that of normal arterioles. After several months, the dog's newly formed collateral vessels have a normal amount of medial smooth muscle, a characteristic used as evidence of "mature" collaterals.

By that criterion, the pig fails to develop mature intercoronary collateral vessels. The consequences of this underdevelopment are a predictable decrease in the vasoconstrictive and autoregulatory potential of these vessels. In fact, "ameroid-occluded" pigs, which exhibit normal exercise-induced hyperemia at moderate exercise levels, have ischemia at strenuous exercise levels. Pigs, in contrast to dogs, have a limited collateral reserve that does not permit blood flow sufficient for the demands of strenuous exercise, even under conditions of vasodilation.

There are at least four ways by which angiogenic changes can be quantified: counting of blood vessels in tissue sections from the hearts of animals examined at different times after occlusion; measurement of collateral flow with flow probes inserted at the time of surgery; detection of the incorporation of radiolabeled thymidine as an indicator of nucleic acid synthesis; and measurement of the density of injected radiolabeled microspheres, to assess flow. Endocardial collateral flow increases over 14-fold in the 3 weeks following ameroid occlusion of the left circumflex in pigs, from 60 l/min/g to 860 l/min/g (White et. al., 1992). Morphometric analysis of the number and sizes of blood vessels and physiologic data on blood flow suggests that collateral development in the pig reaches a plateau 8 weeks after placement of the ameroid constrictor on the left circumflex coronary artery. Incorporation of [^{3}H] thymidine suggests a similar time course, with the labeling index (a direct measure of cell division in the vessels) achieving a maximum at 2 to 3 weeks after ameroid placement. The labeling indices then decreased, more rapidly in the pig than in the dog. There was a 50–70-fold increase in the labeling index of both endothelial and smooth muscle cells in the pig ameroid model. In the dog, the overall time course is similar, but the labeling index is three times greater than in the pig (White et al., 1992; Schaper, 1971; Pasynck et al., 1982). This finding reflects the large angiogenic response of the dog, with newly synthesized or expanding collateral vessels providing nearly complete restoration of blood flow in the region of the ameroid occluder. Revascularization in the pig heart is much more limited and, importantly, resembles that in the human heart. The molecular, cellular, and hormonal bases for the different extents of angiogenesis following occlusion in various species are areas of active research. Although bromodeoxyuridne (BrdU) labeling is a common measure of rapidly dividing cells, few studies have examined whether it is a useful index in the ameroid model. BrdU labeling has been used to determine the degree of angiogenesis occurring after gene transfer into the ameroid model (Giordano et al., 1996). Since control animals in that study also had ameroid constrictors, there are no comparative data available from sham animals without ameroid occluders, and thus the background level of DNA synthesis is not known.

Within 3 weeks of the onset of ameroid occlusion, there is a significant increase in the number of capillaries in the ischemic region, shown by an increase in density of nearly 20% above control (White and Bloor, 1992), which returns to normal levels several weeks later. More importantly from a functional viewpoint are the changes that occur in the arterioles of the ischemic region. The density of arterioles also increases at 3 weeks after the onset of ameroid occlusion, but remains increased above normal levels at later time points. The cross-sectional area of the arteriolar bed shows a 25% increase above control at 3 weeks, but by 8 weeks it increases further after the onset of ameroid occlusion to 154% of control. This increase in the cross-sectional area of the arteriolar bed has a large effect on collateral blood flow to the ischemic region. Taken together, the changes in the capillary and arteriolar beds suggest that the early angiogenic changes occur in the capillaries and with time then affect the arteriolar bed with resultant further remodeling.

One surprising feature of the swine heart is that extracardiac conduits of blood flow can be important for myocardial perfusion (White et al., 1989). These extracardiac collaterals extend mainly from the internal mammary and bronchial arteries and from the lung, if it is permitted to adhere to the surface of the heart. Such collaterals appear along a time course similar to that of the intercoronary collaterals and have a smooth muscle mass intermediate between that of normal vessels and that of the thinner-walled coronary collaterals. Extracardiac coronary collaterals may provide complete restoration of coronary blood flow to an ischemic region and can represent a large portion of overall oxygen delivery, especially during ischemia, in which extracardiac collateral flow may contribute 30% of the total collateral flow. It is possible that extracardiac vessels could be similarly important in humans, especially with increasing age or in the presence of coronary stenosis.

There is relatively little information regarding changes in gene expression induced by ischemia produced by the ameroid occlusion model. This reflects the variability of closure times by ameroid occluders of various designs. The window of changes in gene expression may be narrow; thus it is critical that the selected ameroid occluder causes reproducible results in dependable times of occlusion so that tissue samples can be obtained at the optimal times. The expression of extracellular matrix metalloproteinases and tissue plasminogen activators increases in the ameroid model (Tyagi et al., 1996), which suggests that upregulation of vascular remodeling mechanisms occurs during chronic ischemia, and thus may play a critical role in collateral development. Also, urokinase type plasminogen activator activity increases in the ischemic region in the heart subjected to ameroid occlusion (Knoepfler et al., 1995). Its expression reaches a peak at 6 days after the onset of ameroid occlusion and 1 week later has returned to control levels, reaffirming the transient nature of increased gene expression.

REPETITIVE ISCHEMIA MODEL

Periodic, brief occlusion of coronary flow, repeated for several weeks, will induce an angiogenic response. The procedure is usually carried out on a chronically instrumented animal in which occlusion can be accomplished by remote activation of a pneumatic occluder cuff. The left circumflex artery is generally the vessel chosen, since its brief occlusion is less frequently lethal than is compared to occlusion of the left anterior descending (LAD) and because it is more accessible from an opening in the chest. Repetitive ischemia has been used most successfully in dogs

(Mohri et al., 1989; Fujita et al., 1987; Franklin et al., 1981). The devices are inserted via a left thoracotomy at the fourth intercostal space in the anesthetized dog, as described above for insertion of an ameroid constrictor. A portion of the left circumflex artery is dissected. Around the free section a pneumatic cuff occluder is placed as well as a flow probe, so that changes in flow through the left circumflex can be monitored (Fig. 10.3). A variety of instruments can be inserted while the chest is open, such as piezoelectric crystals to measure regional wall motion by segment shortening, catheters for assessing ventricular pressure development, and electrodes for monitoring epicardial electrocardiograms. Wires and tubing are passed through the skin near the base of the neck and secured between the scapulae (Mohri et al., 1989). The animals are permitted to recover for 10–14 days before the start of the occlusion regimen. This recovery period is a significant advantage over the ameroid model, in which expansion of the ameroid begins immediately, while the animal is recovering from major surgery.

In principle, the pneumatic cuff occluder offers full control over the onset, extent, and duration of occlusion. In practice, researchers do not

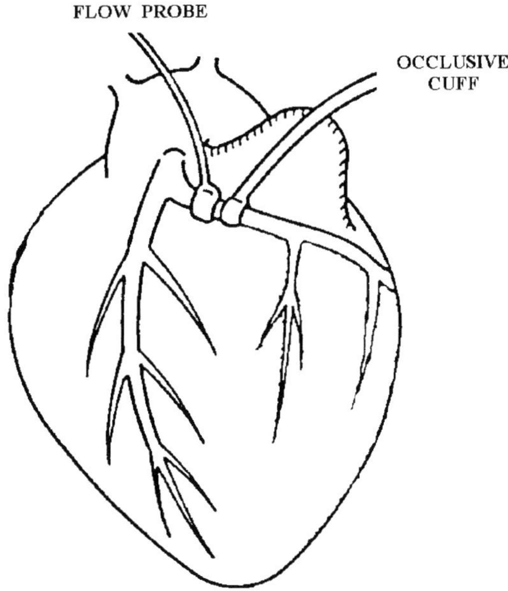

Figure 10.3. Intermittent ischemia with a cuff occluder. A cuff occluder is implanted on the left circumflex artery. The occluder can be attached to servomechanisms to provide controlled occlusions of precise duration and frequency. As noted in the text, a series of 2-minute occlusions interspersed by 30-minute periods of normal flow will stimulate angiogenesis. A flow probe is attached proximal to the cuff to monitor flow and to assess the level of reactive hyperemia after a constriction. Cessation of reactive hyperemia indicates development of collateral blood supply.

attempt reproducible partial occlusion but rather choose brief periods of total occlusion followed by restoration of normal flow. Experiments have established the appropriate duration and frequency of occlusion to induce an angiogenic response. For instance, 90 minutes of occlusion per day has been applied as 15-second bursts every 4 minutes and as 2-minute occlusions every 32 minutes (Mohriet et al., 1989). Even though the total time of occlusion is 90 minutes in each 24-hour period for either schedule, only the regimen with the 2-minute periods was associated with physiologic responses that indicated the development of collaterals.

It is instructive to think about the physiologic data that distinguish between a lack of collateral flow in the control animal and the presence of a robust angiogenic response in a subject in which the response has been properly induced. In the above experimental comparison of 15-second and 2-minute periods of ischemia, the first 2-minute occlusion of the left circumflex produces reduced shortening of muscle segments in the region supplied by the left circumflex artery, a modest reduction in $|\pm dP/dt|$, an increase in left ventricular end diastolic pressure (i.e., the heart is emptying less completely), and a decrease in mean aortic pressure (i.e., the heart is not pumping as effectively and is thus not developing the same pressure per unit time). Moreover, when the occlusion is released, there is a profound increase in flow beyond control levels, which is termed *reactive hyperemia.* After 5 days of periodic 2-minute occlusions, regional hypokinesia is modest and reactive hyperemia is slight, compared to that in control animals. By 10–14 days of periodic ischemia (2 minutes, 45 times a day, equally spaced), all of the hemodynamic and contractile assessments of ventricular function mentioned above are not distinguishable from values in control animals and reactive hyperemia is slight, presumably because the region had developed alternate effective blood flow. By all measures, repetitive occlusions of 15 seconds, even though repeated to give the same total occlusion time per day, were ineffective in producing collateral development (Mohri et al., 1989). It is notable, however, that during a regimen of repetitive ischemia, reactive hyperemia is attenuated before regional contractility is restored (Fujita et al., 1987), so the measure of effective collateral circulation must be chosen carefully. One effective regimen for inducing angiogenesis via periodic repetitive ischemia, arrived at empirically, involves occlusion for 2 minutes at 30–60 minute intervals; the coronary artery is occluded for 2 minutes, then normal flow is restricted for 30–60 minutes; this sequence can be repeated for as long as desired, usually at least 10 days, and frequently as long as 21 days (Mohri et al., 1989; Fujita et al., 1987; Franklin et al., 1981; Yamamoto et al., 1984; Rugh et al., 1987). Comparison of 1-and 2-minute periods of ischemia indicates that the more severe ischemia produced by a 2-minute period is more effective in creating the desired effect; that is, a 2-minute period of ischemia produced hourly is more effective than is a 1-minute period every 30 minutes (Yamamoto et al., 1984). This protocol may have to be varied according to the species employed. Transient ischemia has been successfully applied to ponies, a species with a poorly developed endogenous coronary collateral circulation, and in which occlusion of the left anterior descending coronary artery produces an ischemic zone that is supplied by collaterals as early as 8 days into the occlusion protocol (Rugh et al., 1987).

A serious problem with the repetitive ischemia model that leads to consideration of alternatives is the high rate of death of the experimental animal. In one study (Mohri et al., 1989), 10 of 34 dogs died from ventricular fibrillation resulting from the occlusion. Loss of one-third of instrumented animals in which one has invested considerable time is unacceptable to many investigators. Another problem is fixed stenosis, resulting from a lack of reversibility of the cuff-induced occlusion; five of 18 dogs in the group subjected to frequent short, (15-second) occlusions developed a 90%+ luminal reduction as diagnosed by angiography. These results also illustrate the need to monitor parameters of cardiovascular function and to confirm, by angiography, the patency of the coronary vessels being studied, since the model assumes such patency except for the short periods when the cuff is inflated. Clearly, induction of repetitive ischemia via a pneumatic occluder is not as simple as one might hope, despite its several advantages.

The ineffectiveness of oft-repeated, very short periods of ischemia, such as the 15-second periods discussed above, contrasts sharply with the time course by which metabolic intermediates such as adenosine are accumulated. Following occlusion, maximal vasodilation occurs within about 7 seconds in resistance vessels (Olsson & Gregg, 1965); intramyocardial adenosine rises fivefold after 15 seconds of coronary occlusion (Olsson et al., 1978). Adenosine, as well as other factors, might need to be present at effective concentrations longer than 5 to 10 seconds every 4 minutes to stimulate angiogenesis. It seems likely that an angiogenic response would require a more substantial and longer reduction of oxygen before angiogenic factors can be induced or secreted.

The transient repetitive ischemia model mimics vasospasm to some extent. Indeed, physiologic findings in the model are similar to those of vasospasm. Patients with vasospastic disease develop coronary collaterals; however, angiographic studies in these patients reveal that the collaterals are sufficiently filled with blood to be detectable by angiographic techniques only during a spasm. Thus, intermittent myocardial ischemia, a pressure gradient between intact and occluded coronary arteries, or both, can probably stimulate the development of collateral coronary vessels if the extent and duration of ischemia are sufficient.

MICROEMBOLIZATION: OCCLUDING THE VESSELS WITH CALIBRATED BEADS

Another common method for occluding the coronary circulation is by the injection of plastic microspheres of a known size into a discrete vascular bed. The diameter of the beads can be selected to correspond roughly to the approximate diameter of vessels of different types, ranging from arteries to capillaries (see Table 10.1). In practice, larger beads will block a capillary bed substantially, whereas small beads will lead to incomplete or partial blockage. Thus, by using microspheres from seven to 75 μm, occlusion and subsequent ischemia can be introduced in the coronary circulation either gradually (small beads, administered repeatedly) or abruptly (large beads). Microembolization was originally performed as a single administration of large microspheres; however, the repeated administration of smaller microspheres has become the method of choice and is referred to as *repetitive microembolization* (Chilian et al., 1990; Sabbah et al., 1991).

Both regimens of microembolization stimulate the growth of collateral vessels; the angiogenic response is undoubtedly caused by occlusion of vascular flow. As comparison of the sizes of ameroid occluders, pneumatic cuffs, and microspheres demonstrates (compare Figs. 10.1, 10.3, and Table 10.1), the site of the occlusion with microspheres is "downstream" from the sites occluded by ameroid and inflatable cuff occluders. As a consequence, microspheres can produce a localized or regional ischemia that is lesser in severity than does complete blockage of the coronary artery at a more proximal point. This aspect of microembolization produces a condition similar to that likely to occur in human heart disease. An advantage of the microembolization model is that the investigator has the option of increasing the size of the microspheres to target larger branches of the coronary arteries. Additionally, the microspheres can be administered as often as needed to titrate to a desired diminution of flow and accompanying ischemia.

Microspheres or "beads" are most often administered via precisely placed catheters while the animal is under anesthesia. The left atrium, left ventricle, and left main and left circumflex coronary arteries have all been used for injection of the microspheres to measure flow or occlude capillaries and arterioles. For the purposes of occlusion, it is best to inject the beads as near to the desired ischemic zone as is feasible, thereby achieving a discrete and circumscribed region of ischemia. The left circumflex and left main coronary arteries are most frequently used for microembolization (Chilian et al., 1990; Sabbah et al., 1991; Zimmermann et al., 1997). Many more microspheres must be used to induce microembolization than is the case for flow studies. Concentrations ranging from 10^4 to 10^6 microspheres per ml are necessary to introduce the millions of beads required to produce tissue ischemia. The beads, usually about 15 μm in diameter, can be made of glass, polystyrene, or other plastics; such a relatively concentrated suspension of particles should contain a surfactant such as Tween-80 to prevent the beads from clumping together.

Although the injection of microspheres is invasive, it is far less so than the thoracotomies required for ameroid and cuff occluder placement. Thus, a long recuperative period is not required, nor is significant mortality expected (although a physiologic method of assessing the extent of angiogenesis to correlate findings with function is necessary, which may entail surgical insertion of, e.g., flow probes, depending on the experimental protocol). The small size of the microspheres reduces the probability of an acute occlusion of a major coronary artery and thus the consequent morbidity and mortality.

The microembolization model has been used to show that stimulated capillary growth can be measured within 24 hours of embolization (Zimmermann et al., 1997) and also in long-term (10-month) studies to assess LV diastolic and systolic function following microembolization (Sabbah et al., 1991; Zimmermann et al., 1997). Thus, time courses can be constructed to fit the needs of a particular study. Concerning reproducibility, the timing decreases in left ventricular ejection fraction in dogs subjected to microembolization vary. Five to nine microembolizations done 1–3 weeks apart and for 9–19 weeks appears to be necessary to reduce LV ejection fraction to less than 35% of controls (Kono et al., 1992), representing a significant animal-to-animal variability. Thus, in using this model, one must set parameters that will be monitored to quantify the heart function and the extent of angiogenesis that follows microembolization. A defined endpoint of altered function or reduced/restored flow must be established rather than assuming that a series of applications of microspheres will produce identical results in a series of animals. Presumably, variations in extent of vascularization, size of vessels, and factors such as preexisting coronary disease could contribute to this variability among animals.

Microembolization has been used most often to study ischemia in dogs and pigs. These animals are relatively affordable, provide hearts that are sufficiently large to study with relative ease, and are acceptable models for the study of human angiogenesis. The pig is similar to the human in two respects: It has an anatomically similar coronary circulation and a relatively low capacity for collateral growth. Although studies using primates might provide a more appropriate model for humans, the high cost per animal together with the large numbers of animals required for studies of this nature has prevented their widespread use. It seems more likely that future studies will involve smaller animals such as mice, since microsurgical techniques have been developed and since cardiac development and the function of expressed or deleted gene products can be studied in transgenic mice.

A strength of the microembolization model is the flexibility with which the investigator can alter experimental parameters of bead size and frequency and quantity of injection to produce a wide range of cardiovascular effects. As expected, injection of large beads (> 75 μm) can induce acute infarctions, often leading to the death in as many as 50% of the subjects. Alternatively, one can choose smaller beads and perform repetitive embolizations to produce significant and lasting LV dysfunction, while at the same time reducing the risk of morbidity and mortality. Multiple embolizations can produce focal areas of ischemia in small coronary vessels, and the angiogenic growth that ensues appears to occur independently of pressure changes between major coronary arteries (Sabbah et al., 1991).

It is possible to study the effects of exogenous growth factors on angiogenesis in animals subjected to microembolization. An intracoronary balloon has been used to deliver microspheres either with or without exogenous fibroblast growth factor-2 (FGF-2) into the LAD of pigs (Battler et al., 1993). Ventricular wall motion can be measured by echocardiography (or other methods) to produce an index of cardiac performance, which is depressed immediately following microembolization and at least 3 hours thereafter. Improvement in cardiac performance is seen 2 days following the infarct; however, no further improvement is observed throughout the remainder of the 14-day study. Angiogenesis can be assessed at day 14 by sectioning the hearts and quantifying new vessel growth by a standard immunoperoxidase technique employing antibodies to human factor VIII. Coadministration of FGF-2 with the microspheres leads to a significant enhancement of angiogenesis, more than threefold over that seen with microspheres alone.

The gradual blockade of a coronary artery with repeated microembolization very likely mimics that produced by human coronary atherosclerosis. The time course over which angiogenesis can be stimulated with microbeads makes the model especially useful for studying angiogenesis. Injections of beads need not be confined to the coronaries; the beads can be administered systemically to mimic increased vascular resistance, or to a particular organ to mimic a chronic reduction in perfusion. The great utility of microembolization lies in its flexibility and control and the variety of pathophysiologic conditions that it can create, including depression of left ventricular systolic and diastolic function, left ventricular hypertrophy and dilation, reduced cardiac output, increased vascular peripheral resistance, and enhanced sympathetic activity.

MYOCARDIAL INFARCTION MODEL

One alternative to the above models of slow and progressive occlusion is to ligate a coronary vessel. Ligation has the advantages of simplicity, and of certainty about the onset of ischemia, the extent and location of the change in perfusion, and reproducibility. Dogs and rats will survive this procedure, but pigs will not. Important features of the rat heart's response to left coronary artery ligation and postinfarction angiogenic responses have been described. The findings in this model vary according to where (with respect to the infarct zone and the endocardial surface) one looks for angiogenesis, as well as the time of coronary artery ligation, and the techniques one uses to detect an angiogenic response. Within the infarct region, the appearance of the myocardium can be complicated by cell death, myocyte hypertrophy, and fibroblastic growth. In the border areas and nonischemic myocardium, data are easier to interpret.

Evidence of angiogenesis in the rat coronary artery ligation model has been presented (Xie et al., 1997); an elevation of the angiogenic molecule FGF-2 that was apparent and widespread 24 hours postligation has been demonstrated by immunohistochemical staining and persisted as punctate staining for 30 days. Substantial increases in capillary density in the subendocardium 30 days postinfarction could be demonstrated in the nonischemic zone with further increases in the border zone.

Reliance only on counting the number of capillaries may give a misleading view of angiogenesis when there is simultaneous death of vascular tissue, such as near an infarct. A variety of biochemical techniques that specifically target the cells engaged in an angiogenic response can provide clarity. The left anterior descending artery of rats has been ligated to study the temporal and spatial expression of VEGF and its putative receptors, flt-1 and flk-1, in the postinfarction period. One hour following an acute infarction, VEGF expression rises throughout the left ventricle (+175% over control), as does flk-1 (+275% over control) and flt-1 (300% over control). These diffuse increases in VEGF expression persist for about a week but are succeeded by focal increases in border areas around the infarct. By 6 hours postinfarction, myocytes adjacent to the infarct zone express increased amounts of VEGF mRNA. At 6 and 24 hours postinfarction, small vessels at the edge of the infarct express mRNAs for flk-1 and flt-1, and that expression persists up to 6 weeks as vessels infiltrate into the infarct zone (Li et al., 1996). It seems likely that this model, along with the baseline data provided by Li et al. (1996), will prove useful in future studies of pathophysiologic interactions of different cell types and growth factors in the angiogenic response to myocardial infarction.

HYPERCHOLESTEROLEMIC MODELS

As mentioned earlier in this chapter, atherosclerotic disease leads to a decrease in the radius of vessels, with a concomitant increase in resistance that decreases blood flow and increases pressure. As described earlier, restriction of oxygenation and flow can stimulate angiogenesis. Some of the pathophysiologic conditions that contribute to atherosclerotic disease, however, do not enhance angiogenesis. Examples that illustrate this point are the findings in dietary hypercholesterolemia and rats with genetic hypercholesterolemia. Hypercholesterolemia not only does not enhance, but actually reduces, growth of endothelial cells and their response to angiogenic signals (Henry, 1993). The general nature of the experimental condition and, in the case of the genetic disease, the influence of the underlying metabolic disease, render it difficult to determine the cause for this inhibition. It is clear, however, that factors associated with atherosclerosis other than hypercholesterolemia are responsible for the increase in collateral vessels.

HIND LIMB ISCHEMIA, A MODEL OF PERIPHERAL ANGIOGENESIS

New capillary formation can be studied in the ischemic hind limb. In this experimental model, a portion of the femoral artery to one hind limb is dissected, ligated, and completely excised. Thus, the distal limb of the animal becomes almost entirely dependent upon collateral arteries for continued perfusion and viability. The model has several advantages over those based in the heart. First, the surgical technique is relatively simple and results in minimal morbidity and mortality. Second, several indices of collateral development are easily measured in this model, including blood pressure ratios between the ischemic limb and the contralateral normal limb, pressure gradients across the obliterated portion of femoral artery, and labeling of endothelial cells and smooth muscle cells that are undergoing DNA synthesis as collateral vessels develop. In addition, high-resolution angiograms are easily obtained from the site of collateral development. In these angiograms, the major zones of the collaterals—the stem, midzone, and reentry portions (Fig. 10.4)—are readily defined. Thus, tissue samples can be harvested from these well-defined zones and analyzed for their respective characteristics in terms of genesis of collaterals.

The sequence of collateral development in the ischemic limb appears to be similar to that described for collateral development in other vascular beds. The initial feature of angiogenesis is the activation of endothelial cells within a parent vessel, followed by disruption of the basement membrane and subsequent migration of the endothelial cells into the interstitial space, usually in the direction of an ischemic stimulus. Endothelial cell proliferation, intracellular-vacuolar lumen formation, pericyte capping, and production of new basement membrane follow. With appropriate labeling of the endothelial cells, the rate of collateral development can be quantified and regionalized.

A few general features have been noted about the development of collaterals in the ischemic hindlimb; first, endothelial cell proliferation is nearly nonexistent in normal arteries; second, peak endothelial cell proliferation varies between species, and is, for example, three- to fourfold greater in dogs than in pigs; third, as is the case with other vascular beds, proliferation of smooth muscle cells is a key component; fourth, the highest proliferative activity of both endothelial and smooth muscle cells occurs in the region of the smallest-diameter collateral vessels; and finally, proliferation of endothelial and vascular smooth muscle cells is associated with angiogenesis.

Investigators have used this model to study the potential effects of ther-

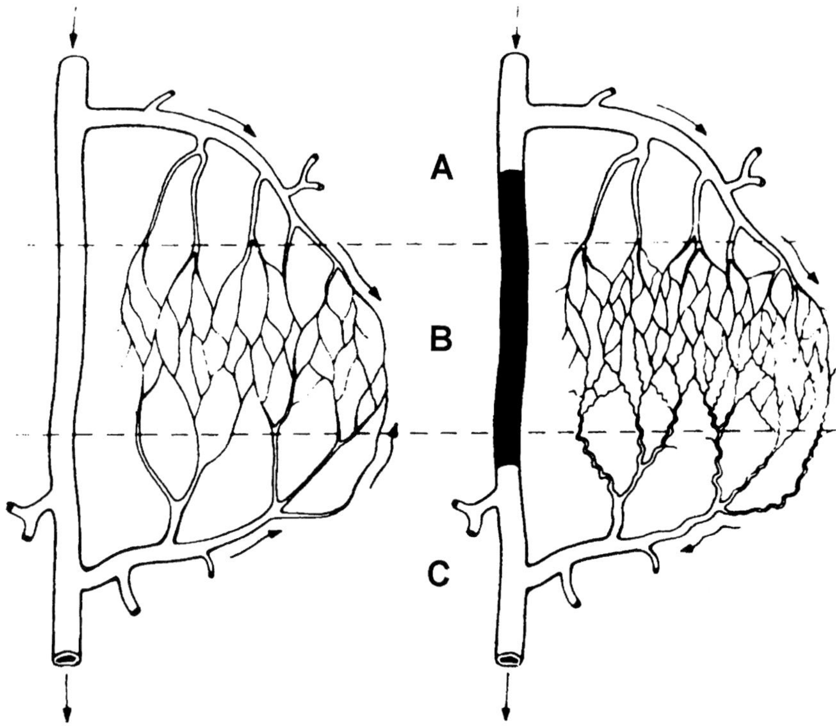

Figure 10.4. Arterial blood flow in the ischemic hind limb preparation. The left panel shows the existing collateral channels under normal conditions. The right panel shows the increase in collateral circulation that develops after ligation of or removal of a portion of the main artery (the blackened segment). In each panel, the arrows indicate the direction of blood flow. The vascular bed can be subdivided into three regions: A the proximal stem zone; B the midzone, in which collaterals increase in number and size under the influence of an angiogenic stimulus; and C the distal reentrant zone. In zone B of the left panel (normal), there is a hypothetical point at which incoming pressures from the arterial branches are equal; this equality is disrupted by the ligation of the main artery (right panel) such that the direction of flow in the distal segment reverses, a process facilitated by collateral formation.

apeutic angiogenesis. For example, VEGF has been infused into the rabbit ischemic hindlimb and the collateral development has been contrasted with that seen in animals with ischemic hind limbs without therapy, showing that augmented cellular proliferation induced with the mitogen enhances collateral development (Takeshita et al., 1995). Additional useful studies to follow up this observation include those to optimize collateral development by examining the effect of timing or choice of agent on cellular proliferation and migration of endothelial cells and the associated lysis of the extracellular matrix.

RELATIONSHIP OF THE MODELS TO INFARCTED, STUNNED, HIBERNATING, AND PRECONDITIONED MYOCARDIUM

The models of cardiac angiogenesis discussed thus far rely on reductions in flow and oxygenation to stimulate the angiogenic response. The extent, duration, and reversibility of the effects of the reduced flow vary among the models and may be important to the observed functional changes. Furthermore, it is possible that variations in severity of ischemia may produce myocardium that is either stunned, or hibernating, or ischemically preconditioned. These states can be defined by the severity and persistence of myocardial dysfunction:

Infarction: permanent dysfunction resulting from prolonged ischemia and cell death

Hibernating myocardium: persistent depression of function resulting from chronic ischemia and hypoperfusion; coronary flow remains low (Rahimtoola, 1989)

Stunned myocardium: prolonged dysfunction caused by an ischemic episode followed by reperfusion; slowly reversible; coronary flow is restored to normal (Braunwald & Kloner, 1982).

Preconditioned myocardium: a paradoxical state in which myocardium reversibly injured by brief ischemia is more tolerant of subsequent ischemic episodes (Murry et al., 1986)

Transient ischemia: brief periods of ischemia and dysfunction, such as occurs in periodic angina

Thus, contractile dysfunctions of distinct character occur in response not only to infarction and transient ischemia, but also to the intermediate states (Vroom and van Wezel, 1996). Understanding these concepts is necessary to interpret the effects of angiogenic growth factors on ischemic myocardium if the contractile state of the ventricle is a major endpoint of the study.

Ligation of a coronary artery clearly corresponds to the ischemia produced by a clinically defined myocardial infarction. At the other end of the spectrum, the transient ischemia model could mimic periodic angina, perhaps generating some of the protective effects associated with ischemic preconditioning, or producing a stunned myocardium. The mechanism of ischemic preconditioning may involve diffusible messengers; regional preconditioning seems to benefit remote areas of the myocardium (Vroom and van Wesel, 1996), but whether angiogenic factors are among the factors responsible is not clear.

Whether the effects of ameroid occlusion and of microembolization fit into the above spectrum (infarction/hibernation/stunning) has generated considerable interest and debate. The microembolization model would be expected to produce multiple microischemic zones as capillaries are blocked. These blockages are permanent but relatively sparse (compared to ligation of a coronary artery) unless large quantities of microspheres are used, and thus avoid cell death and necrosis. The overall effect is that of reduced regional blood flow, which has certain features that correspond to hibernating myocardium.

The model of ischemia that has been more thoroughly investigated is that of ameroid constriction; as the ameroid swells, flow is progressively reduced until complete closure of the vessel, which occurs within 14–20 days in most cases. Thus, the consequences of ameroid constriction are thought to be the sequelae of regional ischemia. The available data are supportive but not conclusive, however. Tritiated thymidine labeling data obtained from other models indicate that vascular DNA synthesis is apparent 36 hours after occlusion and peaks four days postocclusion (Pasynck et al., 1982); thus, the angiogenic response is rapid. In "ameroid occluded" dogs, however, the first available cell labeling data are a 3-week time point, at which point the labeling index has increased from zero to almost four (Schaper et al., 1971). A 3-week "postameroid" time point is probably 1–7 days after occlusion, but the exact temporal relationship between occlusion and an angiogenic response is unknown; nor is it known whether the angiogenic response occurred before occlusion as a consequence of reduced flow or after occlusion as a consequence of no flow.

In the pig model, virtually no thymidine labeling of nuclei is found in sham-operated animals, but a burst of labeling 2 weeks following ameroid placement (labeling index, 0.7) is noted that drops to control levels by 6 weeks (White et al., 1992). The peak at 2 weeks likely occurs at or near the time of cessation of blood flow. Measurements of flow and contraction have been taken only at 3 weeks, so an exact correlation is not possible. Perhaps reduced (but measurable) flow occurring as the ameroid swelled provoked an angiogenic response, but that is not yet established.

The effect of ameroid constriction in the pig on regional function has been documented with daily measurements (Shen and Vatner, 1995; Camici et al., 1997). Wall thickening distal to the ameroid is significantly lowered (by 30%) at 17 days and maximally lowered (by 56%) at 20 days. Subendocardial blood flow distal to the ameroid is not substantially reduced at the time of maximal wall thickening; thus, complete occlusion may not have been achieved. These data argue against this ameroid model inducing either myocardial ischemia or hibernation, both of which are defined by reduced flow. The "ameroid-occluded" pigs appeared to suffer significant stenosis that, during periods of spontaneous physical activity, produced an imbalance of oxygen supply and demand. Thus, the reduced function following ameroid-induced stenosis appears to reflect an accumulation of the effects of repeated episodes of myocardial stunning rather than the primary and prolonged hypoperfusion that characterizes hibernating myocardium (Shen and Vatner, 1995). Ameroid occlusion of the left circumflex artery of the pig has been found not only to stimulate an angiogenic response but also to provide a stable model of persistent exercise-induced ischemia (White et al., 1989). The fact that progressive depression of function and the ensuing recovery occur without significant reduction of flow (Shen and Vatner, 1995) may also indicate significant concurrent formation of collateral vessels, even without obliteration of the flow distal to the ameroid.

The issue of whether ameroid-mediated occlusion of the coronary artery is a model of ischemia or of multiple episodes of stunning has yet to be resolved (Camici et al., 1997). For successful resolution of this controversy, daily measurements of function and flow, along with monitoring of cellular and molecular markers of angiogenesis, must be performed in animals that can be shown to have complete occlusion following ameroid implantation. It is clear that different animal models respond differently to reduced blood flow. Stunning induced by short (10-minute) coronary artery occlusions is less severe in pigs and primates than in dogs, who demonstrate a "preconditioning effect" in response to serial occlusions, an effect that is absent in pigs (Shen and Vatner, 1996). Such a preconditioning-like effect reduces the utility of the dog model for studies of stunning and of interventions that could ameliorate its effects. On the other hand, understanding the cellular and molecular bases of these species differences could elucidate the basic mechanisms of reduced contractile function and of the beneficial effects of ischemic preconditioning.

SUMMARY AND CONCLUSIONS

Table 10.2 compares some of the features of the major models of cardiac angiogenesis presented above. All have strengths and weaknesses and should be evaluated for specific research protocols, as described earlier in this chapter. Many of these models can be used to address multiple questions; for instance, several protocols for inducing angiogenesis resemble those to assess preconditioning and subsequent reduction of ischemic damage.

As methodology and technology improve, the use of smaller animals such as rabbits, rats, or mice may provide viable alternatives to dogs and pigs as models for collateral flow. With the use of genetically altered mice to study cardiovascular development and pathophysiology, interest in developing mouse models of collateral flow will increase. Surgical techniques and microelectronics have been developed and can be applied to the study of cardiovascular angiogenesis. The disadvantage of the expected increase in surgical mortality is easily outweighed by the lower cost and ready availability of smaller animals. One must remember, however, that the extensive catalog of cardiovascular measurements that have been performed on larger animals does not yet exist for mice. Thus, establishing and verifying that these models mimic cardiovascular conditions in smaller

Table 10.2 Comparison of Angiogenic Models

	Means of Occlusion[a]		
Criterion	*Ameroid*	*Cuff*	*Microbeads*
Simple?	+++	+	++
Reproducible?	++	+++	+
Applicable to which species?	Pigs, dogs, and ponies	Pigs, dogs	Pigs, dogs, rats, and mice
Morbidity?	+++	+++	++
Mortality?	+++	+++	+++
Mimics a human disease/condition?	++	++	+++
Inflammation at site of constriction?	+++	+++	+
Major strengths	Gradual occlusion[b]	Precise control of vessel closure	Gradual occlusion of smaller vessels; localized ischemia
Major weaknesses	Variable time of vessel closure[b]	Requires extensive instrumentation; lack of cuff durability	Extended time course for collateral growth, temporal variability among subjects

[a] +++ = most applicable; + = least applicable.
[b] Closure is highly dependent on ameroid design (see Fig. 10.1).

animals will be necessary first steps. Much remains to be learned about smaller animals and their cardiovascular systems, including whether they demonstrate properties that relate to human pathophysiology.

REFERENCES

Battler, A., Scheinowitz, M., Bor, A., Hasdai, D., Vered, Z., DiSegni, E., Varda-Bloom, N., Nass, D., Engelberg, S., Eldar, M., Belkin, M., and Savion, N. (1993). Intracoronary injection of basic fibroblast growth factor enhances angiogenesis in infarcted swine myocardium. J. Am. Coll. Cardiol. 22: 2001–2006.

Braunwald, E. and Kloner, R. A. (1982). The stunned myocardium: prolonged, postischemic ventricular dysfunction. Circulation 66: 1149–1149.

Camici, P. G., Wijns, W., Borgers, M., De Silva, R., Ferrari, R., Knuuti, J., Lammertsma, A. A., Liedtke, A. J., Paternostro, G., and Vatner, S. F. (1997). Pathophysiological mechanisms of chronic reversible left ventricular dysfunction due to coronary artery disease hibernating myocardium. Circulation 96: 3205–3214.

Carroll, S. M. (1997). Enhancement of coronary collateral development by therapeutic agents. Cardiovasc. Pathobiol. 2: 12–24.

Chilian, W. M., Mass, H. J., Williams, S. E., Layne, S. M., Smith, E. E. and Scheel, K. W. (1990). Microvascular occlusions promote coronary collateral growth. Am. J. Physiol. 258: H1103–H1111.

Franklin, D., McKown, D., McKown, M., Hastley, J. and Caldwell, M. (1981). Development and regression of coronary collaterals induced by repeated, reversible ischemia in dogs. Fed. Proc. 40: 339–345.

Fujita, M., McKown, D., McKown, M., Hartley, J. and Franklin, D. (1987). Evaluation of coronary collateral development by regional myocardial function and reactive hyperemia. Cardiovasc. Res. 21: 377–384.

Giordano, F. J., Ping, P., McKirnan, M. D., Nozaki, S., DeMaria, A., Dillmann, W. H., Mathieu-Costello, O., and Hammond, H. K. (1996). Intracoronary gene transfer of fibroblast factor-5 increases blood flow and contractile function in an ischemic region of the heart. Nat. Med. 2: 534–539.

Henry, P. (1993) Hypercholesterolemia and angiogenesis. Am. J. Cardiol. 72: 61C–64C.

Knoepfler, P. S., Bloor, C. M. and Carroll, S. M. (1995). Urokinase plasminogen activator activity is increased in the myocardium during coronary artery occlusion. J. Mol. Cell. Cardiol. 27: 1317–1324.

Kono, K., Sabbah, H. N., Rosman, H., Alam, M., Stein, P. D. and Goldstein, S. (1992). Left atrial contribution to ventricular filling during the course of evolving heart failure. Circulation 86: 1317–1322.

Li, J., Brown, L. F., Hibberd, M. G., Grossman, J. D., Morgan, J. P., and Simons, M. (1996). VEGF, flk-1, and flt-1 expression in a rat myocardial model of angiogenesis. Am. J. Physiol. 270: H1803–H1811.

Mohri, M., Tomoike, H., Noma, M., Inoue, T., Hisano, K., and Nakamura, M. (1989). Duration of ischemia is vital for collateral development: repeated brief coronary occlusions in conscious dogs. Circ. Res. 64: 287–296.

Murry, C. E., Jennings, R. B. and Reimer, K. A. (1986). Preconditioning with ischemia: a delay of lethal cell injury in ischemic myocardium. Circulation 74: 1124–1136.

Olsson, R. and Gregg, E. (1965). Myocardial reactive hyperemia in the unanesthetized dog. Am. J. Physiol. 208: 224–230.

Olsson, R., Snow, J., and Gentry, M. (1978). Adenosine metabolism in canine myocardial reactive hyperemia. Circ. Res. 42: 358–362.

Pasynk, S., Schaper, W., Schaper, J., Pasyk, K., Miskiewicz, G., and Steinseifer, B. (1982). DNA synthesis in coronary collaterals after coronary artery occlusion in conscious dog. Am. J. Physiol. 242: H1031–H1037.

Rahimtoola, S. H. (1989). The hibernating myocardium. Am. Heart J. 117: 211–221.

Rugh, K., Garner, H., Hatfield, D., and Miramonti, J. (1987). Ischemia-induced development of functional coronary collateral circulation in ponies. Cardiovasc. Res. 21: 730–736.

Sabbah, H. N., Stein, P. D., Kono, T., Gheorghiade, M., Levine, T. B., Jafri, S., Hawkins, E. T., and Goldstein, S. (1991). A canine model of chronic heart failure produced by multiple sequential coronary microembolizations. Am. J. Physiol. 260: H1379–H1384.

Schaper, W. (1971). Pathophysiology of coronary circulation. Prog. Cardiovasc. Dis. 14: 275–296.

Schaper, W., Schaper, J., Xhonneux, R. and Vandesteene, R. (1969). Morphology of intercoronary anastomoses in chronic coronary artery occlusion. Cardiovasc. Res. 3: 315–323.

Schaper, W., De Brabander, M., and Lewi, P. (1971). DNA synthesis and mitoses in coronary collateral vessels of the dog. Circ. Res. 28: 671–679.

Shen, Y.-T., and Vatner, S. F. (1995). Mechanism of impaired myocardial function during progressive coronary stenosis in conscious pigs. Circ. Res. 76: 479–488.

Shen, Y.-T., and Vatner, S. F. (1996). Differences in myocardial stunning following coronary artery occlusion in conscious dogs, pigs, and baboons. Am. J. Physiol. 270: H1312–H1322.

Takeshita, S., Rossow, S., Kearney, M., Zheng, L., Bauters, S., Ferrara, N., Symes, J., and Isner, J. (1995). Time course of increased cellular proliferation in collateral arteries after administration of vascular endothelial growth factor in a rabbit model of lower limb vascular insufficiency. Am. J. Pathol. 147: 1649–1660.

Tyagi, S. C., Kumar, S., Cassatt, S., and Parker, J. L. (1996). Temporal expression of extracellular matrix metalloproteinases and tissue plasminogen activator in the development of collateral vessels in the canine model of coronary occlusion. Can. J. Physiol. Pharmacol. 74: 983–995.

Vroom, M. B. and van Wezel, H. B. (1996). Myocardial stunning, hibernation, and ischemic preconditioning. J. Cardiothorac. Vasc. Anesth. 10: 789–799.

White, F. C. and Bloor, C. M. (1992). Coronary vascular remodeling and coronary resistance during chronic ischemia. Am. J. Cardiovasc. Pathol. 4: 193–202.

White, F. C., Roth, D. M., McKirnan, M. D., and Bloor, C. M. (1989). The importance of extra-coronary sources of coronary collaterals during exercise-induced ischemia. Circulation 80 Suppl. II: II–548.

White, F. C., Carroll, S. M., Magnet, A., and Bloor, C. M. (1992). Coronary collateral development in swine after coronary artery occlusion. Circ. Res. 71: 1490–1500.

Xie, Z., Gao, M., Batra, S., and Koyama, T. (1997). The capillarity of left ventricular tissue of rats subjected to coronary artery occlusion. Cardiovasc. Res. 33: 671–676.

Yamamoto, H., Tomoike, H., Shimokawa, H., Nabeyama, S., and Nakamura, M. (1984). Development of collateral function with repetitive occlusion in a canine model reduces myocardial reactive hyperemia in the absence of significance coronary stenosis. Circ. Res. 55: 623–632.

Zimmermann, R., Arras, M., Ullmann, C., Strasser, R., Sack, S., Mollnau, H., Schaper, J., and Schaper, W. (1997). Time course of mitosis and collateral growth following coronary microembolization in the porcine heart. Cell Tissue Res. 287: 583–590.

11

Growth Factor Delivery Strategies

CHUN YU, ANTHONY ENGLISH, AND ELAZER R. EDELMAN

Growth factors are essential compounds in a wide variety of pathological and physiological states, not the least of which are vascular diseases. Elucidation of their mechanism of action would aid immensely in understanding a number of disease processes and biological phenomena including atherosclerosis. For the pharmacologists and controlled release engineers, these compounds are interesting for additional reasons. They are active in minute quantities (picograms–nanograms) with disparate effects at different concentrations, and despite recombinant technology in some instances they remain available in limited quantity or at some expense. In addition, they are often not as stable as other proteins. Prolonged storage may be accompanied by denaturation, degradation, or simply adhesion of the compound to container walls with actual or effective loss in material or biological activity. Moreover, growth factors are rapidly degraded when injected or ingested and, therefore, have very short biological half-lives. The intravenous biological half-lives of fibroblast growth factor-2 (FGF-2): bFGF, transforming growth factor-beta (TGF-β) and platelet-derived growth factor (PDGF), for example, are 3 minutes, 5 minutes, and 2 minutes, respectively. Large potentially toxic systemic doses are, therefore, required to elicit the desired biological effect. The cellular response to growth factors is also highly dose dependent. In addition, the cellular response is dependent on the cell location, type, and the cell cycle state. Furthermore, the cellular response to growth factors can change dramatically with the delivery timing.

Intravascular delivery of therapeutic agents to the arterial wall has been performed using intravenous injection, intravascular catheters, and implanted stents. Polymer-based drug delivery devices have a tremendous potential for the controlled release of growth factors from extravascular devices. These polymer-based controlled-release devices have the unique capacity to deliver therapeutic agents locally while minimizing systemic side effects. Recent applications of polymer devices as cell scaffoldings have shown promising preliminary results for controlling cardiovascular disease.

INTRAVASCULAR DELIVERY STRATEGIES

The earliest reports of the elucidation of growth factor biology involved intravascular injection (Yangisawa-Miya et al., 1992). It is interesting to note that there are an abundance of reports of biological effects after intraarterial and even intravenous administration. Yet, compounds like bFGF bind so tightly to tissue that little of the growth factor injected intravenously is observed within arterial tissue (Edelman et al., 1992). So much of the injected growth factor binds to intervening vascular structures that only a small portion of the original material can be expected to actually be delivered to the desired target. Thus, a number of devices have been proposed for site-directed intravascular application. These include the use of specific catheters and implanted stents. While few of these have been used with growth factors, they may well be adapted in the near future and are worthy of mention.

Porous Balloon Catheters

The porous balloon catheter was first used for the intravascular delivery of heparin (Wolinsky and Thung, 1990) and has been used with a number of different compounds since then. Drug solutions delivered into a balloon under pressure are injected into the artery wall through small perforations that typically measure 25 mm in diameter. The efficacy of this catheter design depends critically on the infusion pressure. A certain minimum pressure is necessary to fully inflate the balloon and position it against the arterial wall so that the downstream distribution and dilution of the drug does not occur. The maximum pressure, which usually varies from 2 to 5 atmospheres, determines the penetration depth and transmural drug deposition in the artery wall.

In canine brachial arteries immediately following artery infusion, flourescently labeled heparin was detected throughout the media and occasionally in the inner aspect of the adventitia. However, when the animals were sacrificed 24–72 hours after infusion, nuclear fluorescence was confined only to the outer 20%–25% of the media with marked necrosis of the inner media and prominent polymorphonuclear cell infiltration. The necrotic damage was observed when either commercial heparin or normal saline solution was infused, implying that the balloon and the high-pressure infusion cause significant damage to the blood vessel. A beneficial biologic effect has so far not been reported following intravascular delivery of standard heparin from balloon catheters. Gimple et al. (1992)

found that while chronic subcutaneous delivery of heparin reduced intimal hyperplasia in denuded femoral arteries of hypercholesterolemic rabbits, intramural delivery of heparin showed no effect.

Intramural delivery via porous balloon catheters has similarly been attempted for a host of other drugs including angiopeptin (Hong et al., 1993), antineoplastic agents such as methotrexate (Muller et al., 1990) and doxorubicin, and antimitotic compounds such as colchicine (Wilensky et al., 1992). A significant decrease in intimal hyperplasia between drug-treated and control animals has, however, not been observed in any of these cases. Trauma caused by drug delivery using porous balloon catheters may mask any relative benefit resulting from the local administration of the drug itself. High infusion pressures and high-velocity fluid jets can lead to vessel perforation or dissection, increasing the stimulus for proliferation or creating a nidus for thrombus formation. In addition, large volumes of drug solution infused into the arterial wall will displace essential structures, alter vascular compliance, and increase overall damage. The infusion of smaller volumes of more concentrated solutions may be less traumatic but expose the artery to greater potential for local drug toxicity. A nonuniform drug distribution within the arterial wall and an inadequate duration of antiproliferative therapy could also have contributed to the inefficacy of intramural drug therapy (Riessen and Isner, 1994).

Several modifications of the single porous balloon have been designed to reduce tissue injury caused by fluid jets. Microporous balloons covered by a permeable polycarbonate membrane with 0.8 mm pores reduce jet-induced injury. Channel balloons infuse drug through small perforated channels located on the surface of an angioplasty balloon (Lambert et al., 1993). A different system for the low-pressure drug infusion using an expandable stent within the balloon to position the balloon against the arterial wall has also been studied (Wilensky et al., 1993). The optimal delivery protocol for each of these device is, however, yet to be determined. The biggest challenge with the porous balloon catheter is to combine efficient drug delivery with minimal tissue damage so that the beneficial effects of local drug delivery outweigh the potentially negative consequences of the delivery procedure (Riessen and Isner, 1994).

Nonetheless, the channel balloon catheter has been successfully employed for the controlled release of vascular endothelial growth factor (VEGF) (Van Belle et al., 1997a,b). Rabbit iliac arteries were denuded of endothelium and implanted with endovascular balloon expandable stainless steel stents. Although local catheter delivery (of vehicle control) itself mildly retarded the extent of stent endothelialization, local channel balloon delivery of 100 μg of VEGF overcame this catheter effect. By day 7, stent endothelialization was nearly complete (91.8 ± 3.8%) ($p < 0.0001$ versus no local delivery). Consequently, stent thrombus and intimal hyperplasia were reduced in the VEGF-treated group.

Hydrogel Coated Balloon Catheter

Normal angioplasty balloon catheters can be coated with a hydrophilic polyacrylic acid polymer that can elute drug within a blood vessel with minimal trauma and without the need for special catheters (Fram et al., 1994; Riessen et al., 1993). The hydrogel coating has a thickness of only 5–20 μm when dry and swells by a factor of three when exposed to an aqueous environment. A thin layer of therapeutic agent is applied to the hydrogel-coated balloon and allowed to dry. Balloon inflation against the arterial intimal surface results in the passive diffusion of agents from the polymer into the vessel wall.

In one particular study, heparin eluted from a hydrogel catheter was deposited in the arterial wall with a mean average penetration depth of 1.4 ± 0.7 mm and mean maximal penetration depth of 1.9 ± 0.9 mm independent of the contact time or hydrogel thickness (Fram et al., 1994). Local delivery of a specific antithrombin D-Phe-Pro-Arg choromethylketone (PPACK) in vivo from such a hydrogel balloon was found to inhibit platelet-dependent thrombosis on thrombogenic dacron porcine arteriovenous shunts (Nunes et al., 1992). The drug was dip-coat incorporated onto the balloon and approximately 50% of it was transferred to the thrombus. Inhibition of radiolabeled platelet deposition was greater than that obtained when the same drug was infused intravenously at a 100-fold greater overall dose. The hydrogel system, however, has limited use. Because the drug is rapidly washed off the balloon after exposure to the bloodstream (Sheriff et al., 1993), a protective sheath must be used and the time between sheath removal and balloon inflation has to be minimized.

Iontophoresis Catheters

To augment the deposition and penetration of drugs to the vascular wall, electric currents have been applied in the form of iontophoresis. Iontophoretic drug delivery involves controlling the movement of drugs by externally modulating the electrical driving force across a rate-limiting medium of the transported drug. Although iontophoresis has been used to increase the rate and depth of drug penetration into arterial walls, drugs have still been observed to be rapidly cleared from the vessel wall.

Drug Release From Stents

Intravascular drug delivery via catheters is short term while indwelling devices may serve as endovascular scaffoldings for drug release over a more prolonged period of time. Endovascular stents have already been used to maintain luminal patency in the setting of abrupt closure of an angioplastied artery and to combat restenosis in the 6 months that follow

(Levin et al., 1990; Serruys et al., 1991; Sigwart et al., 1987, 1988; Urban et al., 1989). Despite the 95%–100% success rate in stent placement (Levin et al., 1990; Urban et al., 1989), long-term efficacy is limited by thrombosis and intimal hyperplasia. Aggressive antithrombotic regiments have reduced thrombosis within the first 2 weeks following implantation (Puel et al., 1987; Serruys et al., 1991) but have not altered restenosis and are accompanied by complications that include transfusion requiring hemorrhage (Levin et al., 1990), thrombocytopenia, electrolyte and intravascular volume shifts, allergic reactions, and the need for indwelling vascular access for drug infusion.

The continuous release of antithrombotic or antiproliferative drugs can be effective from stents coated either directly with drugs or with drug-eluting biodegradable polymer materials. Two compositions of heparin coating applied to slotted-tube stainless-steel stents reduced thrombosis when compared to uncoated stents after implantation in the left anterior descending (LAD) coronary artery of young pigs. Similarly, polymer-bound heparin coated on Nitinol stents was shown to inhibit occlusive thrombosis to a greater extent than bare metal stents in a rabbit model of subacute thrombosis (Sheth et al., 1994). However, the elimination of thrombosis by heparin released from stents has not been accompanied by a decrease in neointimal hyperplasia. Cox et al. (1991) have reported no benefit from the local delivery of heparin and methotrexate on neointimal proliferation in a model involving oversized stenting of porcine coronary arteries (Cox et al., 1991, 1992). Like the perfusion balloon, stents can induce such significant injury as to mask or dwarf the benefit for the drug they might deliver.

We have taken advantage of this heparin binding feature of stents to bind bFGF to heparin-immobilized stents. The growth factor was released with rapid first-order kinetics. When placed within normal or denuded rabbit iliac arteries, no demonstrable effect was achieved. These results highlight the major problem with stent based release. At the outset the geometry of the stent is less than ideal. The optimal stent is expected to have an almost infinite surface-area-to-volume ratio or minimal volume to maintain luminal patency. As drug loading is proportional to volume and drug release to surface area, the ideal stent presents a less than favorable platform for drug reservoir and release. At the same time, turbulence imposed by the stent and the arteriosclerotic lesion, the large circulating blood volume, and the resistance to transport into the injured arterial wall all create further impedance to full mural deposition of stent-released drug.

POLYMER-BASED DRUG DELIVERY DEVICES

To minimize the potential side effects of a molecular intervention, growth factors should be administered at a definite dose rate, for a specific period of time, and target a specific biologic site. Compared to traditional intravenous injection, catheter- and stent-based drug release offer much better control over the release rate and local drug concentration. As noted above, however, these compounds will still be degraded shortly after release within the blood vessel and be rapidly cleared out of circulation. Also, there is no control over drug circulation to other parts of the body that can cause undesired side effects.

Polymer-based drug delivery systems offer the potential for the quantifiable sustained and controlled drug release from minute devices that can be implanted adjacent to target tissues. In contrast to most intravascular release devices, drugs can be incorporated in dry form within polymer-based delivery devices. As a result, the device size is much smaller and drugs are more stable and better protected. Therapeutic agents can be delivered locally to minimize systemic side effects, metabolic inactivation, and poor tissue absorption that are associated with other forms of bolus delivery. Polymer-based delivery devices have been used for the preservation and release of unstable growth factors, tumor growth inhibition, angiogenesis, and the suppression of prosthetic heart valve calcification. This section provides the necessary background for understanding polymer-based drug delivery devices and their potential application to cardiovascular pathology and growth factor biology.

Hydrogels

Different polymer-based drug delivery strategies have been considered depending on the drug substance and targeted biological environment. Hydrogels fabricated from acrylamide (AAm) or hydroxyethylmethacrylate (HEMA), for example, are usually considered for short-term release systems. The high water content of these materials makes them tissue compatible but provides minimal barriers to diffusion and so the embedded or encapsulated drug is rapidly released. Freeze–thaw photopolymerization of a mixed solution of 2-hydroxyethyl methacrylate (HEMA), ethylene glycol dimethacrylate (EDM), and either glucose oxidase (GOx) or interleukin 2 (IL-2) at a low temperature has been used to fabricate slow release devices. Polymerization around frozen ice crystals is used to generate a bead-formed macroporous hydrophilic matrix with the potential for immobilization and sustained release (Atkins et al., 1994). Similarly, VEGF has been incorporated into the slow-release polymer Hydron (Phillips et al., 1994). VEGF-PBS solution was mixed with Hydron solution and dried under vacuum to form pellets. The VEGF-incorporated pellets were implanted into the vascular rabbit cornea. Capillary formation in the cornea was visually analyzed on a daily basis and examined with histology, transmission electron microscopy, and scanning electron microscopy of vascular corrosion casts on days 2 and 7 postimplantation. VEGF implants consistently stimulated angiogenesis in a dose-responsive way. The neovascularization occurred in the absence of inflammation. VEGF acts directly on endothelial cells, initiating and mediating the formation of the capillaries.

Porous Polymers

Passive diffusion through hydrogels is generally too rapid to be of value when drug release is required over long periods of time. If the hydrophobicity of the polymer is increased, the water content and the drug release rate fall. A mixture of macromolecules with hydrophobic polymers can thus prolong the release rate. Some of the earliest methods for preparing slow controlled-release devices involved adding the macromolecule in powdered form to a solution of polymer material. The resulting mixture was then cast in a mold and dried to specific shapes and dimensions (Langer and Folkman, 1976). The polymer and the protein can also be mixed in their dry powder forms and then heated and molded into films, fibers, or pellets (Edelman et al., 1991). In this system, proteins move through connected porous paths in the polymer matrix. When hydrogels or hydrophilic polymers are used, proteins can also be released by diffusion through the polymer matrix. The degradation rate of certain types of polymers can also affect the drug release kinetics. The release kinetics can also be controlled by the protein particle size, the protein-to-polymer ratio, the protein solubility and molecular weight, and the matrix dimensions and shape.

Ethylene-vinyl acetate(EVAc) copolymers have been used for the sustained and localized release of biologically active substances. This material is easily processed and immunologically inert. Ethylene-vinyl acetate matrices have been used in a multitude of drug delivery applications (Langer, 1990). Sheets of this copolymer are normally impermeable to compounds over 300 daltons. If the copolymer is melted or dissolved and the drug to be released is added as a dry powder, the resultant slurry can be recast into any form to create a monolithic matrix of drug and copolymer (Rhine et al., 1980). The drug displaces the copolymer material, creating a tortuous network of long channels connecting reservoirs of drug. The relative drug-to-polymer concentration determines the number of reservoirs and channels while the dry drug aggregate size determines the reservoir size. The tortuousity and porosity of the matrix in turn determines the release kinetics. The release of large drug molecules, such as growth factors, can be facilitated by incorporating bovine serum albumin (BSA) as a carrier molecule. The growth factor is uniformly mixed together with the BSA in ratios of 1:500 to 1:1,000, and the two compounds can then be incorporated within polymer matrices. In the most common commercially available form, the EVAc material is washed in ethanol and water or extracted with acetone to remove impurities added for transport and packaging purposes. The purified polymer can then be dissolved in a solvent such as dichloromethane. The powdered mixture of compounds is suspended as a slurry and cast at low temperatures. A film instantaneously hardens as a monolithic matrix of drug surrounded by polymer material. The BSA carrier forms a hydrophilic network throughout the polymer matrix. As water penetrates and dissolves the BSA, the incorporated growth factor is released. The release rate can be controlled by growth factor loading, BSA loading, and particle size in the release device. Using this technique, EVAc, BSA, and nerve growth factor (NGF) were made into cylindrical rods for controlled release (Hoffman et al., 1990). To stimulate bone cell growth, EVAc, BSA, and platelet-derived growth factor B chain (PDGF-BB) were also combined and used to coat stainless-steel Kirschner wire used as an intramedullary nail for small fractures in rats (Nimni, 1997).

Murray et al. (1983) demonstrated the controlled release of epidermal growth factor (EGF) using ethylene-vinyl acetate copolymer (EVAc) matrices. When only microgram quantities of EGF were placed in such an EVAc matrix, this minute quantity of material could only displace a small amount of copolymer material, and a matrix with a sparse network was created. Many, if not all, of the reservoirs were isolated and virtually none of the EGF was released. In contrast, when the EGF was first mixed with a few milligrams of BSA and then combined with mg quantities of EVAc, a matrix was formed with a well-defined network. More importantly, EGF was released in a controlled fashion over time with kinetics proportional to the BSA release. Because the BSA was in great excess, the EGF was transported out along with the BSA in a manner related to their relative concentrations. It was further demonstrated that the released EGF was capable of stimulating endothelial cell proliferation in tissue culture.

Silberstein and Daniels used this technique to investigate the effects of TGF-β controlled release in vivo. The growth factor was coincorporated with BSA into an EVAc matrix which was then placed in front of the mammary end buds of subadult virgin mice. Bud growth and morphogenesis were inhibited twofold (Siberstein et al., 1987). TGF-β is one growth factor that has been successfully incorporated into EVAc-BSA microspheres. First-order release kinetics were observed and approximately 12% of the compound was released within the first 8 days (Fig. 11.1) (Dinbergs et al., 1996). Released TGF-β_1 also retained its biological activity throughout the experiment. When implanted within a murine model of mammary tumors, prolonged control of tumor growth was demonstrated (Silberstein and Daniel, 1987).

Microspheres

Although smaller pieces can be cut from the slabs or films that are produced as previously described, there has been an increasing interest in the fabrication of microspheres (Arras et al., 1998). The size of the microspheres can vary from 1.0 μm to 1,000 μm. They can be small enough to be lodged in tissues without disrupting the total tissue flow. Like other polymer delivery devices, microspheres can be surgically implanted. Microspheres can also be injected or introduced into specific vessels with a

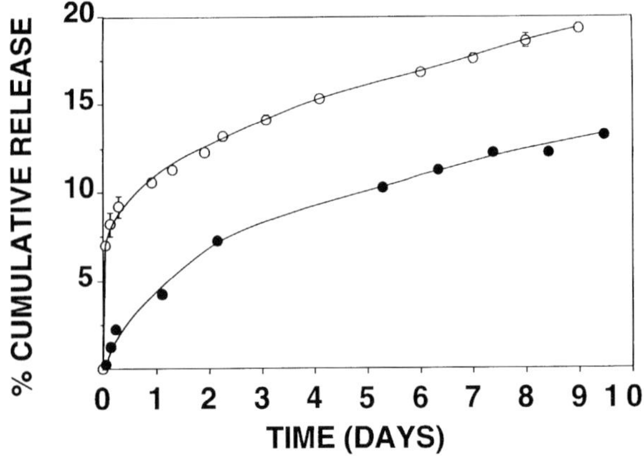

Figure 11.1. Controlled release of bFGF from alginate/heparin-Sepharose microspheres and TGF-β_1 from EVAc microspheres. Percent cumulative release of ^{125}I-bFGF (◯) from alginate/heparin-Sepharose microspheres and ^{125}I-TGF-β_1 (●) from EVAc microspheres during a 9-day time period. Physical release of bFGF was determined by measuring the presence of ^{125}I-bFGF in the release buffer of three alginate/heparin-Sepharose microspheres. Physical release of TGF-β_1 was determined by measuring the presence of ^{125}I-TGF-β_1 in the release buffer of five to 10 EVAc-BSA-^{125}I-TGF-β_1 microspheres. Each data point represents the average ± standard error about the mean of three identical vials. After Dinbergs et al., (1996.)

catheter to avoid the surgical procedures commonly used to implant other polymer delivery devices.

Ethylene-vinyl acetate microspheres can be easily prepared (Sefton et al., 1984). As with slabs, commercially available EVAc must be washed thoroughly in water and ethanol and then dissolved in dichloromethane. Bovine serum albumin can be weighed out and dissolved in a small amount of water to provide the desired loading which usually ranges between 20% and 40% weight BSA/weight EVAc. Growth factor is added to the BSA solution and then the solution is lyophilized to a dry powder. The powder is then crushed fine and added to the EVAc solution to form a suspension. The mixture is then dropped into cold ethanol (−40 °C) cooled by a dry ice-ethanol bath. Hard, spherical pellets form immediately as the mixture enters the cold ethanol solution. The ethanol must be changed and the microspheres allowed to cure overnight at ambient temperature. The next day the ethanol can be decanted and any residual ethanol removed by lyophilization. Growth factor release kinetics can be followed using EVAc-BSA microspheres loaded with radio-labeled growth factor in phosphate-buffered saline.

The above system demonstrated two of the most critical issues with the controlled release of growth factors. First, the controlled release of TGF-β was not as effective at inhibiting vascular endothelial and smooth muscle cells as bolus administration. When the same amount of growth factor was provided to cells in one dose the inhibitory effect was maximized and when released over the course of the 7-day experiment no significant effect beyond control was demonstrated (Fig. 11.2) (Dinbergs et al., 1996). Second, when bFGF was incorporated within the same devices using the same technique virtually all of the biological activity of the growth factor was lost. Encapsulated ^{125}I-bFGF in EVAc matrices follows expected release kinetics, indicating no loss of physical material. Yet, no effect on cells could be obtained. In subsequent experiments, it was determined that

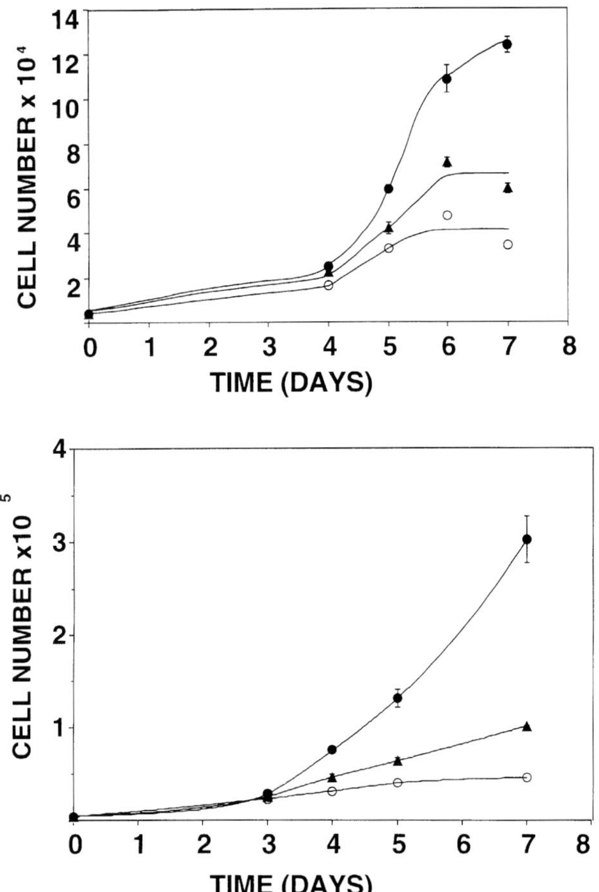

Figure 11.2. Controlled release of bFGF provides optimal endothelial and smooth muscle cell proliferation. Endothelial (A) and smooth muscle (B) cells were plated at 4 × 103 cells/ml/well and grown to near confluency in medium alone (○), or exposed to 8.9 ng of bFGF administered as a single bolus (▲), or released in a sustained fashion from alginate/heparin-Sepharose microspheres (●) over 7 days. Each data point represents the average ± standard error about the mean of four identical wells. Differences between control, microsphere, and bolus groups are all significant for both cell types ($p<.00001$). After Dinbergs et al., (1996.)

virtually all (>94.1%) of the bFGF was denatured by the organic solvents used to fabricate EVAc matrix devices (Nugent et al., 1992). Solvent and temperature conditions are believed to inactivate the protein during matrix fabrication. To solve this problem, methods with milder process conditions needed to be developed.

These two observation are essential in dealing with the controlled release of growth factors. Not every growth factor must be control released and those that are or should cannot necessarily be placed in any system without regard to the impact that the fabrication process may have on the factor biology.

Controlled Release of bFGF

It is worth dwelling upon the experience with bFGF as this has become a classic issue in controlled-release technology. The EVAc matrices, thought to be the gold-standard devices for controlled release, were not appropriate for the storage and release of bFGF. EVAc matrices fabricated as described above using milligram quantities of BSA, and micrograms quantities of bFGF released the growth factor physically intact but biologically inert. Subsequent studies demonstrated that the steps involved in the fabrication of the controlled release device inactivated the growth factor. Gospodarowicz had already shown that heat and acidic pH were particularly potent at reducing the activity of bFGF (Gospodarowicz and Cheng, 1986). We further demonstrated that organic solvents had much the same effect. bFGF is a folded compound (Zhu et al., 1991) and these extremes quite possibly led to conformational changes that did not effect the detection of radiolabeled factor but rendered the released bFGF inactive. When a vial containing 1 mg/ml of the factor was exposed to 50 °C or fumes from the organic solvent dichloromethane, much of the mitogenic activity of the released material was lost. The loss in growth factor activity under these condition is particularly problematic as these are precisely the environments required in the course of controlled release device fabrication.

To circumvent these problems we and others have attempted to use techniques that avoid such harsh conditions. In these alternative methods, the bFGF is absorbed by a controlled-release structure and released with time. Hayek and investigators incubated bFGF over agarose beads and then deposited the beads onto Gelfoam (Hayek et al., 1987). It was estimated that 75% of the bFGF was embedded in this fashion and subsequently released over the next 96 hours. Others have used gelfoam alone as a sponge to soak up bFGF and confirmed (Thompson et al., 1988) the angiogenic potential of released bFGF after implantation in vivo. Gelfoam is a synthetic gelatin matrix and as such bFGF release from this material is remarkably similar to in vivo mechanisms of bFGF storage and release from extracellular matrix. Unfortunately, the use of Gelfoam is limited by the substantial amount of bFGF released within the first 12–24 hours and the completion of release within the first few days.

We sought to extend the release of this growth factor and more precisely control its release in tissue culture and in vivo (Edelman et al., 1991). This was accomplished by taking advantage of the heparin avidity of the growth factor and using the natural seaweed extract alginate as a containing gel capsule. bFGF has a well defined affinity for heparin and has been characterized and purified by passage over columns with immobilized heparin (Burgess and Maciag, 1989; Klagsbrun, 1989; Rifkin and Moscatelli, 1989). Gospodarowicz and Cheng (1986) have shown that the addition of heparin to solutions of bFGF prevents losses in activity that accompany changes in pH or elevation in temperature. We demonstrated that the addition of heparin (20 μ/ml) to bFGF solutions prevented losses in mitogenic activity with other environmental extremes. We therefore chose to examine whether heparin-immobilized Sepharose might be used as a carrier for the storage and release of bFGF. When the growth factor was incubated for 1 hour with the heparin-Sepharose beads 77% of initial ^{125}I-bFGF in solution bound to the beads. After the beads were placed in saline, periodic aliquots revealed that release commenced immediately and proceeded with rapid first-order kinetics. While the released bFGF had retained 97.5% of its mitogenic potential only 25% of the embedded material was released after 14 days. The remaining material could be removed, still biologically active, by exposing the beads to solutions of high ionic strength. This broke the ionic heparin-bFGF bonds but did not affect the mitogenic potential of bFGF.

To prolong release and to construct a single unit of manageable size, the heparin-Sepharose beads were encapsulated within alginate. A mixed solution of sodium alginate (1.2% in saline) and bFGF-bound heparin-Sepharose beads were dropped through a needle into a beaker containing a hardening solution of calcium chloride (1.5% w/v). Capsules were formed instantaneously as the mixture entered the hardening solution. A 25-gauge needle was used to set the microcapsule size and similarly cross-linked capsule envelopes were obtained by limiting hardening to 5-minute immersion in the calcium chloride bath (Fig. 11.3). In this fashion, only an additional 3%–4% of the growth factor was lost. Release kinetics were markedly prolonged as the burst of activity seen in the first 48 hours was retarded (Fig. 11.4) without reducing the retention of biological activity. The amount of factor detected radiologically and mitogenically were remarkably similar (p = NS) at each point in time with 87.6 ± 2.0% of the bFGF having retained its bioactivity. The Sepharose beads remained intact for the duration of all experiments, under all conditions and in extended storage beyond 3 months.

It is interesting to note how heparin operates in this setting. First, the glycosaminoglycan serves in its classic means to protect bFGF from denaturation, but it also dictates release. Alginate, like other hydrogels, presents no demonstrable barrier to diffusion. The sustained nature of release arises from the fact that once the bFGF compound is released from its immobilized heparin it is then presented with many other heparin moi-

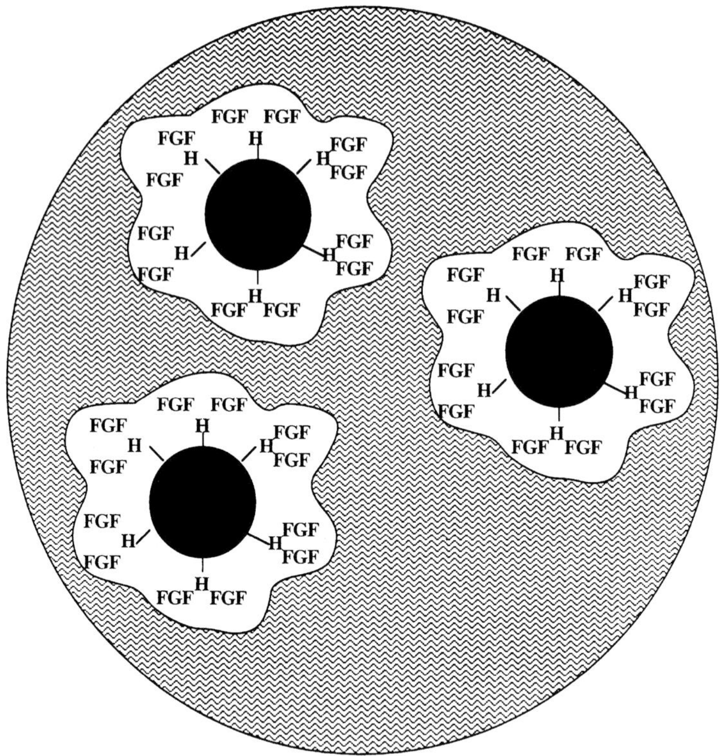

Figure 11.3. Alginate encapsulation of the heparin-Sepharose beads proceeded as follows. The bFGF was incubated over heparin immobilized to Sepharose beads. As milligram quantities of beads were used to bind the micrograms of bFGF, and because one molecule of heparin can bind two molecules of bFGF, bFGF binding to the beads proceeded without saturation and with 77%–80% efficiency. bFGF-laden beads were then suspended in saline and mixed with alginate to a final concentration of 1.2% alginate. This suspension was dropped through a 25-gauge needle into a hardening solution of $CaCl_2$ (1.5%) forming intact capsules 0.5–1 cm in diameter. bFGF release was dictated by the combined kinetics of the dissociation of the heparin-bFGF bonds and the kinetics of bFGF release through the alginate capsule. (After Nugent et al., 1992.)

eties to rebind to. It is this process of release and rebinding that accounts for the sustained nature of release, and it is this effect that most closely mimics the interaction of bFGF with extracellular matrix-bound heparin.

The power of these systems has been demonstrated in a number of in vivo studies and cell culture experiments with fibroblasts, vascular endothelial cells, and smooth muscle cells. Type I collagen, for example, was gelled in 35-mm polystyrene plates and cells added in the presence of Dulbecco's modification of Eagle's medium with 10% calf serum or serum free media containing EGF, insulin, and transferrin. Alginate microcap-

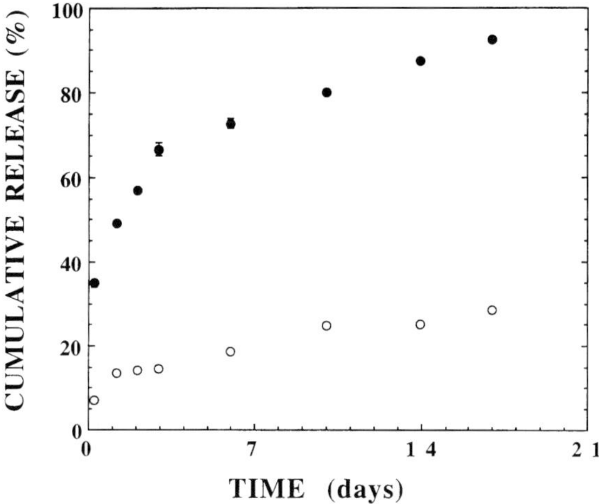

Figure 11.4. Release kinetics from heparin-Sepharose beads demonstrated rapid first-order kinetics, and only a portion of the initially incorporated bFGF was released. When these beads were encapsulated in alginate, release was prolonged but the net amount of growth factor remained unchanged (open circles). The addition of heparinase to the capsules increased net release 2.9-fold (closed circles) (After Nugent et al., 1992.)

sules containing heparin-Sepharose beads with and without bFGF were placed in the gels prior to complete gelation. The capsules continued to secrete bFGF but were immobilized, allowing for cell growth to proceed without danger of mechanical dislocation by capsules rolling freely within the culture plates.

Alginate capsules containing beads without growth factor had little to no effect on cell growth. The collagen gels slow the rate of cell growth observed on plastic alone, yet a constant growth rate was observed. bFGF added to media as a single bolus stimulated cells but the effect was pulsatile and transient. Cell growth increased above the control rates for the first 36–54 hours and then returned to baseline. When identical amounts of bFGF were delivered in a more controlled and sustained fashion the stimulation of cell growth was sustained and more effective (Fig. 11.4). Cells exposed to controlled release of bFGF grew in an almost linear fashion over the course of the experiments. It is possible that the bolus of bFGF exerted its effect early and became progressively less effective as it was degraded or denatured with time. The alginate capsule protected the bFGF from these forces and provided a steady source of the growth factor for cell stimulation. Alginate-heparin-Sepharose-bFGF microspheres implanted into the perivascular space of rat carotid arteries produces a significant increase in vasa vasorum and in intimal mass and proliferation (Edelman et al., 1992), and induced collateral growth when placed over porcine constricted coronary arteries. In these perivascular sites the deposition and distribution of the growth factor is far more favorable than that which can be achieved by means of intravascular injections at a distance or even locally (Edelman et al., 1992).

Variations of this method have been used for a range of growth factors including aFGF, VEGF, TGF-β, and HBEGF. As we have detailed the methodology above we will now only summarize derivative techniques below.

Alginate-a,bFGF Microspheres

Acidic FGF and bFGF growth factors were dissolved in sodium alginate solution and injected into calcium chloride solution to obtain small, uniformly sized microspheres (Downs et al., 1992). The in vivo release of growth factors was shown to depend on charge. When alginate beads were injected subcutaneously into Balb/c mice, neovascularization was observed. Direct subcutaneous injection of angiogenic factors, however, did not cause neovascularization. The same system was also used to entrap tumor cells that release angiogenic factors to induce neovascularization in mice and monkeys (Plunkett and Hailey, 1990). The alginate beads containing tumor cells were injected subcutaneously into animals. The tumor cells are protected from direct contact with the host's immune system and the technique is easy to perform. This model allowed both a qualitative and quantitative assessment of tumor-induced blood vessel growth.

Resin Microspheres

A noninvasive model for growth factor delivery without causing tissue damage was developed by lodging small microspheres in the peripheral circulation (Arras et al., 1998). bFGF was adsorbed to commercially available resin microspheres (size 7 μm, pore size 2 nm) with SO_2 residues which bind bFGF reversibly with a binding efficiency of 96.7%. The microspheres were injected via a coronary catheter into the left circumflex coronary artery (LCX) of closed-chest pigs. bFGF was slowly released from the microspheres within a week and stimulated endothelial cell growth, neovascularization, and improved collateral blood flow to the ischemic heart. About 60% of the injected microspheres had lodged in the targeted perfusion area and 40% of the injected microspheres recirculated without any accumulation in any particular organ. No inflammation or other physiological disturbances were observed after microsphere injection. The method represents a possible precise delivery of angiogenic substance to any selected part of the heart or other organs without causing inflammation or ischemia.

Chitosan-Albumin Microspheres

Chitosan, a biocompatible polysaccharide, was used to form microspheres and fibers with albumin, as potential delivery systems for endothelial cell growth factor (ECGF, an N-terminal extended form of acidic FGF) to stimulate vascularization (Elcin et al., 1996). Chitosan solution with acetic acid was mixed with albumin solution and injected into 0.5 M sodium hydroxide-methanol solution, microspheres or fibres were formed depending on the injection speed. To incorporate the growth factor, the microspheres or fibers were incubated in ECGF solution. The growth-factor-loaded matrices were implanted subcutaneously into rat groin fascia. Chitosan-albumin microspheres and fibers gave similar ECGF release rates. A high degree of neovascularization was observed for both types of implants, starting from 7 days-postimplantation. However, no significant neovascularization was observed for control animals that received ECGF injection.

Collagen

Collagen has been used as a growth factor release vehicle, especially for releasing of growth factors involved in wound healing. Recombinant PDGF (PDGF-BB) was incorporated into a rapidly dissolving collagen type I film (Khouri et al., 1994). Coupled with a syngeneic skin graft, the application of the growth factor led to neovascularization and fibroblast migration and proliferation. Bovine collagen was also mixed with TGF-β to formed a viscous suspension which was easily applied to the cut edge of an incision in a rat model (Beck et al., 1993). The collagen release device provides a prolonged slow release of TGF-β and results in better healing compared to the saline release device, which provides only a short bolus release.

Alternative Materials: Degradable Polymers

No discussion of polymeric controlled-release systems is complete without mention of alternative materials. Degradable controlled-release systems have been proposed for use in place of devices that might require surgical removal (Langer and Moses, 1991). Several polymers have been considered for the fabrication of erodable controlled release devices, including polyesters, polyamides, polyanhydrides, polyurethanes, polyorthoesters, and polyacrylonitriles. Ideally, such polymers should be designed so that the drug will be released as the polymer degrades from the surface, and by the time the drug is all released, the polymer will be degraded and absorbed by the body. To achieve such a surface-degrading polymer requires the hydrolytic degradation on the polymer surface to be much faster than the rate of water penetration into the bulk. Among the many polymer systems studied, only polyorthoesters and polyanhydrides showed surface erosion. Polyorthoesters usually require additives to achieve controlled surface erosion. Polyanhydride copolymers of carbophenoxy propane (CPP) and sebacic acid (SA) erode over a broad range from 1 day to 3 years as determined by the CPP/SA ratio. Drugs are incorporated into these polymer through solvent casting, compression molding, and injection molding.

In one embodiment of degradable systems (Gombotz et al., 1993) TGF-β was incorporated within poly(DL-lactic co-glycolic acid) along with demineralized bone matrix (DBM). Release was further controlled by applying polymeric coatings of varying porosity to the devices. Between 80 and 90% of the TGF releases from the system retained its bioactivity and the devices were sufficiently porous to allow bone growth.

CONCLUSIONS

The controlled release of growth factors has provided us with formulations that enable ready delivery of these compounds to cells and tissues. At the same time we have learned much about growth factor biochemistry, tissue biology, and controlled-release technology. A number of critical issues have come forth:

1. Not all growth factors need to be released in a sustained or controlled fashion. Some growth factors are best delivered as a single bolus. The ability to develop a formulation does not mean that this is the optimum means of administering the compound. As a result, we are obliged to examine whether even the most innovative of release formulations is the most effective means of delivering a compound.

2. Even when dealing with growth factors that are most effectively administered in a sustained fashion, one must be cognizant of the impact of the processing involved in formulation. Exposures to extremes of temperature or to organic solvents might denature the compound and paradoxically eliminate the biologic activity rather than enhance it.

3. The most effective formulations for the sustained and controlled release of growth factors are those that mimic natural means of growth factor metabolism. The use of immobilized heparin within polymer systems is the result of an in-depth understanding of the biochemistry of bFGF and extracellular matrix. Nature has evolved magnificent means of optimizing release effect and we need to strive to understand these mechanisms to create the best devices.

4. The application of these observations and findings to increasingly innovative means of drug delivery that might even include transfected cells, plasmids, and intact or pieces of genetic material will herald a new era in growth factor delivery.

REFERENCES

Arras, M., Mollnau, H., Strasser, R., Wenz, R., Ito, W., Schaper, J., and Schaper, W. (1998). The delivery of angiogenic factors to the heart by microsphere therapy. Nat. Biotech. 16: 159–162.

Atkins, T. W., McCallion, R. L., and Tighe, B. J. (1994). The incorporation and release of glucose oxidase and interleukin 2 from a bead formed macroporous hydrophilic polymer matrix. J. Biomater. Sci. Polym. Ed. 6: 651–659.

Beck, L. S., DeGuzman, L., Lee, W. P.; Xu, Y., Siegel, M. W., and Amento, E. P.

(1993). One systemic administration of transforming growth factor-beta 1 reverses age-or glucocorticoid-impaired wound healing. J. Clin. Invest. 92: 2841–2849.

Burgess, W. H. and Maciag, T. (1989). The heparin-binding (fibroblast) growth factor family of proteins. Annu. Rev. Biochem. 58: 575–606.

Cox, D. A., Anderson, P. G., and Roubin, G. S. (1991). Local delivery of heparin and methotrexate fails to inhibit in vivo smooth muscle cell proliferation. Circulation 84: II–71.

Cox, D. A., Anderson, P. G., and Roubin, G. S. (1992). Effect of local delivery of heparin and methotrexate on neointimal proliferation in stented porcine coronary arteries. Cor. Art. Dis. 3: 237–248.

Dinbergs, I. D., Brown, L., and Edelman, E. R. (1996). Cellular response to transforming growth factor-beta 1 and basic fibroblast growth factor depends on release kinetics and extracellular matrix interactions. J. Biol. Chem. 271: 29822–29829.

Downs, E. C., Robertson, N. E., Riss, T. L.; and Plunkett, M. L. (1992). Calcium alginate beads as a slow-release system for delivering angiogenic molecules in vivo and in vitro. J. Cell Physiol. 152: 422–429.

Edelman, E. R., Mathiowitz, E., Langer, R., and Klagsbrun, M. (1991). Controlled and modulated release of basic fibroblast growth factor. Biomaterials 12: 619–626.

Edelman, E. R., Nugent, M. A., Smith, L. T.; and Karnovsky, M. (1992). Basic fibroblast growth factor enhances the coupling of intimal hyperplasia and proliferation of vasa vasorum in injured rat arteries. J. Clin. Invest. 89: 465–471.

Elcin, Y. M., Dixit, V., and Gitnick, G. (1996). Controlled release of endothelial cell growth factor from chitosan-albumin microspheres for localized angiogenesis: in vitro and in vivo studies. Artif. Cells Blood Substit. Immobil. Biotechnol. 24: 257–271.

Fram, D. B., Aretz, T., and Azrin, M. A. (1994). Localized intramural drug delivery during balloon angioplasty using hydrogel-coated balloons and pressure-augmented diffusion. J. Am. Coll. Cardiol. 23: 1570–1577.

Gimple, L. W., Owen, R. M., and Lodge, V. P. (1992). Reduction in angioplasty restenosis in rabbits by chronic subcutaneous heparin with or without intramural heparin delivery. Circulation 82: III–338.

Gombotz, W. R., Pankey, S. C., Bouchard, L. S., Ranchalis, J., and Puolakkainen, P. (1993). Controlled release of TGF-β1 from a biodegradable matrix for bone regeneration. J. Biomater. Sci. Polym. Edn. 5: 49–63.

Gospodarowicz, D., and Cheng, J. (1986). Heparin protects basic and acidic FGF from inactivation. J. Cell. Physiol. 128: 475–484.

Hayek, A., Culler, F. L., Beattie, G. M., Lopez, A. D., Cuevas, P., and Baird, A. (1987). An in vivo model for the study of the angiogenic effects of basic fibroblast growth factor. Biochem. Biophys. Res. Comm. 147: 876–880.

Hoffman, D., Wahlberg, L., and Aebischer, P. (1990). NGF released from a polymer matrix prevents loss of ChAT expression in basal forebrain neurons following a fimbria-fornix lesion. Exp. Neurol. 110: 39–44.

Hong, M. K., Bhatti, T., and Mathews, B. J. (1993). The effect of porous infusion balloon delivered angiopeptin on myointimal hyperplasia after balloon injury in the rabbit. Circulation 88: 638–648.

Khouri, R. K., Hong, S. P., Deune, E. G., Tarpley, J. E., Song, S. Z., Serdar, C. M., and Pierce, G. F. (1994). De novo generation of permanent neovascularized soft tissue appendages by platelet-derived growth factor. J. Clin. Invest. 94: 1757–1763.

Klagsbrun, M. (1989). The fibroblast growth factor family: structural and biological properties. Prog. in Growth Factor Res. 1: 207–235.

Lambert, C. R., Leone, J. E., and Rowland, S. M. (1993). Local drug delivery catheters: functional comparison of porous and microporous designs. Cor. Art. Dis. 4: 469–475.

Langer, R. (1990). New methods of drug delivery. Science 249: 1527–1533.

Langer, R. and Folkman, J. (1976). Polymers for the sustained release of proteins and other macromolecules. Nature 263: 797–800.

Langer, R. and Moses, M. (1991). Biocompatible controlled release polymers for delivery of polypeptides and growth factors. J. Cell. Biochem. 45: 340–345.

Levin, M. J., Leonard, B. M., and Burke, J. A. (1990). Clinical and angiographic results of balloon-expandable intracoronary stents in right coronary artieries. J. Am. Coll. Cardiol. 16: 332–339.

Muller, D. W. M., Topol, E. J., and Abrams, G. (1990). Intraural methotrexate therapy for the prevention of inimal proliferation following porcine carotid balloon angioplasty. Circulation 82: III–429.

Murray, J. B., Brown, L., and Langer, R. A (1983). A microsustained release system for epidermal growth factor. In Vitro 19: 743–748.

Nimni, M. E. (1997). Polypeptide growth factors: targeted delivery systems. Biomaterials 18: 1201–1225.

Nugent, M. A., Chen, O. S., and Edelman, E. R. (1992). Controlled release of fibroblast growth factor: activity in cell culture. Mat. Res. Soc. Symp. Proc. 252: 273–284.

Nunes, G. L., King, S. B., and Hanson, S. R. (1992). Hydrogel-coated PTCA balloon catheter delivery of an antithrombin inhibits platelet dependent thrombosis. Circulation 86: I–380.

Phillips, G. D., Stone, A. M., Jones, B. D., Schultz, J. C., Whitehead, R. A., and Knighton, D. R. (1994). Vascular endothelial growth factor (rhVEGF165) stimulates direct angiogenesis in the rabbit cornea. In Vivo 8: 961–965.

Plunkett, M. L. and Hailey, J. A. (1990). An in vivo quantitative angiogenesis model using tumor cells entrapped in alginate. Lab. Invest. 62: 510–517.

Puel, J., Rousseau, H., and Joffre, F. (1987). Intravascular stents to prevent restenosis after transluminal coronary angioplasty. Circulation 76: IV–27.

Rhine, W., Hsieh, D., and Langer, R. (1980). Polymers for the sustained macromolecule release: procedures to fabricate reproducible delivery systems and control release kinetics. J. Pharm. Sci. 69: 265–270.

Riessen, R. and Isner, J. M. (1994). Prospects for site-specific delivery of pharmacologic and molecular therapies. J. Am. Coll. Cardiol. 23: 1234–1244.

Riessen, R., Rahimizadeh, H., and Blessing, E. (1993). Arterial gene transfer using pure DNA applied directly to a hydrogel coated angioplasty balloon. Hum. Gene Ther. 4: 749–758.

Rifkin, D. B. and Moscatelli, D. (1989). Recent developments in the cell biology of basic fibroblast growth factor. J. Cell Biol. 109: 1–6.

Sefton, M. V., Brown, L. R., and Langer, R. S. (1984). Ethylene-vinyl acetate copolymer microspheres for controlled release of macromolecules. J. Pharm. Sci. 73: 1859–1861.

Serruys, P. W., Strauss, B. H., and Beat, K. J. (1991). Angiographic follow-up of a self-expanding coronary artery stent. N. Engl. J. Med. 324: 13–17.

Sheriff, M. U., Khetpal, V., and Spears, J. R. (1993). Method of application of local high dose heparin during balloon angioplasty. J. Am. Coll. Cardiol. 21: 188A.

Sheth, S., Park, K. D., and Dev, V. (1994). Prevention of stent subacute thrombosis by segmented polyurethaneurea-polyethylene oxide-heparin coating in the rabbit carotid. J. Am. Coll. Cardiol. 23: 187A.

Sigwart, U., Puel, J., and Mirkovitch, V. (1987). Intravascular stents to prevent occlusion and restenosis after transluminal angioplasty. N. Engl. J. Med. 316: 701–706.

Sigwart, U., Urban, P., and Golf, S. (1988). Emergency stenting for acute occlusion after coronary balloon angioplasty. Circulation 78: 1121–1127.

Silberstein, G. B. and Daniel, C. W. (1987). Reversible inhibition of mammary gland growth by transforming growth factor-β. Science 237: 291–293.

Thompson, J. A.; Anderson, K. D., DiPietro, J. M., Zwiebel, J. A., Zametta, M., Anderson, W. F., and Maciag, T. (1988). Site-directed neovessel formation in vivo. Science 241: 1349–1352.

Urban, P., Sigwart, U., and Golf, S. (1989). Intravascular stenting for stenosis of aortocoronary venous bypass grafts. J. Am. Coll. Cardiol. 13: 1085–1091.

Van Belle, E., Maillard, L., Tio, F. O., and Isner, J. M. (1997b). Accelerated endothelialization by local delivery of recombinant human vascular endothelial growth factor reduces in-stent intimal formation. Biochem. Biophys. Res. Commun. 235: 311–316.

Van Belle, E., Tio, F. O., Couffinhal, T., Maillard, L., Passeri, J., and Isner, J. M. (1997b). Stent endothelialization. Time course, impact of local catheter delivery, feasibility of recombinant protein administration, and response to cytokine expedition. Circulation (DAW) 95: 438–448.

Wilensky, R. L., Gradus-Pizlo, I., and March, K. L. (1992). Efficacy of local intramural injection of colchicine in reducing restenosis following angioplasty in the atherosclerotic rabbit model. Circulation 86: I–52.

Wilensky, R. L., March, K. L., and Gradus-Pizlo, I. (1993). Enhanced localization and retention of microparticles following intramural delivery into atherosclerotic arteries using a new delivery catheter. J. Am. Coll. Cardiol. 21: 185A.

Wolinsky, H. and Thung, S. N. (1990). Use of a perforated balloon catheter to delivery concentrated heparin into the wall of the normal canine atery. J. Am. Coll. Cardiol. 15: 475–481.

Yanagisawa-Miwa, A., Uchida, Y., Nakamura, F., Tomaru, T., Kido, H., Kamijo, T., Sugimoto, T., Kaji, K., Utsuyama, M., and Kurashima, C. (1992). Salvage of infarcted myocardium by angiogenic action of basic fibroblast growth factor. Science 257: 1401–1403.

Zhu, X., Komiya, H., Chirino, A., Faham, S., Fox, G. M., Arakawa, T., Hsu, B. T., and Rees, D. C. (1991). Three dimensional structures of acidic and basic fibroblast growth factors. Science 251: 90–93.

12

Coronary Microcirculation and Angiogenesis

FRANK W. SELLKE AND DAVID G. HARRISON

Because of its obvious importance in terms of delivery of blood and nutrients to the myocardium, there has been a long-standing interest in properties of the resistance circulation of the heart. Prior to the mid-1980s, due to technical limitations, it was difficult to directly study coronary microvessels either in situ or in vitro. Traditionally, therefore, studies of the coronary microcirculation had been limited to indirect assessments using measurements of coronary flow and calculations of coronary resistance. While these provided a great deal of insight into the properties of the intact coronary circulation, significantly more has been learned in the last 10 years as new approaches have been developed for direct study of coronary microvessels. Further, methods have recently been developed for study of the coronary circulation in humans which have increased our understanding of coronary pathology.

As is the case with other vascular beds, the coronary microcirculation is composed of resistance arterioles, capillaries, and small veins (venules). There are unique features of the coronary microcirculation which allow it to function in the setting of a contracting support structure, to interact with the surrounding tissue, and to respond to rather dynamic changes in requirements for nutrients. These features of the coronary microcirculation have been reviewed previously in extensive review articles (Feigel, 1983; Hoffman, 1987) and entire books (Marcus, 1983; Schaper, 1979). Although space does not permit a thorough reanalysis of all facets of coronary physiology covered in these prior reviews, the following paragraphs will be used to discuss and emphasize some of the critical aspects of the physiology of the coronary circulation, in particular, as they relate to the coronary microcirculation. In subsequent paragraphs, we will discuss new information regarding the physiology and pharmacology of the coronary microcirculation and emphasize how these pertain to angiogenesis.

DEFINITIONS: THE CORONARY RESISTANCE CIRCULATION AS DEFINED BY PRESSURE GRADIENTS

By strictest definition, resistance vessels are those vessels over which pressure losses occur. Traditionally, resistance vessels were considered to be precapillary arterioles (25–50 μm), and vessels larger than this were thought to have little, if any role, in regulation of perfusion. For the coronary circulation, this concept was radically changed in the 1980s when first Nellis et al. (1981) and subsequently, Chilian and co-workers (1986) demonstrated that approximately 50% of total coronary vascular resistance is present in vessels larger than 100 μm in diameter. In these studies, it was found that pressure decreases could be observed in vessels as large as 300 μm. As illustrated in Figure 12.1, the distribution of vascular resistance is not static and the size of vessels regulating vascular resistance depends on the tone of the vasculature. The intravenous administration of dipyridamole causes a significant redistribution of microvascular resistance such that larger arteries and veins account for a greater proportion of resistance under conditions of vasodilation, such as during ischemia (Chilian et al., 1989). In fact, up to 30% of resistance may reside in the venous circulation under conditions of maximal vascular dilatation, in contrast to that predicted by older traditional theories of vascular regulation. These observations have led to numerous studies, both in vivo and in vitro, examining properties of these larger (100–300 μm) microvessels.

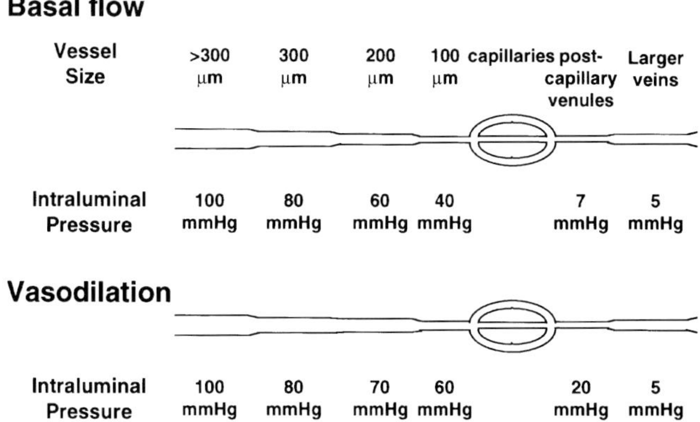

Figure 12.1. Intravascular pressures in the coronary microcirculation under basal conditions and during vasodilation with dipyridamole. Adapted from Chilian et al. (1989).

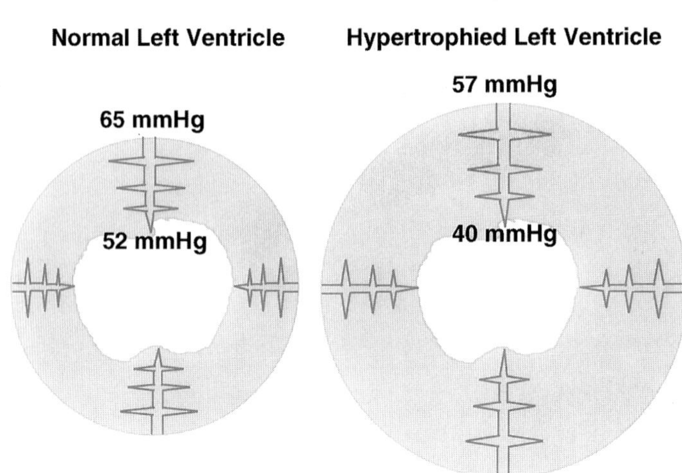

Figure 12.2. Transmural losses of coronary perfusion pressure in normal and hypertrophied hearts. Pressures were measured using micropuncture-servo null techniques in hearts perfused via the left main coronary artery at 100 mmHg. Adapted from Fujii et al. (1992).

Coronary circulation is unique in that there are not only pressure losses as vessel size decreases, but also additional pressure losses in vessels as they penetrate from the epicardium to the endocardium (Chilian, 1991). During maximal vasodilation, this pressure gradient increases from a few millimeters of mercury (8–10) to >20 mmHg. Importantly, in the setting of cardiac hypertrophy, this transmural pressure gradient is increased (Fujii et al., 1992), (Fig. 12.2). This results in a reduction of perfusion pressure in the subendocardium and may explain, in part, the susceptibility of hypertrophied hearts to develop subendocardial ischemia or infarction.

REGULATION OF CORONARY VASOMOTOR TONE. ENDOGENOUS AND EXOGENOUS CONTROL

Vasomotor tone results from the complex interaction of circulating substances, properties intrinsic to the vessel wall, influences from surrounding parenchymal tissue, neuronal influences and extravascular factors. Properties intrinsic to the vessel wall and interactions with adjacent tissues may work together to promote metabolic regulation and autoregulation. In the coronary circulation, there is evidence that all of these play a role in setting the tone of the microvessels. These are summarized in Fig. 12.3.

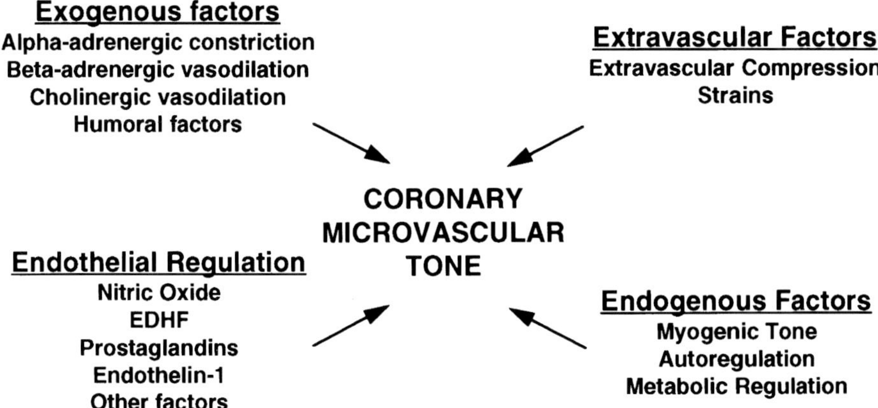

Figure 12.3. Major factors contributing to regulation of coronary microvascular tone.

Myogenic Tone

Myogenic tone is a property of the vascular smooth muscle in most vessels, including coronary microvessels (Kuo et al., 1988). The myogenic response is defined as an increase in wall tension, or a decrease in vessel diameter, in response to an increase in vascular transmural pressure. Myogenic mechanisms importantly contribute to regulation of blood flow and maintenance of basal vascular tone and have been postulated to be one mechanism whereby autoregulation occurs (as discussed below). Increases in myogenic tone, which occur during stretch of vascular smooth muscle, are associated with an increase in inositol 1,4,5-trisphosphate, presumably due to activation of phospholipase C (Osol et al., 1991; Narayanan et al., 1994). Recent evidence in cerebral arteries indicates that a large conductance, calcium-activated potassium channel is opened when the vascular smooth muscle is depolarized, providing a feedback inhibitory mechanism limiting the degree of depolarization and vasoconstriciton (Brayden and Nelson, 1992). Inhibitors of protein kinase C reduce myogenic tone while activators of protein kinase C increase myogenic tone (Osol et al., 1993). Myogenic tone in coronary vessels is not affected by removal of the endothelium. The degree of myogenic tone that has been observed in coronary vessels is variable depending on the preparation used and the species studied. In porcine and primate coronary vessels, spontaneous tone and myogenic responses are often observed, while in canine coronary microvessels, spontaneous and myogenic tone are uncommonly observed. Myogenic responses to increases in pressure are greater in coronary microvessels from the subepicardium than in vessels from the subendocardium (Kuo et al., 1988). Interestingly, exercise training seems to increase the capacity for coronary arterioles to generate myogenic tone (Muller et al., 1993). The physiological relevance of this remains unclear.

Metabolic Regulation and Autoregulation

The tone of the coronary microcirculation and consequently levels of myocardial perfusion are tightly coupled to the state of myocardial oxygen consumption. When myocardial oxygen needs are increased, coronary flow rises accordingly. In part, this is due to the fact that myocardial oxygen extraction is near maximum even under resting conditions. Thus, the ability of the myocardium to extract additional oxygen to meet increased demand is limited.

Autoregulation refers to the ability of a vascular bed to constrict and dilate in order to maintain flow constant during changes in perfusion pressure. In the coronary circulation, autoregulation is most effective between pressures of 40 to 160 mmHg. The range of pressures over which autoregulation can be observed is different for the subendocardium, as compared to the subepicardium. Thus, flow will begin to decrease at pressures < 70–75 mmHg in the subendocardium, as opposed to substantially lower pressures in the more superficial layers of the heart (Boatwright et al., 1980). Importantly, chronic hypertension shifts the range of pressures over which autoregulation occurs in the subendocardium such that flow will begin to decline at even higher pressures. This may be related to changes in subendocardial perfusion pressure (discussed above) and thus may also explain the propensity for the subendocardium to develop ischemia in the setting of myocardial hypertrophy. Of note, during both autoregulation and metabolic regulation, studies using direct observations of the coronary microcirculation indicate that the predominant changes in vasomotion occur in vessels < 100 μm in diameter.

The signaling molecule(s) linking flow to demand and participating in the autoregulation process has been the subject of extensive investigation, but remains poorly defined. Prostaglandins, nitric oxide, tissue levels of oxygen, carbon dioxide, hydrogen ions, and potassium have all been considered as candidates (Olsson and Bunger, 1987). Extensive research spanning 40 years has been devoted to understanding a potential role of adenosine as a mediator of either autoregulation or metabolic regulation. Adenosine was thought to be a likely candidate because it was a potent vasodilator and would accumulate as a result of increased cardiac work or ischemia. Indeed, several studies showed that adenosine levels in the heart and coronary sinus correlated with the state of myocardial work and coronary perfusion (Olsson and Bunger, 1987). Despite this, antagonists of the adenosine receptor and degradation of adenosine using adenosine deaminase were found, in most studies, to have only minor effects on myocardial perfusion at rest or during a variety of interventions (for review see Marcus, 1993). Subtle changes in myocardial perfusion in intact animals have been observed during adenosine deaminase infusion (which serves to degrade interstitial adenosine) (Gewirtz et al., 1986) and in isolated hearts. This intervention has been shown to markedly alter reactive hyperemia, metabolic regulation, and autoregulation (Serban et al., 1989). Recently, a role for ATP-sensitive potassium channels in regulation of myocardial perfusion has been discovered. Kamoru and co-workers showed that blockade of these channels with glibenclamide inhibited the vasodilation of coronary microvessels less than 100 μm in diameter caused by reduction in perfusion pressure (Komaru et al., 1993). Likewise, blockade of these channels reduce basal coronary perfusion in vivo (Duncker et al., 1993). A very attractive concept regarding regulation of myocardial perfusion has recently been put forth by Dunker and colleagues (Duncker et al., 1996). These investigators have observed that two separate pathways, potassium channel opening and adenosine receptor activation, seem to interact to modulate myocardial flow during exercise and during changes in myocardial perfusion pressure. The concept that there is redundancy in terms of control of such an important process as coronary metabolic and autoregulation is extremely important, and may explain why previous studies, in which these individual pathways were examined alone, were, in general, negative.

Recently, it has been suggested that an arachidonic acid metabolite of cytochrome P_{450}, 20-HETE, may be important in local regulation of blood flow in response to oxygen, at least in the renal circulation (Harder et al., 1996). This molecule is a potent vasoconstrictor and an inhibitor of large-conductance potassium channels in renal arterioles (Zou et al., 1996). Immunoblotting and reverse-transcription polymerase chain reactions have shown that renal and cremasteric arterioles express mRNA and protein for the cytochrome P_{450} 4A2 enzyme. Further, 20-HETE can be detected as being produced by these tissues. Interestingly, the production of 20-HETE is dependent on oxygen, and it has been suggested that 20-HETE may serve as an oxygen sensor in renal arterioles (Harder et al., 1996). Whether this occurs in other vascular beds remains to be established. However, if 20-HETE can serve as an oxygen sensor, it is easy to visualize a role for it in modulating local flow in response to oxygen demand and supply.

Extravascular Forces

The coronary circulation is particularly unique in that it is exposed to a large number of extravascular forces produced by contraction of adjacent myocardium and intraventricular pressures. Extravascular influences may become more evident during ischemia or in the setting of other pathologic processes leading to decreased tissue compliance or increased tissue edema. For example, collateral perfusion is particularly sensitive to changes in heart rate (more frequent extravascular compression) and ventricular diameter (stretch) (Schaper, 1979; Conway et al., 1988).

Of relevance to the concept of extravascular pressures is the idea that extravascular pressure might collapse coronary vessels under certain circumstances. In 1978, Bellamy reported that flow through the epicardial coronary arteries halted when aortic pressure fell to values ranging from 25 to 50 mmHg (Bellamy, 1978). This observation, and others like it, raised the possibility that extravascular forces might be sufficiently high to collapse vessels when intraluminal pressures declined to values below this "critical closing pressure." It soon became apparent, however, that flow in the coronary microcirculation continued even when the arterial driving pressure was minimally higher than coronary venous pressure. Based on modeling and various experimental interventions, it was determined that the decrease of antegrade blood flow in larger upstream vessels associated with continued forward flow in microvessels was likely due to capacitance in the coronary circulation (Eng et al., 1982). Kanatsuka and colleagues used a floating microscope to visualize epicardial capillaries and were able to show that red cells continued to flow, even after perfusion had stopped in the more proximal vessels. Using this approach, they were able to show that the "stop-flow" pressure in the epicardial coronary microvessels was within a few mmHg higher than right atrial pressure (Kanatsuka et al., 1990). Furthermore, they did not observe closure of epicardial coronary microvessels at any pressure. It, therefore, seems likely that the concept of "critical closing pressure" is not applicable to all vessels in the coronary circulation. It is conceivable, however, that vessels deeper in the subendocardium might be made to collapse by pressure transmitted from the ventricular chamber, particularly when left ventricular diastolic pressure is very high.

Neurohumoral Control of the Circulation

In the past three decades, there has been an enormous amount of research devoted to understanding the role of the sympathetic and parasympathetic nervous systems in regulation of coronary perfusion (Young et al., 1987). In vivo, in awake animals, α-adrenergic stimulation produces rather marked reductions in coronary flow, suggesting constriction of coronary resistance vessels (Eng et al., 1982). Administration of β-adrenergic stimuli results in marked coronary vasodilation, due both to a direct effect on the β-adrenergic receptors on the coronary microvessels and an increase in myocardial metabolic demand. During direct sympathetic nerve stimulation, in general, coronary vasodilation occurs. If β-adrenergic antagonists are administered, a transient vasoconstriction can be observed. When coronary microvessels are studied in vitro, α-adrenergic stimulation has minimal contractile effects (Wang et al., 1994). When selective α_{2}-adrenergic stimulation is applied using pharmacological stimuli, there is rather potent vasodilation of all sized coronary microvessels, predominantly due to a release of endothelium-derived nitric oxide (NO$^{\bullet}$). β-adrenergic stimulation produces a potent relaxation of all coronary arteries, but especially small resistance vessels (Wang et al., 1994). It appears that the β_2-adrenergic receptor-subtype predominates in vessels less than 100 μm in diameter in in vitro studies (Wang et al., 1994), whereas a mixed β_1-or β_2-adrenergic receptor population controls vascular resistance in in vivo studies. Larger coronary vessels are regulated by a mixed β_1-and β_2-adrenoceptor subtype population, or a predominant β_1-adrenergic mechanism.

Activation of cholinergic receptors by either vagal stimulation or by the infusion of acetylcholine produces a uniform vasodilation of coronary vessels (Lamping et al., 1992a). This vasodilation is predominantly mediated by endothelium-derived NO•, although release of a hyperpolarizing factor (discussed below) (Hammarstrom et al., 1995) and the release of prostaglandin substances (Sellke and Dai, 1993) may also play a role in the response of vessels to many vasoactive substances. The role of endothelium-derived factors in regulation of coronary microvascular tone is discussed more thoroughly in later paragraphs in this chapter.

Effects of Humoral Agents on the Coronary Microcirculation

The response of the coronary microcirculation to a variety of humoral agents is very heterogeneous. For example, serotonin (Lamping et al., 1989) constricts vessels greater than 100 μm in diameter whereas it causes potent vasodilation of smaller arteries. In contrast, vasopressin produces greater constriction of microvessels less than 100 μm in diameter than it produces in larger microvessels (Lamping et al., 1989; Sellke et al., 1990c). In the larger epicardial coronary arteries, vasopressin causes predominantly vasodilation. Endothelin-1 produces vasoconstriction when administered to the adventitial surface of coronary microvessels. The degree of constriction produced by endothelin-1 is inversely related to the size of the vessels. Paradoxically, when endothelin-1 is administered intraarterially, vasodilation occurs, presumably, by via release of nitric oxide (Lamping et al., 1992). Activation of other receptors, such as the thromboxane receptor (Sellke and Dai, 1993), results in uniform constriction of all coronary arterioles and veins.

ENDOTHELIAL REGULATION OF THE CORONARY MICROCIRCULATION

In addition to direct influences on the vascular smooth muscle, numerous neurohumoral stimuli modulate coronary vascular tone via their effect on the endothelium. As in all other circulations, in the coronary circulation, the endothelium releases a variety of substances which modulate tone of the resistance vessels. These substances include nitric oxide (NO•), prostaglandins, a hyperpolarizing factor, endothelin, and reactive oxygen species. Among these various factors, NO• plays a predominant role. The enzyme responsible for production of NO• is a 133-kDa protein constitutively expressed by endothelial cells which is known as the *endothelial nitric oxide synthase (eNOS or NOS-3)*. The biochemical mechanisms responsible for function of the NO synthases have recently been elucidated. For all isoforms, an electron donor, NADPH, binds to a site at the carboxyl terminus of the protein. Electrons are then transferred from NADPH to the flavins, flavin adenine dinucleotide (FAD) and flavin mononucleotide (FMN) noncovalently bound within the reductase domain. For the neuronal NOS and eNOS, electrons are stored on the flavins until the enzyme is activated by calcium/calmodulin (Ca/CaM). When calmodulin binds to the enzyme, electrons are transferred to a prosthetic heme group in the oxygenase domain. Upon heme reduction, catalysis of arginine to citrulline and nitric oxide occurs. The NO˙ formed diffuses to underlying vascular smooth muscle, where it (among other actions) stimulates soluble guanylate cyclase, increasing cGMP, and prompting vasodilation via activation of cGMP-dependent protein kinase (Murad, 1986). There is substantial evidence that NO˙ may undergo reactions which other molecules, such as thiol containing compounds, to form biologically active nitroso intermediates (Myers et al., 1990). While binding of calcium/calmodulin is a prerequisite for activity of the enzyme, there is evidence that other phenomena, such as phosphorylation (Corson et al., 1996), membrane binding (Venema et al., 1995), and association with the integral membrane protein caveolin (Michel et al., 1997), can also modulate NOS activity. The eNOS is constitutively expressed; however, its expression is subject to modest, and yet likely important, degrees of regulation. Thus, factors such as shear stress (Uemetsu et al., 1995), the state of endothelial cell growth (Arnal et al., 1994), hypoxia (McQuillan et al., 1994), exposure to oxidized low density lipoprotein, and exposure to cytokines have been shown to affect expression of eNOS. In some instances, factors known to decrease eNOS expression are associated with decreases in eNOS mRNA half-life rather than changes in the rate of its transcription. In the coronary circulation, the release of NO˙ confers a state of basal vasodilation, and administration of NO synthase antagonists produces an increase in resting coronary resistance (Amezcua et al., 1989). When substances such as acetylcholine and bradykinin are administered, coronary microvessels of all sizes dilate.

There is also evidence, particularly in smaller vessels both in the coronary and peripheral circulations, that factors other than NO˙ can modulate endothelium-dependent vascular relaxation. One such factor is the endothelium-derived hyperpolarizing factor (EDHF). Even before the endothelium was found to be critical in modulating vascular tone, it was known that certain relaxing substances would hyperpolarize vascular smooth muscle. It was subsequently shown that this phenomenon was endothelium-dependent (Taylor and Weston, 1988). This hyperpolarizing effect occurs via opening of vascular smooth muscle potassium channels, and the channel type involved has been the subject of substantial interest. These have largely been characterized using pharmacological means. In cerebral vessels, a voltage-regulated potassium channel has been implicated in endothelium-dependent hyperpolarization (Petersson et al., 1997), whereas others have suggested that the EDHF acts on large conductance potassium channels. When the vascular smooth muscle is hyperpolarized, voltage-sensitive calcium channels are closed, leading to a reduction in intracellular calcium. There is debate as to the nature of the hyperpolarizing factor, and some investigators have suggested that it is simply $NO^{\bullet}$ acting in a fashion independent of guanylate cyclase. Recent data supports the concept that the hyperpolarizing factor is a cytochrome P_{450} fatty acid metabolite (Campbell et al., 1996), although this remains controversial (Fulton et al., 1997). In the coronary circulation, the importance of the hyperpolarizing factor in modulating endothelium-dependent vascular relaxation seems to increase as vessel size decreases (Shimokawa et al., 1996).

Prostaglandin synthesis by the endothelium also contributes to modulation of tone in the coronary microcirculation. Interestingly, the production of prostaglandins seems to inhibit production of nitric oxide during hypoxia (Xu et al., 1995), although the mechanism for this has not been clarified.

CONSIDERATIONS REGARDING THE CORONARY VENULES IN MODULATION OF OVERALL CORONARY VASCULAR RESPONSIVENESS

While the arterial microcirculation is considered to be the predominant regulator of coronary blood flow, venules may have a considerable importance under conditions of vascular dilation, as noted above (Chilian et al., 1989), such as during exercise, metabolic stress, or during reperfusion after myocardial ischemia. The venous circulation may also influence myocardial stiffness and diastolic properties of the heart. Veins may respond differently to agonists and neuronal stimulation compared to arteries in the same vascular bed (Sellke and Dai, 1993; Klassen and Armour, 1982). Thus, a consideration of the venous circulation apart from the arterial circulation may be warranted under certain physiologic and clinical conditions.

Not only is vasomotor regulation differentially controlled between the venous and arterial microcirculations, but certain reactions to pathologic stimuli occur preferentially on one side of the capillary bed. For example, postcapillary venules are the initiating site of neutrophil adherence and transmigration (Yuan et al., 1995), whereas arterioles seldom manifest these initial changes in the inflammatory response. In addition, complement fragment C5a causes neutophil adherence in venules but not in arterioles, suggesting that different mechanisms mediate neutrophil–endothelial adherence in the two vessel types. However, while ischemia reperfusion has been determined to cause endothelial dysfunction in veins (Lefer et al., 1992), under similar conditions, arterioles appear to be more susceptible to a reduction in endothelium dependent relaxation than are coronary venules (Piana et al., 1996), despite the fact that leukocytes preferentially adhere to venular as compared to arterial endothelial cells.

THE ROLE OF ENDOTHELIAL FACTORS IN VASCULAR GROWTH, DEVELOPMENT, AND RESPONSE TO INJURY

Relevant to a role of endothelial mediators in the coronary microcirculation is the recent interest in the role of nitric oxide and nitric oxide-related factors on the growth of vascular cells and blood vessels. This research was largely spurred by an observation made in 1989 by Garg and Hassid. These investigators reported that nitrovasodilators and NO˙ donors, such as sodium nitroprusside and S-nitrosopenacillamine, reduced growth of vascular smooth muscle cells and fibroblasts in culture (Garg and Hassid, 1989). This observation, subsequently, prompted a large number of studies examining the effect of NO˙ on vascular development and cell growth. In Garg and Hassid's initial studies, very large concentrations of the nitrovasodilators seemed to be necessary to produce this effect, and there was initially some skepticism regarding the physiological importance of this finding. Subsequent studies have largely supported their premise, implicating NO˙ as a inhibitor of smooth muscle growth. In rabbits, treatment with L-nitroarginine methyl ester L-NAME, which inhibits NO˙ formation) markedly increases the neointimal development following vascular balloon injury (Cayatte et al., 1994). Likewise, local transfection of the rat carotid artery with the eNOS cDNA reduces the intimal proliferation which follows balloon injury (von der Leyen et al., 1995). Recently, it has been reported that the vascular response to injury is enhanced in mice deficient in eNOS (Moroi et al., 1996). This effect of NO˙ on vascular smooth muscle growth is mediated by cGMP and can be mimicked by cGMP analogs (Yu et al., 1997). Interestingly, atrial natriuretic factor (which increases cGMP via activation of a particulate guanylate cyclase) shares this property of nitric oxide (Itoh et al., 1992). Of relevance to intact vessels, C-type natriuretic peptide (CNP), which is produced by endothelial cells, can also inhibit smooth muscle growth (Yu et al., 1997). There is some debate as to whether the antigrowth effects of NO˙ or the natriuretic peptide are mediated by cAMP-cGMP-dependent protein kinases (Yu et al., 1997; Cornwell et al., 1994). Recent data indicate that a portion of the effect of NO˙ on vascular smooth muscle is not only to inhibit growth, but also to promote apoptosis (Pollman et al., 1996).

These effects of NO˙ on smooth muscle cell growth have obvious implications for neointimal formation in atherosclerosis and following vessel injury. Thus, there has been substantial interest in using nitric oxide donors, or organic nitrates, as an approach to modify the atherosclerotic process or to prevent restenosis following angioplasty. Studies to date using these drugs have not shown any obvious benefit. However, the potential use of these agents as modulators of mitogenesis and proliferation may not be as yet realized.

While NO˙ and cyclic GMP elevating agents inhibit the growth of fibroblasts and vascular smooth muscle, they do not alter the rate of growth of endothelial cells as assessed by cell number or [^{3}H]-thymidine incorporation (Arnal et al., 1994). This is important, because, as discussed above, one of the most potent stimuli for increasing expression of the endothelial NO synthase is proliferation. Proliferating cells express about sixfold as much eNOS mRNA as confluent cells (Arnal et al., 1994). An example of this is shown in Fig. 12.4. This is associated with a threefold increase in eNOS protein and nitric oxide production by the proliferating cells as compared to nongrowing cells. If one considers this in terms of the ability of the vessel to respond to injury, it makes teleological sense. Following endothelial denudation, the proliferating endothelial cells, as

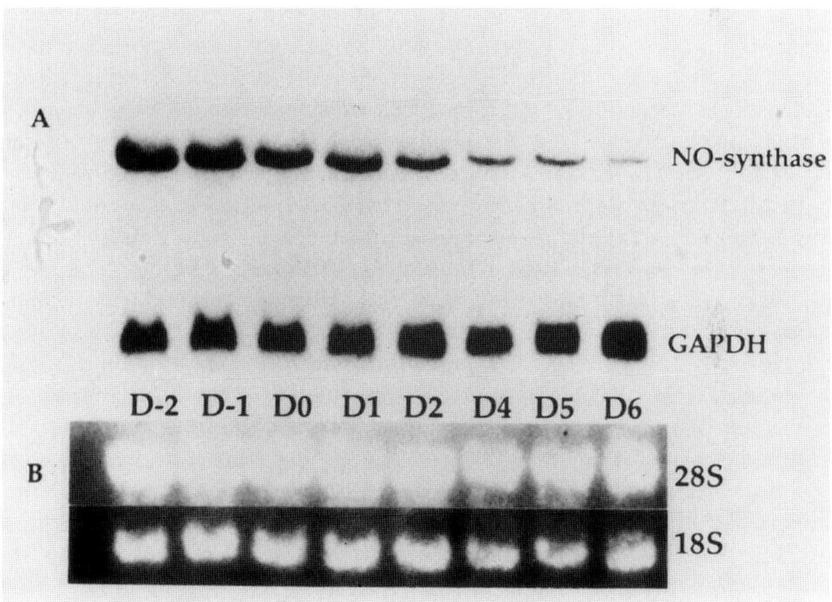

Figure 12.4. The effect of endothelial cell growth state on expression of NO synthase. Endothelial cells were seeded so that they reached confluence after 3 days in culture (D0). Cells were harvested and total RNA extracted on the various days from 2 days before confluence (D−2) to 6 days postconfluence (D6). Northern analysis was performed for eNOS and the housekeeping gene GAPDH. Shown below is the ethidium bromide stain of the blot for appearance of the 28 and 18s rRNA bands. The data from the GAPDH and the ethidium bromide stain indicate that the gel was equally loaded for all lanes. Note the dramatic decrease in eNOS mRNA as the cells reach confluence in culture. From Arnal et al. (1994).

they grow back to re-cover the exposed intima, produce large amounts of nitric oxide to make up for the paucity of endothelial cells in this area. This would tend to minimize platelet adhesion and vascular smooth muscle proliferation in the area. It is also advantageous that endothelial cells do not seem to be sensitive to the growth inhibitory effects of nitric oxide. This would permit them to rapidly reendothelialize a denuded region, even while producing large quantities of nitric oxide.

ROLE OF NITRIC OXIDE IN THE ANGIOGENIC PROCESS

In addition to the effect of nitric oxide in influencing the rate of vascular smooth muscle growth and the vascular response to injury is its effect on new vessel growth. The process of blood vessel formation involves several distinct steps, including increased vascular permeability and dissolution of the bond between the endothelium and basement membrane, migration, reattachment of endothelial cells, proliferation and migration, and finally the formation of a tubule which is the rudimentary vascular structure (Ware and Simons, 1997). The cellular and molecular changes required for the angiogenic process and the exact roles of growth factors and nitric oxide are as yet relatively poorly understood and at times seem contradictory, a fact that is not surprising considering the seemingly divergent effects of nitric oxide on the growth of endothelial cells and vascular smooth muscle cells. Almost universally, pathological conditions such as tissue hypoxia and inflammation that may lead to angiogenesis are associated with the production and release of growth factors, suggesting that these substances are critical to the formation of new blood vessels. Not only is the increased expression of growth factors seemingly critical to the initiation of collateral development, but their respective growth factor receptors must be upregulated and inhibitory factors must themselves be inhibited if the growth factors are to play a role in the initiation and later steps of vessel development. Indeed, increased expression of FGF receptor-1 and the VEGF receptors flt-1 and flk-1 is known to occur in both acute (Li et al., 1996) and chronic (Sellke et al., 1996) myocardial ischemia (Fig. 12.5).

There is also a strong relation between the release of NO with subsequent activation of guanylate cyclase and the regulation of blood vessel growth and development. But again, the relationship is not well defined and at times seems contradictory. For example, substance P and growth factors such as VEGF and FGF, all of which stimulate release of NO (Sellke et al., 1996; Wu et al., 1996; Ziche et al., 1994), induce new vessel formation in vivo in addition to increasing the permeability, migration, and proliferation of postcapillary endothelial cells in tissue culture (Wu et al., 1996; Morbidelli et al., 1996). Inhibitors of NO synthase suppress angiogenesis and the proliferative effect of VEGF is decreased in the presence

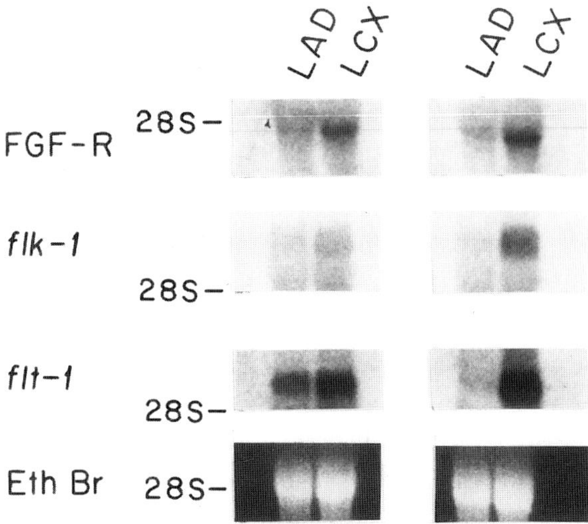

Figure 12.5. Expression of FGF-2 (FGFR1) and VEGF (flt-1, flk-1) receptors in chronically ischemic myocardium (Sellke et al., 1996).

of NO synthase inhibitors. It has also been demonstrated that tube development by growing endothelial cells in three-dimensional gels in response to transforming growth factor-β is dependent on nitric oxide and inhibited by antagonists of NO synthase (Papapetropoulos et al., 1997). The stimulated synthesis and release of endothelium-derived NO by VEGF and FGF-2 has been shown to be largely regulated by tyrosine kinase (Sellke et al., 1996), further implicating the role of NO in blood vessel formation. In a recent study using the rabbit corneal angiogenesis model, however, NOS was found to be involved in VEGF-induced angiogenesis, but not in angiogenesis induced by FGF-2 (Ziche et al., 1997). In addition, others have observed that the NO donor sodium nitroprusside and the NOS substrate L-arginine inhibit, while inhibitors of NO synthase increase, angiogenesis as assessed by protein synthesis and vascular density in the chick embryo chorioallantoic membrane (Pipili-Synetos et al., 1994) Likewise, in mice transplanted with Lewis lung carcinomas, tumor development and vascularity were inhibited by treatment with either isosorbide mononitrate or isosorbide dinitrate (Pipili-Synetos et al., 1995).

Overall, the exact roles of NO in the different stages of angiogenesis have not been determined with certainty, and may differ between species and vascular beds within species. Furthermore, NO and the cyclic GMP pathway are not the only mediators and modulators of the various stages of vessel development. For example, adenosine and increased tissue concentrations of cyclic AMP have been implicated in increased proliferation from studies of cultured endothelial cells (Meininger and Granger, 1990).

Thus, the coupling of humoral mediators with the development of collateral vessels appears redundant, complex, and as yet still poorly understood, with no single unifying mechanism or pathway.

To summarize, the ultimate effect of nitric oxide on vascular cellularity and growth is complex. Experimentally, nitric oxide clearly suppresses vascular thickening and intimal proliferation following balloon injury, and inhibits growth of vascular smooth muscle cells in culture. The ultimate effect on vessel growth of nitric oxide and related molecules seems to depend on the model employed and on whether a separate stimulus for angiogenesis is applied. The therapeutic benefit of NO donors on microcirculatory development in a clinical setting (for example, to stimulate new vessel growth in the heart) remains questionable. A major problem with the use of the currently available nitric-oxide-generating compounds in humans is that they cannot be used for prolonged periods of time due to the development of tolerance (in the case of the organic nitrates), toxicity (in the case of sodium nitroprusside), or generation of reactive oxygen species (in the case of molsidimine like drugs).

THE CORONARY MICROCIRCULATION IN DISEASE STATES:

A variety of systemic and cardiac diseases affect the coronary microcirculation. These may be considered functional alterations involving changes in responsiveness of the coronary microvessels, and structural effects, such as alterations of the number and diameter of the coronary microvessels.

Pathophysiological Alterations of Functional Properties of the Coronary Microcirculation

A particularly important aspect of endothelial regulation of vasomotion is that endothelial-mediated vasodilation is abnormal in a variety of pathological conditions. These include atherosclerosis, hypercholesterolemia, diabetes, hypertension, cigarette smoking, and aging. The mechanisms underlying these abnormal endothelium-dependent responses have been the subject of substantial debate. Deficiencies of the substrate for eNOS, L-arginine, and the cofactor tetrahydrobiopterin have all been implicated. Abnormalities of G-protein signaling, resulting in reduced activation of eNOS in response to endothelial cell receptor activation, have also been shown to occur. A substantial body of data suggests that in some of these conditions (hypercholesterolemia, hypertension and diabetes), increased production of vascular superoxide ($\bullet O_2^-$) occurs. Superoxide reacts very rapidly with NO$^\bullet$, leading to the formation of the toxic peroxynitrite anion. While peroxynitrite can produce vasodilation, it is a very weak vasodilator and as a result of this reaction, much, if not all of the vasodilator capacity of NO$^\bullet$ is lost.

The initial studies demonstrating abnormal endothelium-dependent vascular relaxation in various disease models were performed in larger vessels. Subsequent experiments have shown that most, if not all, of these disease processes also affect the coronary microcirculation in a similar fashion. This is of particular interest in the case of hypercholesterolemia and atherosclerosis. One of the first examples of an alteration in coronary microvessels in atherosclerosis was made in vessels from monkeys fed a high cholesterol diet for 18 months (Sellke et al., 1990a). These animals develop advanced atherosclerotic lesions in larger vessels, and had previously been shown to have abnormal vasodilation in response to acetylcholine, the calcium ionophore A23187, and thrombin in larger vessels. In coronary microvessels from monkeys fed a high cholesterol diet for 18 months, relaxations to the same acetylcholine, bradykinin, and the calcium ionophore A23187 were dramatically impaired, and in some cases, these agents produced paradoxical constrictions (Fig. 12.6). Similar findings have been made in other animal models of diet induced atherosclerosis. Subsequent studies performed using in vivo techniques showed that

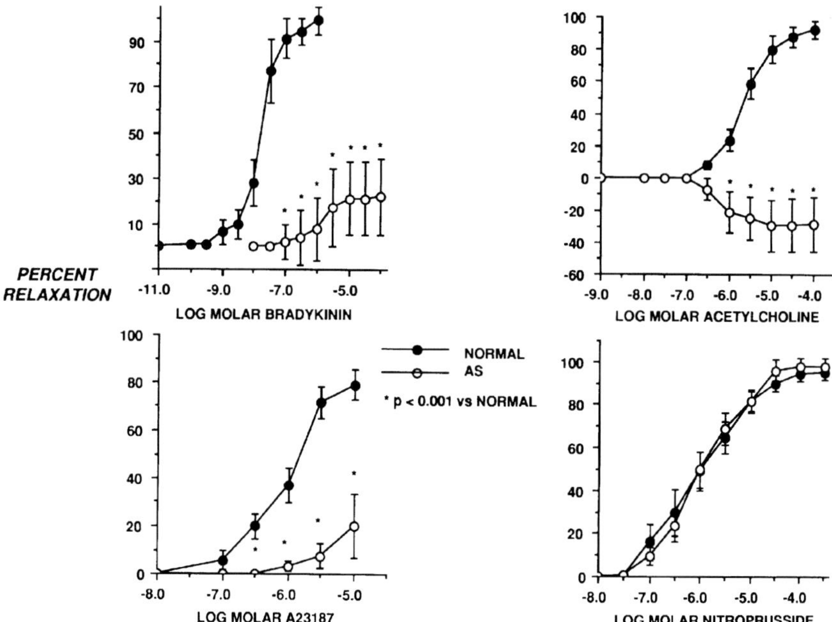

Figure 12.6. Effects of atherosclerosis on endothelium-dependent and endothelium-independent vasodilation. Cynomolgus monkeys were made atherosclerotic by being fed a high-cholesterol diet for 18 months. Coronary microvessels ranging from 70 to 140 μm in diameter were studied in a pressurized state using video microscopy. Following preconstriction, the various vasoactive agents were added in a cumulative fashion. Relaxations were expressed as a percent of preconstricted tension. Data are from Sellke et al. (1990a).

vasoconstriction caused by serotonin and ergonovine (both known to be modulated by the endothelium) was markedly enhanced in the coronary microcirculation of hypercholesterolemic monkeys (Chilian et al., 1990). These findings are striking because the coronary microcirculation is spared from the development of overt atherosclerosis. Thus, vessels that have been exposed to a high cholesterol milieu, even in the absence of atherosclerosis, develop abnormal vasomotion. While it is difficult to perform such studies in human vessels, investigators have used Doppler techniques to measure coronary flow in humans. Diminished flow responses to acetylcholine have been demonstrated in humans with hypercholesterolemia (Drexler et al., 1991). Importantly, this abnormality of vascular function has been corrected by reduction of serum cholesterol (Drexler et al., 1991). Similar observations have been made in either humans or experimental models of hypertension (Treasure et al., 1993), ischemia followed by reperfusion (Piana et al., 1996; Quillen et al., 1990), and diabetes (Matsunaga et al., 1996). Indeed, altered endothelial regulation of vasomotion has been found in the coronary arteries of patients with chest pain and normal coronary arteries, and it is thought that, at least in some instances, this might contribute to their clinical symptoms.

A particularly important clinical setting in which endothelial function is altered in the coronary microcirculation is following cardioplegic arrest and extracorporeal circulation (Sellke et al., 1993). This abnormality persists for some time after cardiopulmonary bypass and normalizes thereafter. Obviously, such a deficit in endothelial function may have important clinical implications because of the frequency in which cardioplegia is used in cardiovascular surgery. It is not uncommon for patients undergoing coronary artery bypass grafting, with seemingly complete coronary revascularization, to exhibit signs of myocardial ischemia during the hours following surgery. It is conceivable that alterations of endothelial function may contribute to this alteration in cardiac function. In addition, it is likely that the arteriopathy ofter observed after cardiac transplantation is in part related to endothelial injury as a result of inadequate vascular preservation.

A condition that rather strikingly alters coronary vascular reactivity is the development of collateral vessels. When a coronary artery is gradually occluded, flow to the subtended myocardium does not cease, but persists via perfusion through collateral vessels. As discussed in other chapters in this text, when these vessels fully develop, they are capable of providing normal resting perfusion to the region previously served by the occluded vessel, albeit at a lower perfusion pressure. Because collateral vessels represent "new" vessels, and because of their obvious pathophysiological importance, there has been interest in factors that might modulate their reactivity. To perform such studies, investigators have used ameroid constrictors to produce gradual occlusion of coronary arteries in dogs and pigs and have removed mature collateral vessels weeks to months later. For the most part, these vessels have demonstrated normal endothelium-dependent vascular relaxation and normal responses to most agents studied in vivo. In mature canine collateral vessels, however, constrictions to vasopressin are markedly enhanced when compared to the effect of vasopressin on similar sized native coronary arteries (Sellke et al., 1990c). In vivo, vasopressin has been shown to markedly reduce perfusion to collateral-dependent myocardium in doses that have no effect on normally perfused myocardium (Peters et al., 1989). This effect may be limited to pharmacologic properties of vasopressin, because studies of pigs with developed collaterals have failed to demonstrate an effect of a vasopressin antagonist on collateral perfusion during exercise (Symons et al., 1993). Interestingly, the coronary arterioles nourished by collaterals develop markedly abnormal vascular reactivity characterized by impaired endothelium-dependent vascular relaxations and enhanced constrictions to vasopressin (Fig. 12.7) (Sellke et al., 1990c). These observations were originally made in vitro in microvessels from a canine model of collateral development, but have since been repeated in a porcine model of chronic ischemia (Harada et al., 1996; Sellke et al., 1994).

The mechanism of the impaired microvascular endothelium-dependent relaxation in the collateral-dependent region has not been determined, but it may be related to increased local levels of NO due to increased expression of inducible nitric oxide synthase (iNOS) leading to reduced activity of eNOS (Ravichandran et al., 1995). Recent studies have demonstrated a marked increase in iNOS expression in chronically ischemic

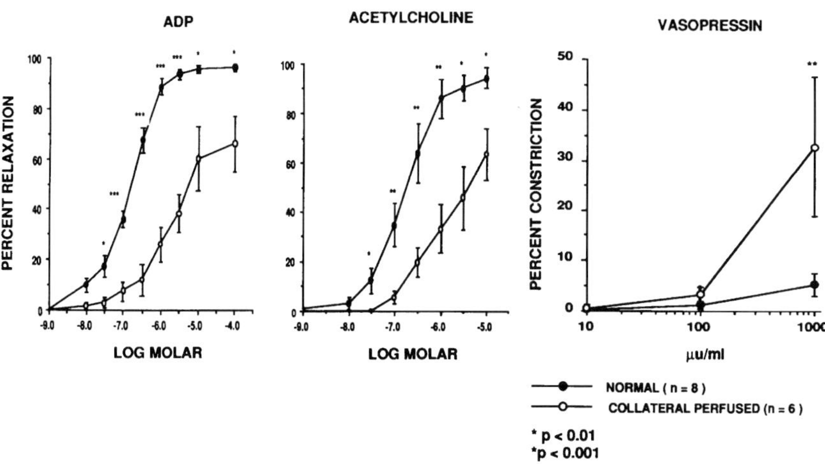

Figure 12.7. Alternations of vascular reactivity in microvessels from collateral-perfused myocardium. Collaterals were produced by placement of an ameroid constrictor on the circumflex coronary artery of dogs for 3–6 months. Following this, coronary microvessels ranging from 100 to 220μm were studied in vitro as described in Figure 12.6. Of note, vasodilation in response to the calcium ionophore A23187 and nitroglycerine was not altered in these vessels. Data are from Sellke et al. (1990c).

myocardium (Laham et al., 1998). Alternatively, changes in strear stress or pulsatile flow in the collateral dependent microvasculature may contribute to the altered vascular reactivity (Uemetsu et al., 1995). Finally, changes in intracellular calcium mobilization have been observed in collateral vessels (Rapps et al., 1997) which may impact on changes in vascular tone and responses.

Recent studies have addressed the possibility that collateral growth and coronary microvessel function might be altered by the direct perivascular application or infusion of angiogenic growth factors such FGF-1 or FGF-2, or VEGF. Indeed, such studies have shown that these therapeutic interventions are not only associated with improved myocardial function and improved perfusion in chonic ischemic models, but also with normalization of endothelium-dependent relaxation in the collateral-dependent vasculature (Bauters et al., 1995; Harada et al., 1996; Sellke et al., 1994) The cause of this enhancement of endothelium-dependent relaxation is not fully understood but several mechanisms may be involved. Both FGF-2 and VEGF release nitric oxide (Sellke et al., 1996), which may improve collateral perfusion and decrease tissue ischemia. As stated earlier, expression of receptors for both FGF-2 and VEGF are selectively increased in chronically ischemic myocardium (Sellke et al., 1996), suggesting that these growth factors are functionally upregulated. This may also explain why enhanced endothelium-dependent relaxation only occurs in the collateral-dependent region and not in the normally perfused myocardium after the perivascular exogenous administration of VEGF or FGF-2. Alternatively, FGF-2 and VEGF may counteract the effects of substances detrimental to vascular function or stabilize nitric oxide or NOS. Another possibility is that the growth factors induce enough collateral formation to prevent a reduction in myocardial blood flow or in pulsitile perfusion. In summary, treatment of collateral-dependent vessels with angiogenic growth factors may enhance endothelium-dependent relaxation, in addition to improving other aspects of cardiac performance. This may, at least in theory, be the basis for a clinical improvement in patients after therapeutic angiogenesis suffering inoperative myocardial ischemia.

ACUTE MICROVASCULAR EFFECTS OF GROWTH FACTORS

One potential problem associated with the intravascular administration of VEGF, FGF-2, and other angiogenic growth factors is the peripheral vasodilation. The angiogenic potential of FGF-2 is largely independent of the release of NO, while VEGF-induced vessel formation is potently coupled to the release of NO (Ziche et al., 1997). The intravascular infusions of FGF-2 and VEGF are poorly tolerated, owing to a potent release of NO (Sellke et al., 1996; Lopez et al., 1997) and systemic hypotension. Profound hypotension is obviously not well tolerated by patients with severe and inoperable coronary artery disease. VEGF-induced relaxation may be inhibited by the concomitant administration of L-NAME, suggesting a possible method to counter the vasodilatory effect of acute administration of VEGF. Interestingly, VEGF produces a rapid tachyphylaxis to subsequent bolus injections of the growth factor, and also to the injection of other endothelium-dependent vasoactive agents such as serotonin. The relaxations to sodium nitroprusside and adenosine are not affected, suggesting a selectively acquired defect in the endothelial vasodilatory mechanism (Lopez et al., 1997). Examples of these vascular effects are shown in Figure 12.8.

While the predominant effect of VEGF may lie in the NO-guanylate pathway, other pathways may also be important. Relaxation of vessels by VEGF is not affected to the same degree by the tyrosine kinase inhibitor genistein as it is by an inhibitor of NOS, nor is VEGF-induced relaxation totally inhibited by N^Gnitro-L-arginine (Sellke et al., 1996). This suggests that VEGF-induced relaxation may have an endothelial component independent of NO, or that it may release NO through a mechanism unrelated to its two different tyrosine kinase receptors (Lopez et al., 1997). The VEGF-induced release of platelet activating factor (PAF), which may cause vasodilation in low concentrations, has recently been reported to increase vascular permeability in intact vessels and cultured aortic endothelial cells (Sirois and Edelman., 1997). An understanding of the acute vascular effects of growth factors may increase our understanding of the initial steps in blood vessel development and growth and also help clinicians deal with

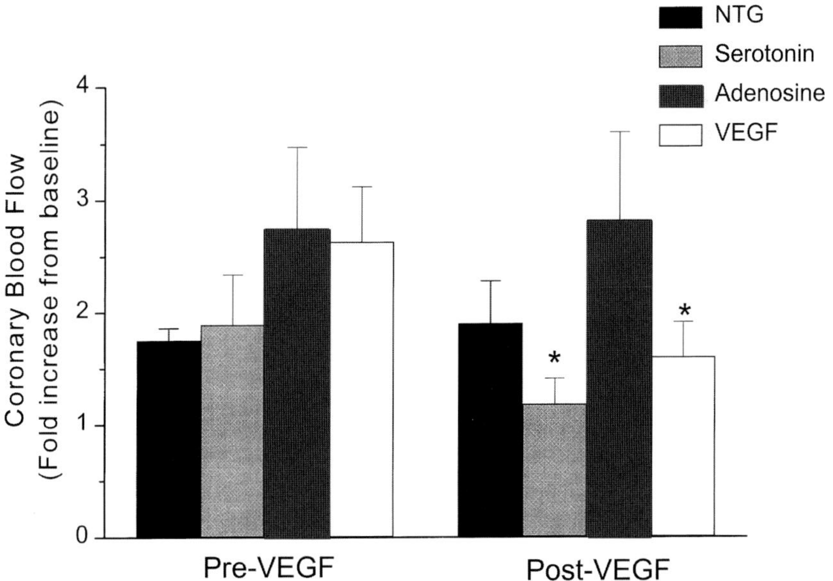

Figure 12.8. Coronary vascular effects of VEGF and altered vascular responsiveness after exposure of vessels to exogenous. From VEGF and Lopez et al. (1997).

hypotension associated with the intravascular administration of VEGF and other growth factors.

Structural Changes in the Coronary Microcirculation

For years it has been observed that patients with cardiac hypertrophy, due to a variety of causes, have chest pain suggestive of myocardial ischemia. This has led to an extensive body of research examining potential alterations of structure of the coronary microcirculation in a variety of conditions associated with cardiac hypertrophy. In both experimental animals and humans with cardiac hypertrophy, there is a reduction in the maximal capacity of the coronary circulation to dilate in response to either reactive hyperemia or pharmacological stimuli (Marcus, 1983; Marcus et al., 1987). Two hypotheses have been proposed to explain this defect in vasodilator function. One is that, as the myocardium hypertrophies, the coronary resistance circulation does not increase to keep pace with the larger myocardial mass. Thus, peak flow normalized to myocardial mass is reduced because of this relative paucity of coronary arterioles. A second structural alteration of the microcirculation, which occurs in hypertension, is actual loss of coronary resistance vessels.

It has been assumed that these studies examining a loss of maximal vasodilator reserve reflect a structural alteration of the coronary microcirculation, because they are observed during maximal pharmacological stimulation, and thus, the resultant flow must reflect the driving pressure for perfusion and the cross sectional area of the coronary resistance circulation. The pharmacological agents employed in these studies have largely been agents such as adenosine, dipyridamole, or papaverine. Many of these observations were made prior to understanding the importance of the endothelium in modulation of vasodilation, but in fairness, it is likely that most of these changes in maximal vasodilation were not due to altered release of vasodilator substances from the endothelium. The vasodilation caused by adenosine and papaverine is not greatly influenced by the endothelium. Further, loss of endothelial function is not always associated with an impaired maximal vasodilation to adenosine. Nevertheless, it is possible that some of impaired vasodilator responses, attributed to losses of vascular cross sectional area, were in fact due to changes in endothelial function.

There are structural changes in the coronary microcirculation that occur with hypertension and myocardial hypertrophy which alter autoregulation and the perfusion pressure in the subendocardium, as discussed above.

PHARMACOLOGY OF THE CORONARY MICROCIRCULATION

As discussed above, the response of the coronary microcirculation to a variety of neurohumoral stimuli is heterogeneous. Similarly, a variety of pharmacologic agents such as organic nitrates, adenosine, dipyridamole, and certain inhalation anesthetics exert heterogeneous effects on the coronary microcirculation.

The organic nitrates represent a diverse groups of compounds which contain a nitrate ester moiety. Unlike many other nitrovasodilators, the organic nitrates do not spontaneously release nitric oxide but must undergo a three electron reduction of the nitrogen atom which eventually is released as NO˙. Both enzymatic and nonenzymatic mechanisms for this "biotransformation" have been implicated; it is thought that enzymatic processes predominate in vivo. The enzyme systems involved have only been partially characterized. The importance of this is that it appears that only certain tissues are capable of this enzymatic process. This is true in the coronary circulation. It was noted as early as the 1960s (Winbury et al., 1969; Fam and McGregor., 1968) that the organic nitrates produced prolonged vasodilation of the larger, epicardial coronary arteries while producing only minimal and short-lived increases in coronary flow. In keeping with these findings, recent studies, both in vitro and in vivo, have shown that coronary microvessels >200 μm in diameter are potently dilated in response to nitroglycerine, while vessels <100 μm in diameter are dilated only minimally by suprapharmacological concentrations (>1 μmol/l) of the drug (Sellke et al., 1990b; Kurz et al., 1991). This property of nitroglycerine is shared by other organic nitrates and likely is related to the common requirement for biotransformation of the nitrate ester. Nitrovasodilators such as S-nitrosocysteine (a nitrosothiol) and sodium nitroprusside either yield nitric oxide upon a one-electron reduction or spontaneously, potently dilate all-size coronary microvessels; thus, it seems that the smaller coronary microvessels (<100 μm in diameter) can respond to nitric oxide but are simply incapable of biotransforming nitroglycerine to the free NO˙ gas. Subsequent studies have shown that this biotransformation process likely requires glutathione and that differences in the ability of large but not small coronary microvessels to respond to nitroglycerine may be related to variations in intracellular glutathione levels in different sized microvessels (Wheatley et al., 1994). Figure 12.9 illustrates the responses of coronary microvessels to various nitrovasodilators.

This pharmacological property of the organic nitrates—the ability to to dilate larger coronary arteries preferentially while having minimal effect on the smaller coronary microvessels—is likely extremely important in terms of their antianginal properties. Drugs that dilate the smaller (<100 μm) coronary microvessels have been implicated in producing the coronary steal phenomenon. Thus, by sparing coronary microvessels <100 μm in diameter, the organic nitrates avoid this untoward effect while having the beneficial effects of dilating venous capacitance vessels (reducing cardiac preload), epicardial coronary arteries (sites of coronary stenoses), and coronary collateral vessels. This profile of vascular activity may explain the tremendously beneficial effect these drugs and other agents that have

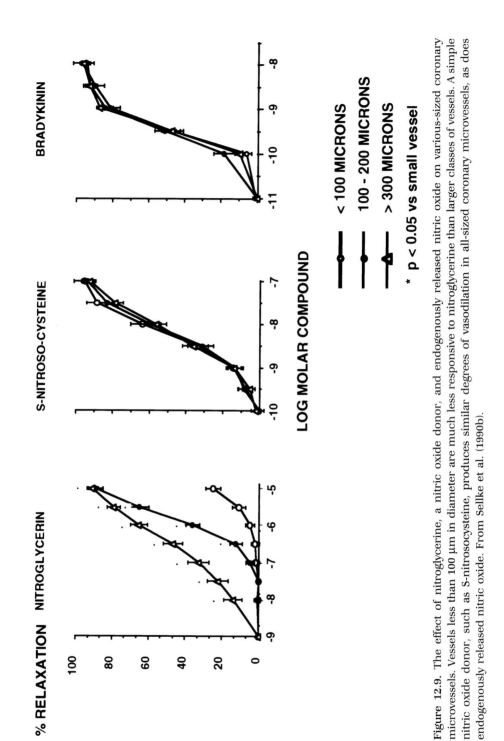

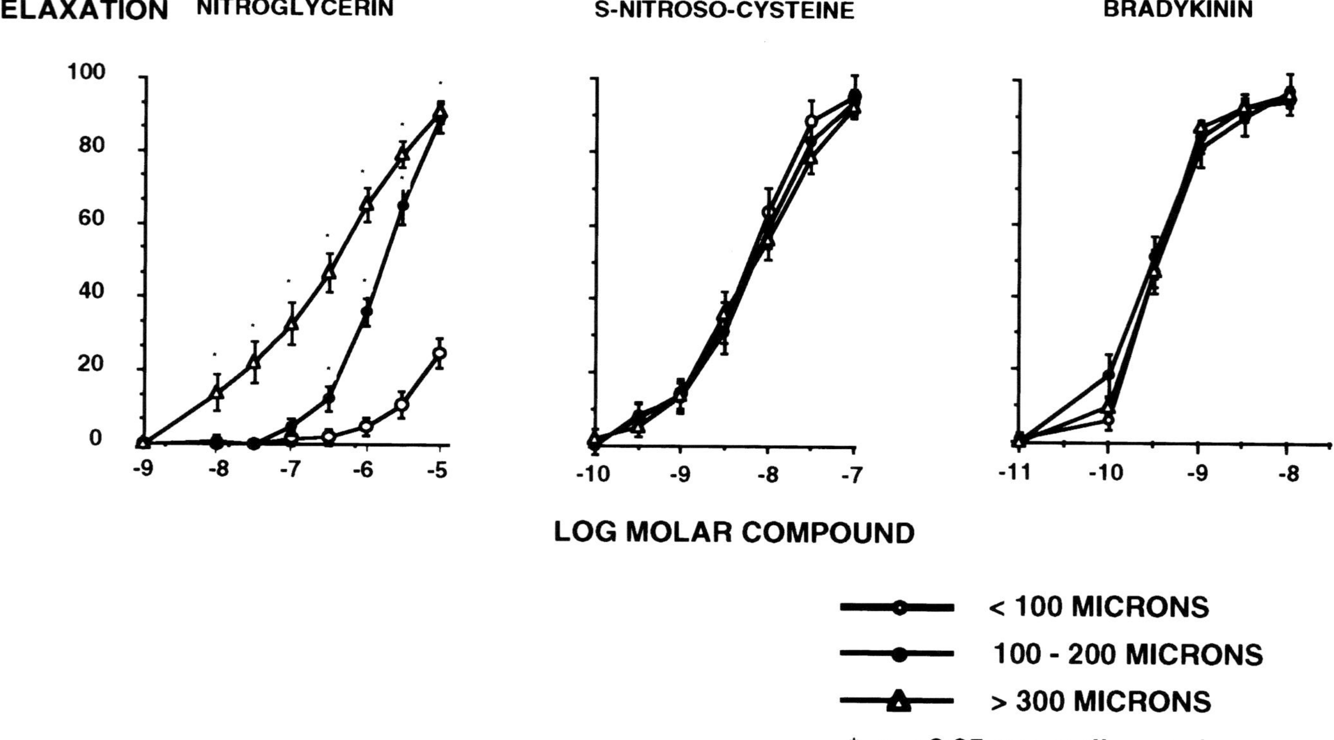

Figure 12.9. The effect of nitroglycerine, a nitric oxide donor, and endogenously released nitric oxide on various-sized coronary microvessels. Vessels less than 100 μm in diameter are much less responsive to nitroglycerine than larger classes of vessels. A simple nitric oxide donor, such as S-nitrosocysteine, produces similar degrees of vasodilation in all-sized coronary microvessels, as does endogenously released nitric oxide. From Sellke et al. (1990b).

a similar heterogeneous vasomotor effect (Park et al., 1994) have in the treatment of myocardial ischemia.

Adenosine has an effect on the coronary microvessels that is precisely the opposite of that caused by organic nitrates. While adenosine is not generally considered a pharmacological agent, it is worth mentioning here because it is used therapeutically for treatment of arrhythmias, and diagnostically to induce myocardial ischemia. Dipyridamole is also often used for this latter purpose, and its effect is mediated by its ability to both enhance adenosine's release and inhibit its degradation. Adenosine produces potent vasodilation of coronary microvessels <100 μm in diameter and only modest dilation of larger vessels.

The dyhydropyridine-type calcium channel antagonists produce uniform vasodilation of all classes of coronary microvessels. There has not been a reported comparison of the effect of the other subtypes of calcium channel antagonists.

As indicated in the section entitled Metabolic Regulation and Autoregulation in this chapter, there is a great deal of interest in the role of potassium channels in modulating coronary flow. A variety of potassium channel opening agents, principally those that affect the K_{ATP} channel, have been studied in terms of their ability to alter coronary hemodynamics. These agents, which include drugs such as cromakalim, lemakalim, and bemikalim, are potent vasodilators of all vessels, and markedly increase coronary flow when administered in vivo. The profile of coronary microvessels dilated by these agents does not seem to have been examined, but they are capable of hyperpolarizing smooth muscle of very small coronary arterioles. A potentially useful therapeutic agent is nicorandil, an organic nitrate with potassium channel opening properties. Not surprisingly, nicorandil dilates all sized coronary microvessels under normal conditions; however, it becomes selective for vessels larger than 100 μm in diameter when K_{ATP} channels are blocked by glibenclamide (Akai et al., 1995).

SUMMARY

In this review, we have summarized some of the newer concepts regarding physiological, pathophysiological, and pharmacological control of the coronary microcirculation. Whenever possible, we have focused on studies that have directly examined the coronary microvessels using some of the newer technology (in vitro preparations or in situ observations). It is not possible, however, to understand these studies without consideration of some of the more classical studies of the intact coronary circulation performed in intact animals or isolated hearts. While these older approaches, in general, employed indirect techniques, they provided a wealth of insight and understanding of coronary blood flow regulation. In reviewing this literature, it is clear that many of the methods used in the last three decades for study of the coronary circulation and microcirculation have largely been abandoned, or are being used in relatively few laboratories. In part, this is due to the fact that the research questions that have arisen regarding vascular function have necessitated the use of more basic techniques, including cell culture and molecular biological approaches. Another reason for this is the difficulty of these studies and the expense of larger animals used in many of the physiological experiments. A relatively recent development has been the ability to make many in vivo measurements of coronary hemodynamics in human subjects in the catheterization laboratory, bypassing the absolute need for large-animal studies of flow. Nevertheless, as vascular biology research examines more fundamental questions, it will be important not to lose sight of the need to take basic observations back to the intact circulation. As emphasized in this chapter, properties of peripheral vessels cannot be extrapolated to the coronary circulation, and properties of one size or class of coronary microvessel may not be present in another size or class of coronary microvessel. Future studies will be most successful when fundamental observations can be tested in intact vessels and circulations, including the coronary circulation.

REFERENCES

Akai, K., Wang, Y., Sato, K., Sekiguchi, N., Sugimura, A., Kumagai, T., Komaru, T., Kanatsuka, H., and Shirato, K. (1995). Vasodilatory effect of nicorandil on coronary arterial microvessels: its dependency on vessel size and the involvement of the ATP-sensitive potassium channels. J. Cardiovasc. Pharmacol. 26: 541–547.

Amezcua, J. L., Palmer, R. M., de Souza, B. M., and Moncada, S. (1989). Nitric oxide synthesized from L-arginine regulates vascular tone in the coronary circulation of the rabbit. Br. J. Pharmacol. 97: 1119–1124.

Arnal, J.-F., Yamin, J., Dockery, S., and Harrison, D. G. (1994). Regulation of endothelial nitric oxide synthase mRNA, protein and activity during cell growth. Am. J. Physiol. Cell Physiol. 267: C1381–C1388.

Bauters, C., Asahara, T., Zheng, L., Takeshita, S., Bunting, S., Ferrara, N., Symes, J., and Isner, J. (1995). Recovery of disturbed endothelium-dependent flow in the collateral-perfused rabbit ischemic hindlimb after administration of vascular endothelial growth factor. Circulation 91: 2802–2809.

Bellamy, R F. (1978). Diastolic coronary artery pressure-flow relations in the dog. Circ. Res. 43: 92–101.

Boatwright, R. B., Downey, H. F., Bashour, F. A., and Crystal, G. J. (1980). Transmural variation in autoregulation of coronary blood flow in hyperperfused canine myocardium. Circ. Res. 47: 599–609.

Brayden, J. E., and Nelson, M. T. (1992). Regulation of arterial tone by activation of calcium-dependent potassium channels. Science 256: 532–535.

Campbell, W. B., Gebremedhin, D., Pratt, P. F., and Harder, D. R. (1996). Identification of epoxyeicosatrienoic acids as endothelium-derived hyperpolarizing factors. Circ. Res. 78: 415–423.

Cayatte, A. J., Palacino, J. J., Horten, K., and Cohen, R. A. (1994). Chronic inhibition of nitric oxide production accelerates neointima formation and impairs endothelial function in hypercholesterolemic rabbits. Arterioscler. & Thromb. 14: 753–759.

Chilian, W. M. (1991). Microvascular pressures and resistances in the left ventricular subepicardium and subendocardium. Circ. Res. 69: 561–570.

Chilian, W. M., Eastham, C. L., and Marcus, M. L. (1986). Microvascular distribution of coronary vascular resistance in beating left ventricle. Am. J. Physiol. 251: H779–H788.

Chilian, W. M., Layne, S. M., Klausner, E. C., Eastham, C. L., and Marcus, M. L. (1989). Redistribution of coronary microvascular resistance produced by dipyridamole. Am. J. Physiol. 256: H383–H390.

Chilian, W. M., Dellsperger, K. C., Layne, S. M., Eastham, C. L., Armstrong, M. A., Marcus, M. L., and Heistad, D. D. (1990). Effects of atherosclerosis on the coronary microcirculation. Am. J. Physiol. 258: H529–H539.

Conway, R. S., Kirk, E. S., and Eng. C. (1988). Ventricular preload alters intravascular and extravascular resistances of coronary collaterals. Am. J. Physiol. 254: H532–H541.

Cornwell, T. L., Arnold, E., Boerth, N. J., and Lincoln, T. M. (1994). Inhibition of smooth muscle cell growth by nitric oxide and activation of cAMP-dependent protein kinase by cGMP. Am. J. Physiol. 267: C1405–C1413.

Corson, M., James, N., Latta, S., Nerem, R., Berk, B., and Harrison, D. (1996). Phosphorylation of endothelial nitric oxide synthase in response to fluid shear stress. Circ. Res. 79: 984–991.

Drexler, H., Zeiher, A. M., Meinzer, K., and Just, H. (1991). Correction of endothelial dysfunction in coronary microcirculation of hypercholesterolaemic patients by L-arginine. Lancet 338: 1546–1550.

Duncker, D. J., Van Zon, N. S., Altman, J. D., Pavek, T. J., and Bache, R. J. (1993). Role of K+ATP channels in coronary vasodilation during exercise. Circulation 88: 1245–1253.

Duncker, D. J., van Zon, N. S., Ishibashi, Y., and Bache, R. J. (1996). Role of K+ ATP channels and adenosine in the regulation of coronary blood flow during exercise with normal and restricted coronary blood flow. J. Clin. Invest. 97: 996–1009.

Eng, C., Jentzer, J. H., and Kirk, E. S. (1982). The effects of the coronary capacitance on the interpretation of diastolic pressure-flow relationships. Circ. Res. 50: 334–341.

Fam, W. M. and McGregor, M. (1968). Effect of nitroglycerin and dipyridamole on regional coronary resistance. Circ. Res. 22: 649–659.

Feigl, E. O. (1983). Coronary physiology. Physiol. Rev. 63: 1–205.

Fujii, M., Nuno, D. W., Lamping, K. G., Dellsperger, K. C., Eastham, C. L., and Harrison, D. G. (1992). Effect of hypertension and hypertrophy on coronary microvascular pressure. Circ. Res. 71: 120–126.

Fulton, D., McGiff, J. C., Wolin, M. S., Kaminski, P., and Quilley, J. (1997). Evidence against a cytochrome P_{450}-derived reactive oxygen species as the mediator of the nitric oxide-independent vasodilator effect of bradykinin in the perfused heart of the rat. J. Pharmacol. Exp. Ther. 280: 702–709.

Garg, U. C. and Hassid, A. (1989). Nitric oxide-generating vasodilators and 8-bromo-cyclic guanosine monophosphate inhibit mitogenesis and proliferation of cultured rat vascular smooth muscle cells. J. Clin. Invest. 83: 1774–1777.

Gewirtz, H., Olsson, R. A., Brautigan, D. L., Brown, P. R., and Most, A. S. (1986).

Adenosine's role in regulating basal coronary arteriolar tone. Am. J. Physiol. 250: H1030–H1036.

Hammarstrom, A. K., Parkington, H. C., and Coleman, H. A. (1995). Release of endothelium-derived hyperpolarizing factor (EDHF) by M3 receptor stimulation in guinea-pig coronary artery. Br. J. Pharmacol. 115: 717–722.

Harada, K., Friedman, M., Lopez, J., Wang, S., Li, J., Prasad, P., Pearlman, J., Edelman, E., Sellke, F., and Simons, M. (1996). Vascular endothelial growth factor administration in chronic myocardial ischemia. Am. J. Physiol. 270: H1791–H1802.

Harder, D. R., Narayanan, J., Birks, E. K., Liard, J. F., Imig, J. D., Lombard, J. H., Lange, A. R., and Roman, R. J. (1996). Identification of a putative microvascular oxygen sensor. Circ. Res. 79: 54–61.

Hoffman, J. I. (1987). Transmural myocardial perfusion. Prog. Cardiovasc. Dis. 29: 429–464.

Itoh, H., Pratt, R. E., Ohno, M., and Dzau, V. J. (1992). Atrial natriuretic polypeptide as a novel antigrowth factor of endothelial cells. Hypertension 19: 758–761.

Kanatsuka, H., Ashikawa, K., Komaru, T., Suzuki, T., and Takishima, T. (1990). Diameter change and pressure-red blood cell velocity relations in coronary microvessels during long diastoles in the canine left ventricle. Circ. Res. 66: 503–510.

Klassen, G. and Armour, J. (1982). Epicardial coronary venous pressure measurements: autonomic responses. Can. J. Physiol. Pharmacol. 60: 698–706.

Komaru, T., Kanatsuka, H., Dellsperger, K., and Takishima, T. (1993). The role of ATP-sensitive potassium channels in regulating coronary microcirculation. Biorheology 30: 371–380.

Kuo, L., Davis, M. J., and Chilian, W. M. (1988). aMyogenic activity in isolated subepicardial and subendocardial coronary arterioles. Am. J. Physiol. 255: H1558–H1562.

and Kurz, M. A., Lamping, K. G., Bates, J. N., Ea tham, C. L., Marcus, M. L., and Harrison, D. G. (1991). Mechanisms responsible for the heterogeneous coronary microvascular response to nitroglycerin. Circ. Res. 68: 847–855.

Laham, R. J., Simons, M., Tofukuji, M., Hung, D., and Sellke, F. W. (1998). Modulation of myocardial perfusion and vascular reactivity by pericardial basic fibroblast growth factor: Insignt into ischemia-induced reduction in endothelium-dependent vasodilatation. J. Thorac. Cardiovasc. Surg. (in press).

Lamping, K. G., Kanatsuka, H., Eastham, C. L., Chilian, W. M., and Marcus, M. L. (1989). Nonuniform vasomotor responses of the coronary microcirculation to serotonin and vasopressin. Circ. Res. 65: 343–351.

Lamping, K. G., Chilian, W. M., Eastham, C. L., and Marcus, M. L. (1992a). Coronary microvascular response to exogenously administered and endogenously released acetylcholine. Microvasc. Res. 43: 294–307.

Lamping, K. G., Clothier, J. L., Eastham, C. L., and Marcus, M. L. (1992b). Coronory microvascular response to endothelin is dependent on vessel diameter and route of administration. Am. J. Physiol. 263: H703–H709.

Lefer, D., Nakanishi, K., Vinten-Johansen, J., Ma, X., and Lefer, A. (1992). Cardiac venous endothelial dysfunction after myocardial ischemia and reperfusion in dogs. Am. J. Physiol. 263: H850–H856.

Li, J., Brown, L., Hibberd, M., Grossman, J., Morgan, J., and Simons, M. (1996). VEGF, flk-1 flt-1 expression in a rat myocardial infarction model of angiogenesis. Am. J. Physiol. 270: H1803–H1811.

Lopez, J., Laham, R., Carrozza, J., Tofukuji, M., Sellke, F., Bunting, S., and Simons, M. (1997). Hemodynamic effects of intracoronary VEGF delivery—evidence of tachyphylaxis and NO dependence of response. Am. J. Physiol. 273: H1317–H1323.

Marcus, M. (1983). The Coronary Circulation in Health and Disease, First Edition. McGraw-Hill, New York.

Marcus, M. L., Harrison, D. G., Chilian, W. M., Koyanagi, S., Inou T., Tomanek, R. J., Martins, J. B, Eastham, C. L., and Hiratzka, L F. (1987). Alterations in the coronary circulation in hypertrophied ventricles. Circulation 75: I 19–I 25.

Matsunaga, T., Okumura, K., Ishizaka, H., Tsunoda, R., Tayama, S., and Yasue, H. (1996). Impairment of coronary blood flow regulation by endothelium-derived nitric oxide in dogs with alloxan-induced diabetes. J. Cardiovasc. Pharmacol. 28: 60–67.

McQuillan, L. P., Leung, G. K., Marsden, P. A., Kostyk, S. K., and Kourembanas, S. (1994). Hypoxia inhibits expression of eNOS via transcriptional and posttranscriptional mechanisms. Am. J. Physiol. 267: H1921–H1927.

Meininger, C. and Granger, H. (1990). Mechanisms leading to adenosine-stimulated proliferation of microvascular endothelial cells. Am. J. Physiol. 258: H198–H206.

Michel, J., Feron, O., Sacks, D., and Michel, T. (1997). Reciprocal regulation of endothelial nitric-oxide synthase by Ca2+-calmodulin and caveolin. J. Boil Chem. 272: 15583–15586.

Morbidelli, L., Chang, C. H., Douglas, J. G., Granger, H. J., Ledda, F., and Ziche, M. (1996). Nitric oxide mediates mitogenic effect of VEGF on coronary venular endothelium. Am. J. Physiol. 270: H411–415.

Moroi, M., Gold, H., Yasuda, T., Fishman, M., and Huang, P. (1996). Mice mutant in endothelial nitric oxide synthase: vessel growth and response to injury [abstract]. Circulation 94: 890.

Muller, J. M., Myers, P. R., and Laughlin, M. H. (1993). Exercise training alters myogenic responses in porcine coronary resistance arteries. J. Appl. Physiol. 75: 2677–2682.

Murad, F. (1986). Cyclic guanosine monophosphate as a mediator of vasodilation. J. Clin. Invest. 78: 1–5.

Myers, P. R., Minor, R. L., Jr., Guerra, R., Jr., Bates, J. R., and Harrison, D. G. (1990). The vasorelaxant properties of the endothelium-derived relaxing factor more closely resemble S-nitrosocysteine than nitric oxide. Nature 345: 161–163.

Narayanan, J., Imig, M., Roman, R. J., and Harder, D. R. (1994). Pressurization of isolated renal arteries increases inositol trisphosphate and diacylglycerol. Am. J. Physiol. 266: H1840–H1845.

Nellis, S. H., Liedtke, A. J., and Whitesell, L. (1981). Small coronary vessel pressure and diameter in an intact beating rabbit heart using fixed-position and free-motion techniques. Circ. Res. 49: 342–353.

Olsson, R. A., and Bunger, R. (1987). Metabolic control of coronary blood flow. Prog. Cardiovasc. Dis. 29: 369–387.

Osol, G., Laher, I., and Cipolla, M. (1991). Protein kinase C modulates basal myogenic tone in resistance arteries from the cerebral circulation. Cir. Res. 68: 359–367.

Osol, G., Laher, I., and Kelley, M. (1993). Myogenic tone is coupled to phospholipase C and G protein activation in small cerebral arteries. Am. J. Physiol. 265: H415–420.

Papapetropoulos, A., Desai, K. M., Rudic, R. D., Mayer, B., Zhang, R., Ruiz-Torres, M. P., Garcia-Cardena, G., Madri, J. A., and Sessa, W. C. (1997). Nitric oxide synthase inhibitors attenuate transforming-growth-factor-beta 1-stimulated capillary organization in vitro. Am. J. Physiol. 150: 1835–1844.

Park, K. W., Dai, H.-B., Lowenstein, E., Darvish, E., and Sellke, F. W. (1994). Heterogeneous vasomotor responses of rabbit microvessels to isoflurane. Anesthesiology 81: 1190–1197.

Peters, K. G., Marcus, M. L., and Harrison, D. G. (1989). Vasopressin and the mature coronary collateral circulation. Circulation 79: 1324–1331.

Petersson, J., Zygmunt, P. M., and Hogestatt, E. D. (1997). Characterization of the potassium channels involved in EDHF-mediated relaxation in cerebral arteries. Br. J. Pharmacol. 120: 1344–1350.

Piana, R. N., Wang, S. Y., Friedman, M., and Sellke, F. W. (1996). Angiotensin-converting enzyme inhibition preserves endothelium-dependent coronary microvascular responses during short-term ischemia-reperfusion. Circulation 93: 544–551.

Pipili-Synetos, E., Sakkoula, E., Haralabopoulos, G., Andriopoulou, P., Peristeris, P., and Maragoudakis, M. E. (1994). Evidence that nitric oxide is an endogenous antiangiogenic mediator. Br. J. Pharmacol. 111: 894–902.

Pipili-Synetos, E., Papageorgiou, A., Sakkoula, E., Sotiropoulou, G., Fotsis, T., Karakiulakis, G., and Maragoudakis, M. E., (1995). Inhibition of angiogenesis, tumour growth and metastasis by the NO-releasing vasodilators, isosorbide mononitrate and dinitrate. Br. J. Pharmacol. 116: 1829–1834.

Pollman, M. J., Yamada, T., Horiuchi, M., and Gibbons, G. H. (1996). Vasoactive substances regulate vascular smooth muscle cell apoptosis. Countervailing influences of nitric oxide and angiotensin II. Circ. Res. 79: 748–756.

Quillen, J. E., Sellke, F. W., Brooks, L. A., and Harrison, D. G. (1990). Ischemia-reperfusion impairs endothelium-dependent relaxation of coronary microvessels but does not affect large arteries. Circulation 82: 586–594.

Rapps, J., Jones, A., Sturek, M., Magliola, L., and Parker, J. (1997). Mechanisms of altered contractile responses to vasopressin and endothelin in canine collateral arteries. Circulation 95: 231–239.

Ravichandran, L., Johns, R., and Rengasamy, A. (1995). Direct and reversible inhibition of endothelial nitric oxide synthase by nitric oxide. Am. J. Physiol. 268: H2216–H2223.

Schaper, W. (1979). The Pathophysiology of Myocardial Perfusion, First Edition. Elsevier/North Holland Biomedical Press, Amsterdam.

Sellke, F. W., and Dai, H. B. (1993). Responses of porcine epicardial venules to neurohumoral substances. Cardiovasc. Res. 27: 1326–1332.

Sellke, F. W., Armstrong, M. L., and Harrison, D. G., (1990a). Endothelium-dependent vascular relaxation is abnormal in the coronary microcirculation of atherosclerotic primates. Circulation 81: 1586–1593.

Sellke, F. W., Meyers, P. R., Bates, J. N., and Harrison, D. G. (1990b). Influence of vessel size on the sensitivity of porcine microvessels to nitroglycerin. Am. J. Physiol. 258: H515–H520.

Sellke, F. W., Quillen, J. E., Brooks, L. A., and Harrison, D. G. (1990c). Endothelial modulation of the coronary vasculature in vessels perfused via mature collaterals. Circulation 81: 1938–1947.

Sellke, F. W., Shafique, T., Schoen, F. J., and Weintraub, R. M. (1993). Impaired endothelium-dependent coronary microvascular relaxation after cold potassium cardioplegia and reperfusion. J. Thorac. Cardiovasc. Surg. 105: 52–58.

Sellke, F. W., Wang, S. Y., Friedman, M., Harada, K., Edelman, E. R., Grossman, W., and Simons, M. (1994). Basic FGF enhances endothelium-dependent relaxation of the collateral-perfused coronary microcirculation. Am. J. Physiol. 267: H1303–1311.

Sellke, F. W., Wang, S. Y., Stamler, A., Lopez, J. J., Li, J., Li, J. Y., and Simons, M. (1996). Enhanced microvascular relaxations to VEGF and bFGF in chronically ischemic porcine myocardium. Am. J. Physiol. 271: H713–720.

Serban, D. N., Salichi, L. I., Branisteanu, D. D., and Haulica, I. D. (1989). Short-time adenosine deaminase interventions upon underperfused rat hearts in vitro—a test for the role of adenosine in the coronary flow control. Physiologie 26: 17–23.

Shimokawa, H., Yasutake, H., Fujii, K., Owada, M. K., Nakaike, R., Fukumoto, Y., Takayanagi, T, Nagao, T., Egashira, K., Fujishima, M., and Takeshita, A. (1996). The importance of the hyperpolarizing mechanism increases as the vessel size decreases in endothelium-dependent relaxations in rat mesenteric circulation. J. Cardiovasc. Pharmacol. 28: 703–711.

Sirois, M. and Edelman, E. (1997). VEGF effect on vascular permeability is mediated by synthesis of platelet-activating factor. Am. J. Physiol. 272: H2746–H2756.

Symons, J. D., Longhurst, J. C., and Stebbins, C. L. (1993). Response of collateral-dependent myocardium to vasopressin release during prolonged intense exercise. Am. J. Physiol. 264: H1644–1652.

Taylor, S. G. and Weston, A. H. (1988). Endothelium-derived hyperpolarizing factor: a new endogenous inhibitor from the vascular endothelium. Trends Pharmacol. Sci. 9: 272–274.

Treasure, C. B., Klein, J. L., Vita, J. A., Manoukian, S. V., Renwick, G. H., Selwyn, A. P., Ganz, P., and Alexander, R. W. (1993). Hypertension and left ventricular hypertrophy are associated with impaired endothelium-mediated relaxation in human coronary resistance vessels. Circulation 87: 86–93.

Uemetsu, M., Ohara, Y., Navas, J. P., Nishida, K., Murphy, T. J., Alexander, R. W., Nerem, R. M., and Harrison, D. G. (1995). Regulation of endothelial cell nitric oxide synthase mRNA expression by shear stress. Am. J. Physiol. 269: C1371–C1378.

Venema, R. C., Sayegh, H. S., Arnal, J.-F., and Harrison, D. G. (1995). Role of the enzyme calmodulin-binding domain in membrane association and phospholipid inhibition of endothelial nitric oxide synthase. J. Biol. Chem. 270: 14705–14711.

von der Leyen, H. E., Gibbons, G. H., Morishita, R., Lewis, N. P., Zhang, L., Nakajima, M., Kaneda, Y., Cooke, J. P., and Dzau, V. J. (1995). Gene therapy inhibiting neointimal vascular lesion: in vivo transfer of endothelial cell nitric oxide synthase gene. Proc. Nat. Acad. Sci. USA 92: 1137–1141.

Wang, S. Y., Friedman, M., Johnson, R. G., Weintraub, R. M., and Sellke, F. W. (1994). Adrenergic regulation of coronary microcirculation after extracorporeal circulation and crystalloid cardioplegia. Am. J. Physiol. 267: H2462–H2470.

Ware, J. and Simons, M. (1997). Angiogenesis in ischemic heart disease. Nat. Med. 3: 158–164.

Wheatley, R. M., Dockery, S. P., Kurz, M. A., Sayegh, H. S., and Harrison, D. G.

(1994). Interactions of nitroglycerin and sulfhydryl-donating compounds in coronary microvessels. Am. J. Physiol. 266: H291–H297.

Winbury, M. M., Howe, B. B., and Weiss, H. R. (1969). Effect of nitrates and other coronary dilators on large and small coronary vessels; an hypothesis for the mechanism of action of nitrates. J. Pharmacol. Exp. Ther. 168: 70–95.

Wu, H., Yuan, Y., McCarthy, M., and Granger, H. (1996). Acidic and basic FGF's dilate arterioles of skeletal muscle through a NO-dependent mechanism. Am. J. Physiol. Heart Circ. Physiol. 271: H1087–1093.

Xu, X. P., Tanner, M. A., and Myers, P. R. (1995). Prostaglandin-mediated inhibition of nitric oxide production by bovine aortic endothelium during hypoxia. Cardiovasc. Res. 30: 345–350.

Young, M. A., Knight, D. R., and Vatner, S. F. (1987). Autonomic control of large coronary arteries and resistance vessels. Prog. Cardiovasc. Dis. 30: 211–234.

Yu, S. M., Hung, L. M., and Lin, C. C. (1997). cGMP-elevating agents suppress proliferation of vascular smooth muscle cells by inhibiting the activation of epidermal growth factor signaling pathway. Circulation 95: 1269–1277.

Yuan, Y., Mier, R., Chilian, W., Zawieja, D., and Granger, H. (1995). Interaction of neutrophils and endothelium in isolated coronary venules and arterioles. Am. J. Physiol. Heart Circ. Physiol. 268: H490–H498.

Ziche, M., Morbidelli, L., Choudhuri, R., Zhang, H., Donnini, S., Granger, H., and Bicknell, R. (1997). Nitric oxide synthase lies downstream from vascular endothelial growth factor-induced but not basic fibroblast growth factor-induced angiogenesis. J. Clin. Invest. 99: 2625–2634.

Ziche, M., Morbidelli, L., Masini, E., Amerini, S., Granger, H. J., Maggi, C. A., Geppetti, P., and Ledda, F. (1994). Nitric oxide mediates angiogenesis in vivo and endothelial cell growth and migration in vitro promoted by substance P. J. Clin. Invest. 94: 2036–2044.

Zou, A. P., Fleming, J. T., Falck, J. R., Jacobs, E. R., Gebremedhin, D., Harder, D. R., and Roman, R. J. (1996). 20-HETE is an endogenous inhibitor of the large-conductance Ca(2+)-activated K+ channel in renal arterioles. Am. J. Physiol. 270: R228–R237.

13

Therapeutic Angiogenesis in Myocardial Ischemia

MICHAEL SIMONS AND ROGER J. LAHAM

Ischemic coronary disease remains the leading cause of morbidity and mortality in the Western world. Available therapeutic approaches aim either at relieving symptoms by reducing myocardial oxygen demand, preventing further disease progression by modifying risk factors, or restoring flow to a localized segment of the arterial tree by means of angioplasty or bypass surgery. However, even with all the recent advances in coronary bypass surgery and percutaneous revascularization, a significant number of patients with ischemic heart disease are not candidates for these therapeutic strategies either due to high procedural risk to or coronary anatomy not amenable to surgery or angioplasty; furthermore, these patients may often be refractory to medical therapy. Therefore, it became clear that an alternative revascularization strategy should be sought in these patients, which, if successful, may become a therapeutic option in many other patients with coronary artery disease. Therapeutic angiogenesis may provide that role.

The availability of various angiogenic growth factors—in particular, vascular endothelial growth factor (VEGF), acidic fibroblast growth factor (FGF-1), and basic fibroblast growth factor (FGF-2)—and implications of their role in developmental, ischemia-induced angiogenesis, and tumor angiogenesis have led to studies of their therapeutic efficacy in animal and clinical studies of myocardial ischemia. In this chapter, the results of these studies in both acute and chronic ischemia will be examined along with the current understanding of growth factor actions in these settings and analysis of side effects associated with angiogenic therapy.

Table 13.1 Outcome Measures for Therapeutic Angiogenesis

ANGIOGRAPHY[a]
Collateral Index
TIMI flow
HISTOCHEMICAL AND MOLECULAR ANALYSIS
Myocardial infarction size
Number of capillaries/HPF (immunohistochemistry)
Quantitative analysis for endothelial cell markers (Western analysis)
MICROSPHERE FLOW ANALYSIS
MICROVASCULAR REACTIVITY
ECHOCARDIOGRAPHY[a]
Global and regional left ventricular function
Myocardial perfusion (using echo-contrast agents)
MAGNETIC RESONANCE ANALYSIS[a]
Global and regional left ventricular function
Myocardial perfusion (using MR perfusion)
NUCLEAR PERFUSION STUDIES (EXERCISE OR PHARMACOLOGIC STRESS)[a]

[a]Denotes outcomes measures applicable to clinical evaluation of therapeutic angiogenesis. HPF, High Power Field; MR, Magnetic Resonance.

STUDY END-POINTS

In evaluating the results of therapeutic angiogenesis studies, it is important to consider various end-points used to evaluate growth factor efficacy and to assess whether the observed results are truly due to induced angiogenesis or some other growth-factor-induced physiologic changes. Since the panoply of effects of growth factors used in these studies is substantial, a variety of end-points should be used to describe thoroughly the results of such therapy. A summary of potential measures of growth factor activity is provided in Table 13.1.

Morphological and Molecular Analysis

In considering growth factor-induced neovascularization, it is important to distinguish intramyocardial collateral development from formation of epicardial collaterals (neoarteriogenesis); this issue is discussed at length in Chapter 9. The process of intramyocardial collateral development (angiogenesis) is characterized by the appearance of thin-walled vessels (Fig. 13.1A) with a poorly developed tunica media that are under 200 μm in diameter and by an increase in the number of true capillaries (< 20 μm in diameter containing only a single endothelial layer). Neoarteriogenesis, on the other hand, is characterized by development of larger vessels (>200 μm in diameter) with well-developed media and adventitia that usually form close to the site of the occlusion of a major epicardial cor-

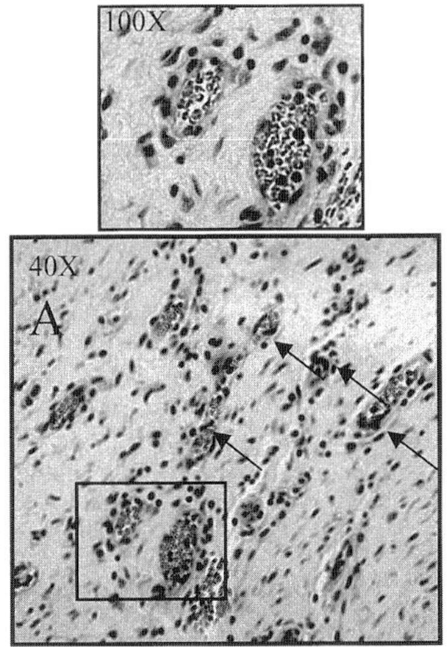

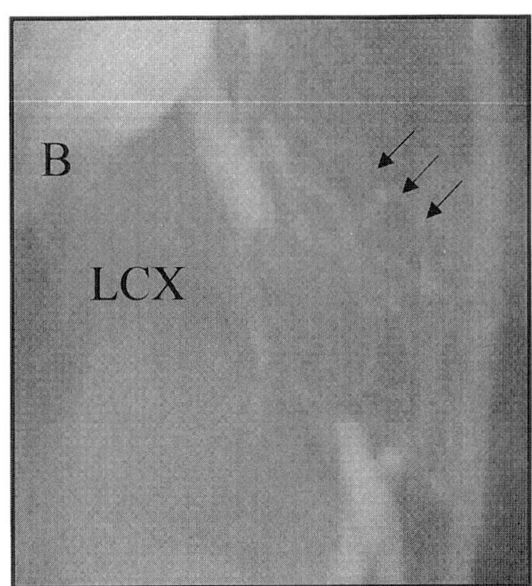

Figure 13.1. The two different types of collaterals: (A) myocardial section showing intramyocardial collaterals with the appearance of thin-walled vessels (<200μm in diameter, shown in the zoom frame) with a poorly developed tunica media and an increased number of capillaries (<20μm, black arrows) (B) left circumflex (LCX) angiography with the ameroid constrictor occluding the LCX. Arrows point to bridging collaterals that bypass the ameroid occlusion to reconstitute the distal vessel.

onary artery (bridging collaterals) or extend from one coronary artery to another (Fig. 13.1B). The distinction between these two groups of newly formed vessels is important not only because of their location, but also because stimuli for their development appear to be quite different and because they exhibit different physiologic properties. (See Chapter 9 for detailed discussion.) Thus, although tissue ischemia may well play a key role in the development of intramyocardial collateral vessels, it is unlikely to be involved directly in the development of epicardial collaterals. The presence of macrophages has been implicated in regulation of both processes, however. Furthermore, the techniques designed to assess the functional impact of collateral development such as assessment of microvasculature or evaluation of coronary flow in large epicardial arteries may produce different outcomes depending on the prevailing process.

Another important factor to consider in immunocytochemical or in situ hybridization analysis of new vessel formation is the time course and spatial heterogeneity of expression of various endothelial cell markers. For example, studies of periinfarct angiogenesis in the rat demonstrate that while all small (<50 μm) and large (50–200 μm vessels) vessels expressed *flk-1* receptor at 7 days postinfarct, only some smaller vessels demonstrated

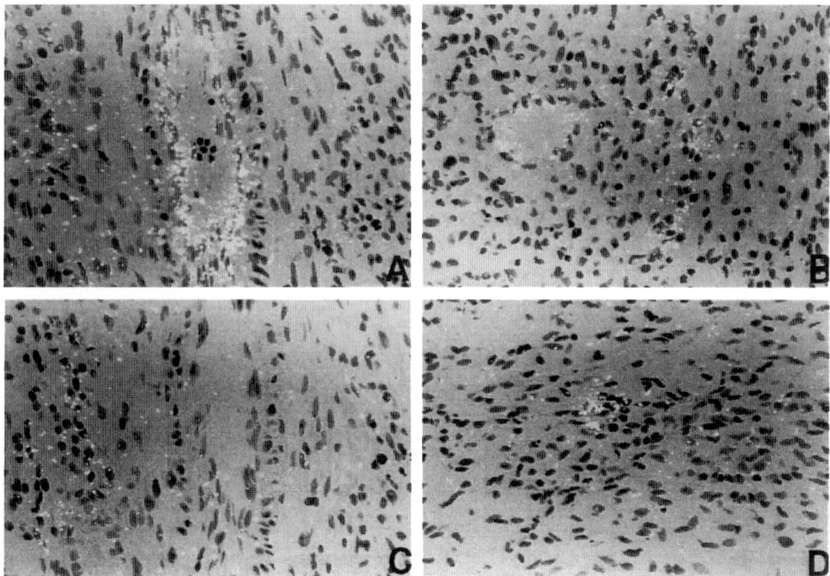

Figure 13.2. In situ hybridization analysis of *flt-1* (A and B) and *flk-1* (C and D) expression in a rat myocardial infarction model. *Flt-1* is strongly expressed in both large vessels (A) and small vessels (B) in healing infarcts. In serial sections, *flk-1* (C) in not expressed by endothelial cells in the same large vessel that showed high *flt-1* expression (A). *flk-1* is expressed by small vessels in healing infarcts (D). (From Li et al, 1996.)

expression of *flt-1* (Fig. 13.2) Thus, the use of *flt-1* as a sole endothelial cell marker would underestimate the number of newly formed vessels (Li et al., 1996). Similarly, expression of vWF-driven Lac Z construct in transgenic mice results in expression only in a subset of cardiac endothelial cells (Aird et al., 1995). Finally, the PDGF-α receptor is expressed only in a small population (~10%) of cardiac endothelial cells (Edelberg et al., 1997).

Additional considerations pertain to uses of other endothelial cell markers. For example, CD-31 (PECAM) is expressed not only on endothelial cells but also on mononuclear cells, platelets, and granulocytes and thus would overestimate the extent of angiogenesis in infarct and other inflammation-dependent models. Furthermore, expression of eNOS, previously considered limited to endothelial cells, has recently been described in myocytes (Kelly et al., 1996), thus complicating the use of this gene product as a marker for endothelial cells.

Evaluation of Coronary Perfusion

While an increase in the number of either epicardial collaterals or intramyocardial blood vessels may result in improvement of myocardial perfusion, another important consideration in evaluating the therapeutic effect of various growth factors is their ability to alter endothelial function. Growth-factor-induced changes in vascular reactivity may by themselves significantly alter coronary flow which may be difficult to differentiate from changes in flow resulting from an increase in vessel numbers. This consideration is particularly relevant in chronic ischemia, since microvessels from chronically ischemic myocardium show increased reactivity to VEGF and FGF-2 administration (Sellke et al., 1996c). As addressed in Chapter 9, improvement in perfusion can result either from development of new epicardial collateral vessels or a small-vessel angiogenic response in the myocardium. It is not clear whether one of these processes is functionally superior to the other. Thus, evaluation of the relative contribution of these two modes of neovascularization could significantly add to rational design of therapeutic strategies.

A number of studies using ischemic pig model have noted an improvement in resting perfusion following growth factor administration (Ware and Simons, 1997). While this change in flow may result from increased vessel number and/or changes in microvascular reactivity, an equally plausible explanation is that functional recovery of hibernating myocardium (see below) resulted in increased coronary perfusion.

Evaluation of Left Ventricular Function

More than any other prognostic parameter, left ventricular function predicts the outcome in patients with ischemic heart disease (Bart et al., 1997; Vandormael et al., 1991). Thus, the ultimate goal of therapeutic angiogenesis should be the restoration of global and regional left ventricular function. Indeed, improvement in left ventricular performance with angiogenic agents has been observed in a number of animal studies and documentation of such improvement both at rest and with stress should be a key element of every study.

Implantation of ameroid occluders in pigs on the left circumflex (LCX) coronary artery results in decreased resting blood flow in the compromised (LCX) compared to the control (LAD) territory; this decline is accompanied by reduced left ventricular wall thickening and radial wall motion. The subsequent recovery of these parameters suggests the presence of hibernating myocardium in this model. The presence of chronically reduced blood flow in the LCX territory in control animals correlates with the previously observed increases in expression of VEGF as well as VEGF and FGF-2 receptors, all of which are induced by ischemia/hypoxia in the LCX but not in normal (LAD) myocardium for as long as 8 weeks after ameroid implantation.

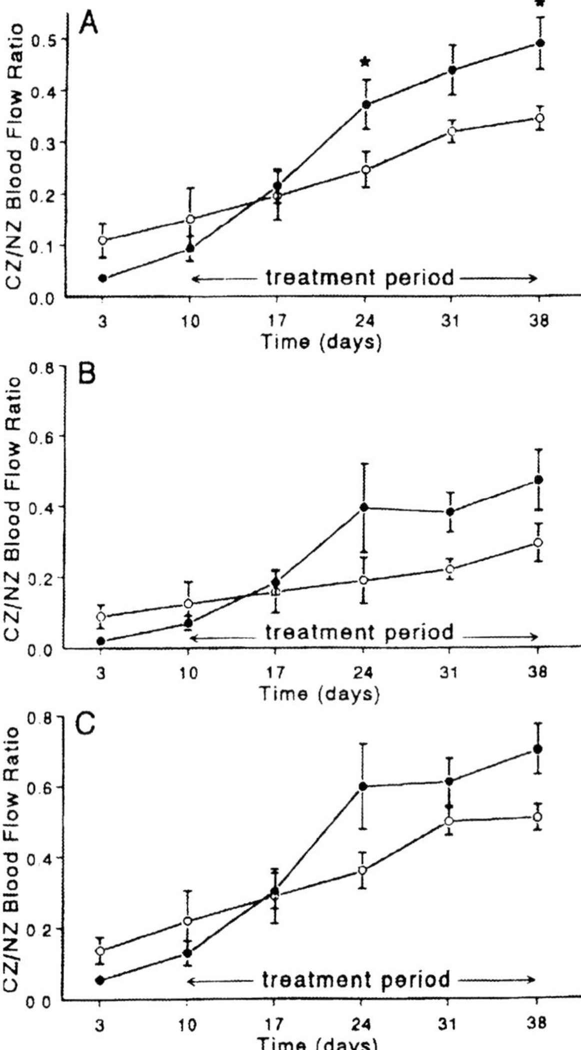
A
CZ/NZ Blood Flow Ratio
treatment period
Time (days)
B
CZ/NZ Blood Flow Ratio
treatment period
Time (days)
C
CZ/NZ Blood Flow Ratio
treatment period
Time (days)

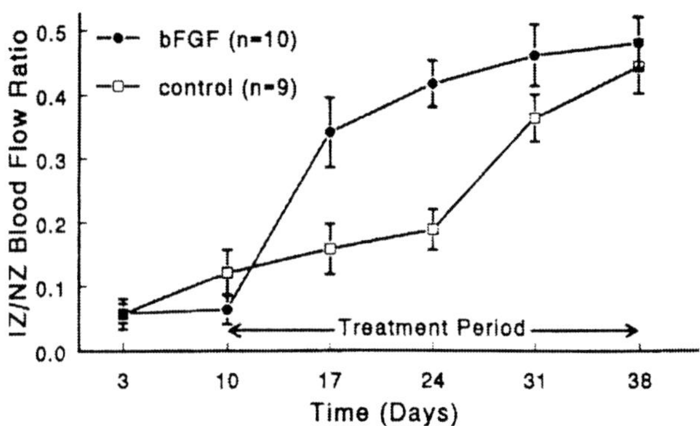
bFGF (n=10)
control (n=9)
IZ/NZ Blood Flow Ratio
Treatment Period
Time (Days)

Microcirculation Studies

The presence of ischemia alters microvascular responses to endothelial receptor-dependent agonists that can be corrected by restoration of normal blood flow; however, both VEGF and FGF-2 (as well as other heparin-binding growth factors) can have a profound effect on microvasculature. Microvessels from ischemic tissues show reduced sensitivity to endothelium-dependent receptor-mediated agonists such as ADP and serotonin (Sellke et al., 1990) while exhibiting greater sensitivity to both VEGF-and FGF-2-induced vasodilation (Sellke et al., 1996*c*). Restoration of microvascular function following growth factor administration, therefore, may reflect a direct effect of these growth factors on microvessels rather than restored myocardial blood flow.

Thus while a variety of physiologic end-points can show beneficial effects of therapeutic growth factor administration, attributing these effects to angiogenesis or neoarteriogenesis per se is much more difficult.

CHRONIC MYOCARDIAL ISCHEMIA

Fibroblast Growth Factor-2

Animal Studies

FGF-2 (basic FGF) is perhaps the most extensively studied growth factor in a variety of angiogenesis models (see Chapter 4). Studies of therapeutic efficacy of FGF-2 in chronic myocardial ischemia have explored a variety of routes of administration in both dog and pig models. The studies of Unger and colleagues have demonstrated that daily injections of 110μg bolus of FGF-2 for 18 days directly into the circumflex coronary artery

---

Figure 13.3. A (left) collateral blood flow as a function of time in a dog ameroid constrictor model. Collateral flow is expressed as collateral-dependent zone to normal zone (CZ/NZ) ratio during maximal vasodilation. Treatment was begun following blood flow measurement at day 10. FGF-2 treated dogs (closed circles) and control dogs (Open circles). During the first 2 weeks of drug administration (days 10–24), the slope of the CZ/NZ vs. time relationship increased significantly in FGF-2 treated dogs compared with control dogs. Transmural collateral flow at days 24 and 38 was significantly higher in FGF-2 treated animals (**A**). Improvement in flow related to FGF-2 was apparent in the endocardium (**B**) as well as epicardium (**C**). **B** (right): line plot of maximal collateral blood flow vs. time for FGF-2 treated animals and controls. Collateral flow was determined with microspheres and expressed as a ration of ischemic zone to normal zone (IZ/NZ). Collateral flow increased markedly in FGF-2 treated dogs during the first 7 days of treatment (days 10–17). However, collateral flow in control dogs caught up with treated animals by day 38. (From Lazorous et al., 1995)

distal to an ameroid occluder hastened restoration of flow in the compromised territory compared to normal saline controls (Unger et al., 1994). Interestingly, the benefit of FGF-2 injections did not appear until 14 days after initiation of treatment and was equally prominent in subendocardial and subepicardial regions of the myocardium (Fig. 13.3A). Analysis of cell proliferation in the collateral-dependent zone showed a nearly fourfold increase in cellular proliferation in FGF-2-treated animals. Morphometric analysis of LCX myocardium demonstrated equal capillary densities in both FGF-2-treated and control animals but a substantial (2-fold) increase in the number of larger (>20μm) vessels (Unger et al., 1994). To examine the effect of systemic FGF-2 administration, the same group of investigators carried out daily left atrial injections of 1.74 mg of the growth factor for 18 days. This mode of FGF-2 administration resulted in early augmentation of coronary flow in the growth-factor-treated animals that was comparable to that seen with direct intracoronary injections (Fig 13.3B) but was lost by day 38 (Lazarous et al., 1995). Prolonged (up to 6 months) infusions of FGF-2 did not result in any further increase in collateral blood flow, which was identical in FGF-2-and saline-treated animals, underscoring the priming role of ischemia for FGF-2-induced collateral development (Shou et al., 1997). In addition, there was no significant structural or vasoproliferative effect of chronic systemic (left atrial) administration of FGF-2, at a dose sufficient to enhance collateral vessel formation, on the nonischemic retina of dogs with myocardial ischemia (Jacot et al., 1996).

While demonstrating beneficial effects of FGF-2 administration on collateral blood flow, these studies are limited by certain characteristics of the animal model, such that brisk natural angiogenic response is sufficient to almost completely restore myocardial blood flow to the ischemic myocardium to normal levels and by the absence of data with regard to functional effects of restoration of coronary perfusion. Furthermore, doses of FGF-2 employed in these studies (1.64 mg intracoronary and 26.1 mg systemically) may result in substantial toxicity and unexpected side effects. Finally, it is difficult to discern whether the observed effects were secondary to neoarteriogenesis around the occluder or the development of intramyocardial collaterals. The absence of a significant increase in the number of capillaries would seem to suggest that most of neovascularization involved larger vessels, although the reliability of such morphologic assessments is subject to considerable error. However, taken together these studies clearly document increased coronary perfusion following FGF-2 treatment that is probably predominately mediated by neoarteriogenesis. At the same time, studies in a porcine microinfarction model demonstrated that when animals received intracoronary injections of 75–150μm Affigel beads, morphometric analysis carried out 2 weeks later demonstrated significantly higher vessel count in animals receiving beads containing FGF-2 compared to control animals (Battler et al., 1993). Thus

FGF-2 was clearly capable of induction of angiogenic response with this mode of delivery in pigs.

To address the functional impact of FGF-2 therapy in chronic myocardial ischemia, we employed a porcine ameroid occluder model taking advantage of slower collateral development in pigs and heparin-alginate polymer to provide sustained release delivery of FGF-2. In addition, FGF-2 was administered perivascularly, with the pellets positioned along the LCX artery below the ameroid occluder. Perivascular delivery of FGF-2 relies on the rich vaso-vasorum network surrounding coronary arteries to effectively distribute the growth factor throughout the vessel wall downstream from the site of deposition (Edelman et al., 1993). The heparin-alginate provides a convenient form of FGF-2 delivery because of a zero-order release kinetics of the growth factor from the polymer over 4–5 weeks, ease of manufacturing, and the absence of any inflammatory reaction associated with polymer placement (Lopez et al., 1996). Furthermore, perivascular delivery has a potential advantage of bypassing the endothelial barrier and avoiding rapid washout of growth factor due to rapid arterial blood flow.

Animals implanted with heparin-alginate pellets containing 8 μg of FGF-2 at the time of ameroid placement (~5 μg released over the course of the experiment—approximately 328-fold less than the dose in the study of Unger et al.) demonstrated significantly better preservation of perfusion of ischemic zone during pacing compared to control animals (Harada et al., 1994). In addition, ventricular function studies demonstrated better preservation of regional left ventricular function in the ameroid-compromised territory at rest and faster recovery following pacing in FGF-2-treated animals (Harada et al., 1994). However, rapid pacing induced equal and significant deterioration in both FGF-2-treated and control groups. Examination of the effect of progressively larger amounts of FGF-2 (10 and 100 μg) delivered in a similar manner in a pig model (Lopez et al., 1997c) demonstrated substantial improvement in resting coronary blood flow in the chronically ischemic myocardium in both FGF-2 groups compared to controls. Combined analysis of animals from both studies demonstrated a dose-dependent decrease in coronary resistance in the ameroid-compromised (LCX) territory, implying improved blood flow (Fig 13.4).

Analysis of left ventricular function demonstrated a higher ejection fraction at rest and during pacing in both 10 and 100 μg FGF-2 groups compared to controls. Similarly, regional wall motion in the ischemic territory was better preserved at rest in both FGF-2 groups although during rapid pacing only the 100 μg FGF-2 group maintained normal wall thickening (Lopez et al., 1997c). Thus, increasing dosages of FGF-2 resulted in a dose-dependent improvement of coronary perfusion and left ventricular function. These studies clearly show, therefore, the feasibility of augmentation of collateral circulation and left ventricular function in pig by FGF-2. Since

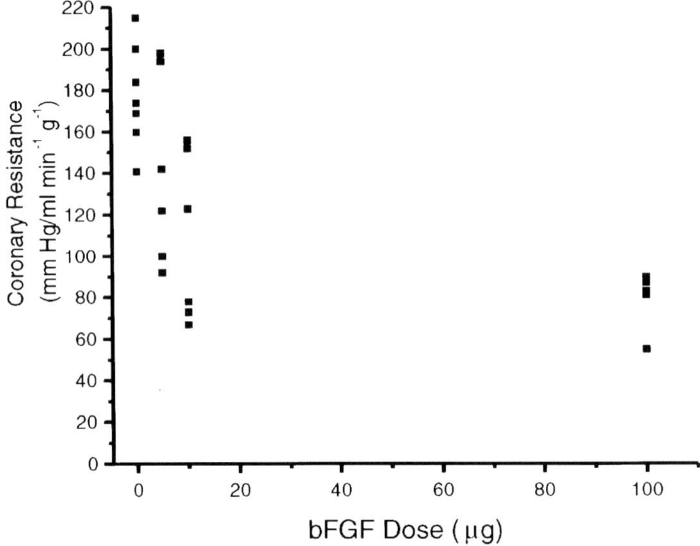

Figure 13.4. Coronary resistance [Resistance (mmHg/ml/min/gm)=MAP/(Sample AU × withdrawal rate/Reference AU × sample wt)] in occluded left circumflex (LCX) territory in ameroid constricted pigs. Data are shown for controls (0µg FGF-2) and 5, 10, and 100 µg FGF-2, with a dose dependent decrease in LCX resistance. (From Lopez et al., 1997c.)

a number of investigators have suggested that angiogenic response in the pig is predominantly of small-vessel type (see Chapter 9), the presence of neoarteriogenesis was examined using coronary angiography. Interestingly, there was a significant increase in angiographically visible collaterals supplying the occluded LCX artery in FGF-2-treated but not in control animals. Furthermore, while there was a significant increase in left-to-left (LAD to LCX and bridging LCX to LCX) collaterals, there was no significant increase in the number of right-to-left (RCA to LCX) collaterals (Lopez et al., 1997c). Given this increase in the number of epicardial collaterals, the observed improvement in coronary blood flow and left ventricular function in these studies may have been equally due to FGF-2-induced neoarteriogenesis as well as true myocardial angiogenesis.

Besides improving both myocardial perfusion and function, FGF-2 administration is associated with significant improvement in receptor-mediated endothelium-dependent relaxation to ADP and serotonin that remained impaired in control animals (Sellke et al., 1994). At the same time, enhanced contraction to acetylcholine seen in control animals was reduced by FGF-2 treatment. Analysis of microvessels from the normal (nonischemic) myocardium of FGF-2-treated pigs showed no effect of growth factor administration on any measured parameters of microvascular function. Thus, FGF-2 administration results in selective improvement of receptor-mediated endothelium-dependent responses in the ischemic, but not normal, myocardium.

In addition to intravascular and perivascular administration, intrapericardial delivery is another means to deliver growth factors. The advantage of this approach derives from the ability to deliver the growth factor to any area of the myocardium regardless of coronary anatomy as well as the absence of systemic side effects associated with administration of these agents (see below). While normal pericardial space contains little fluid, it is nevertheless easily accessible using either a transatrial or a direct percutaneous (subxiphoid) approach. The potential angiogenic efficacy of drugs delivered by this method has been demonstrated in a rabbit model of left ventricular hypertrophy in which infusion of 5 μg of FGF-2 via an implanted minipump led to a significant increase in epicardial vascularity (Landau et al., 1995) that was further increased by a simultaneous induction of left ventricular hypertrophy by angiotensin II infusion. Single intrapericardial administration of FGF-2 (30 μg, 200 μg, and 2 mg) in a porcine left circumflex (LCX) ameroid constrictor model resulted in significant improvement in the presence of angiographically detectable left-to-left collaterals, increased coronary blood flow in the LCX territory, and improved LCX regional wall motion, as well as a significant reduction in the zone of delayed contrast arrival as measured by magnetic resonance perfusion imaging (Fig. 13.5) (Laham et al., 1998b). Thus intrapericardial delivery may represent another approach to growth factor administration.

Clinical Studies

On the basis of these animal data, several clinical studies of FGF-2 in patients with coronary disease are in progress. Unger and colleagues are examining the safety of intracoronary infusion of progressively larger doses of FGF-2 in patients with documented coronary disease (E. Unger, personal communication). In another ongoing trial, the safety of intracoronary and intravenous administration of rFGF-2 is being examined (D. Hung, Chiron Corp. personal communication). Finally an NIH-sponsored double-blind placebo-controlled trial is evaluating the effect of local perivascular rhFGF-2 (10 μg or 100 μg) delivered using heparin-alginate beads implanted at the time of coronary artery bypass surgery in patients who have a viable but underperfused myocardial territory not amenable to bypass grafting. Growth-factor-containing bead implantation added on average 2.8 ± 1.1 minutes to operative time. Interim analysis of the first 12 patients demonstrated no acute or chronic hemodynamic effects following growth factor implantations or significant changes in hematologic

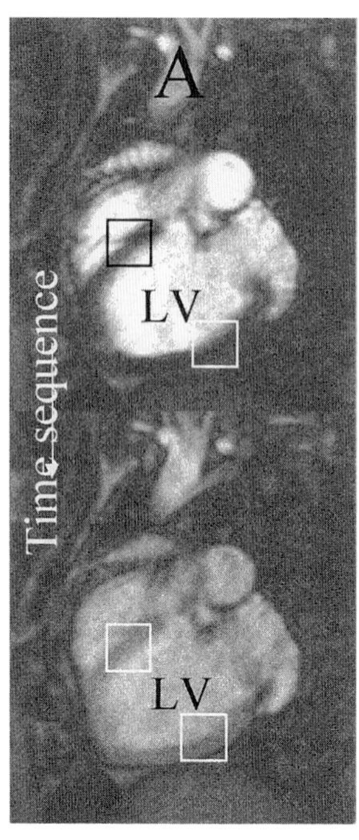
A
LV
Time sequence
LV

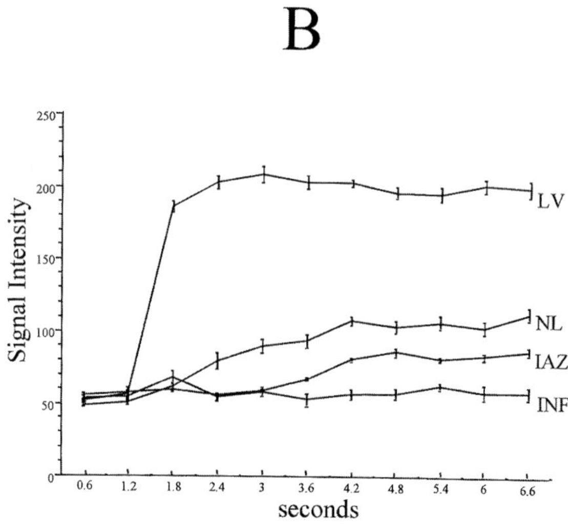
B
Signal Intensity
250
200
150
100
50
0
0.6
1.2
1.8
2.4
3
3.6
4.2
4.8
5.4
6
6.6
seconds
LV
NL
IAZ
INF
LV: left ventricle, NL: LAD territory,
IAZ: Intermediate arrival zone (collateral zone)
INF: Infarcted myocardium

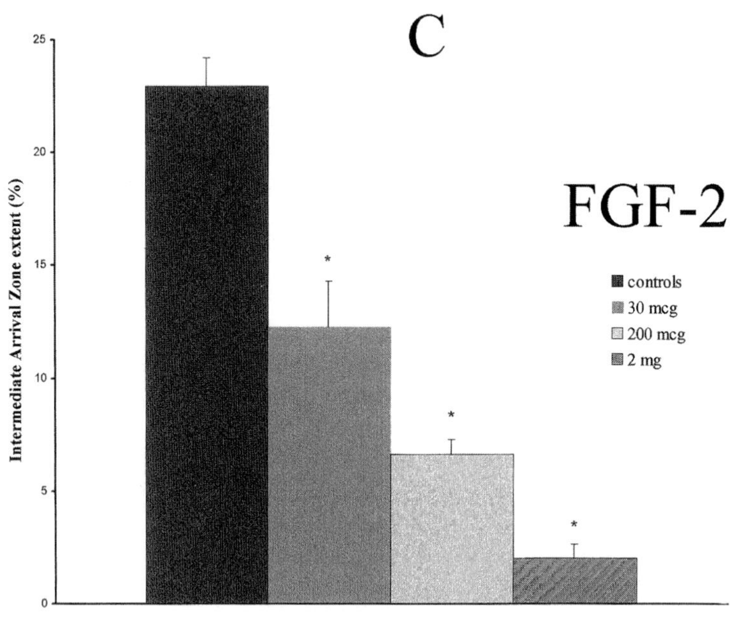
C
Intermediate Arrival Zone extent (%)
25
20
15
10
5
0
FGF-2
controls
30 mcg
200 mcg
2 mg
*
*
*

Table 13.2 Hemodynamic Parameters and FGF-2 Levels in FGF-2 Treated Patients

	Baseline	*1 Day*	*3 Days*	*4 Days*
Mean arterial pressure (mmHg)	91 ± 13	85 ± 18	89 ± 11	93 ± 8
Heart rate (beats per minute)	85 ± 11	100 ± 18	98 ± 11	92 ± 10
FGF-2 level (pg/ml)	17.4 ± 3.3	15.9 ± 1.4	15.9 ± 1.8	16.0 ± 1.8

or chemistry profiles during follow-up; no other adverse events were noted. Plasma FGF-2 levels did not increase above baseline (Table 13.2). Nuclear perfusion scans (Fig 13.6) demonstrated improved perfusion in six of eight FGF-2-treated patients (Laham et al., 1998a; Sellke, 1998).

Fibroblast Growth Factor-1

Animal Studies

Unlike the case with FGF-2, FGF-1 message and protein are abundant in the heart where they are localized predominantly to myocytes (Weiner and Swain, 1989). Hypoxic capillary endothelial cells show a threefold increase in expression of high-affinity FGF receptors in culture along with an increased mitogenic and chemotactic responsiveness to FGF-2 (Shreeniwas et al., 1991). However, while FGF-2 appears to act principally through subset 5 of the FGF receptor, FGF-1 functions efficiently through all seven ligand-selective FGF receptor subtypes generated by alternative splicing of the four known FGF receptor genes. FGF-1 is a potent endothelial cell mitogen and chemotactic factor that is active in animal models of angiogenesis (Thomas, 1992), dermal repair and capillary growth (Mellin et al., 1992), and large vessel re-endothelialization (Bjornsson et al., 1991).

Figure 13.5. Forty magnetic resonance imaging assesment of myocardial perfusion. **(A)** First-pass inversion-recovery turboFLASH magnetic resonance (MR) imaging with sequential arrival of contrast to right ventricle, left ventricle, then left ventricular myocardium. **(B)** In addition to the left ventricle (LV), three distinct zones are observed characterized by either prompt signal appearance (normal myocardium, NL), failure of the signal to increase in intensity (infarction, INF) or delayed signal appearance [delayed arrival zone, Intermediate Arrival Zone (IAZ). On the basis of contrast density data, a 2-D map of contrast intensity vs. time was generated and used to measure the size of the myocardial segments demonstrating impaired myocardial perfusion. **(C)** Dose dependent reduction in the extent of the zone of delayed contrast arrival indicating better myocardial perfusion in the FGF-2 treatment groups.

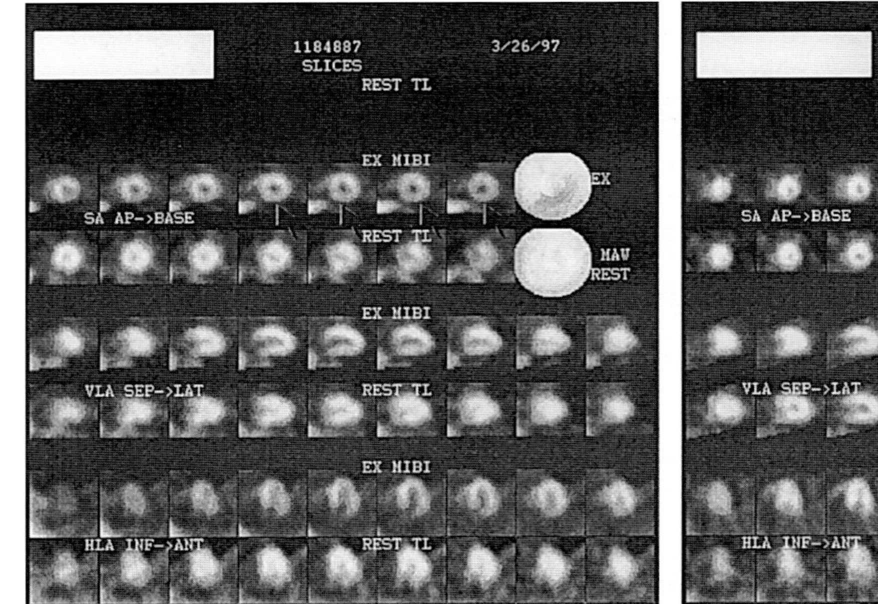

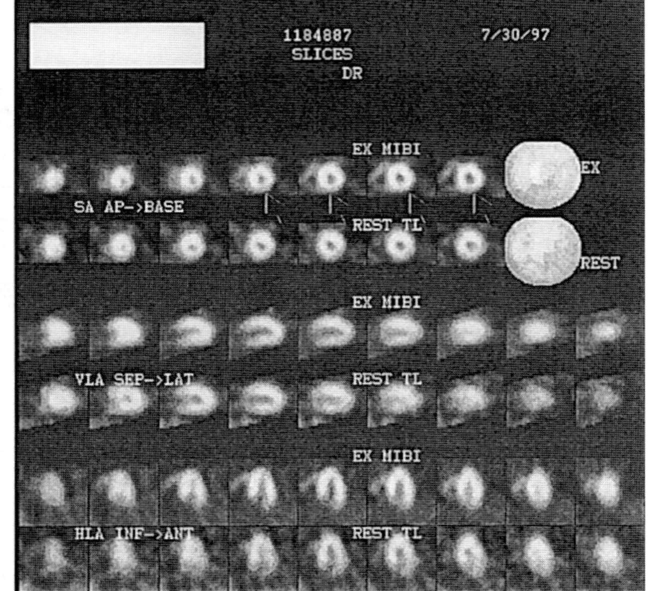

Figure 13.6. *Basic fibroblast growth factor-heparin alginate study*. Shown here is representative nuclear perfusion scans from a patient who underwent coronary artery bypass surgery. However, the right coronary artery (inferior wall) could not be grafted, and FGF-2 heparin-alginate microcapsules were implanted in the epicardial fat of the inferior wall. The scans represent pre-and post-(90 days) treatment nuclear perfusion SPECT imaging (Rest Thallium/Exercise sestaMIBI). Please note the inferior wall defect seen on exercise (left, upper row, *arrows*) but not rest images on the pretreatment scan. The posttreatment scan shows complete resolution of the defect, with a normal scan. Similar results were seen on magnetic resonance perfusion imaging.

Despite these seemingly impressive characteristics, initial experience with therapeutic application of FGF-1 in the setting of chronic myocardial ischemia has been disappointing. In dogs, application of polytetrafluoroethylene (PTFE) fiber or collagen I sponges soaked with up to 800 μg of FGF-1 to an internal mammary artery pedicle positioned over the left anterior descending coronary artery distal to the ameroid occluder failed to stimulate formation of angiographically visible collaterals (Banai et al., 1991). Similarly, infusion of 2.4 mg of FGF-1 with heparin over an 8-week period into an internal mammary artery (IMA) implanted into the myocardium subtended by an ameroid-occluded coronary artery failed to improve IMA flow above that seen with infusion of heparin alone (Unger et al., 1993b). Finally, a 4-week infusion of FGF-1 (30 μg/hour, total dose ~20 mg) with heparin failed to improved collateral zone perfusion to a higher extent than did infusion of heparin alone (Unger et al., 1993a). On the other hand, implantation of 1 μg of *E. coli*-derived FGF-1 in a PTFE sponge between aorta and the left ventricle in rats resulted in appearance of new vessels between the aorta and the myocardium (Schlaudraff et al., 1993). However, given the possible presence of endotoxin in the FGF-1 preparation used in the study, the appearance of aorta-to-LV collaterals may have resulted more from an inflammatory reaction than from FGF-1-induced angiogenesis.

One possible explanation for the failures of FGF-1 to induce vessel formation in chronic myocardial ischemia is that wild-type FGF-1 is rapidly inactivated in vivo. The instability of wild-type FGF-1 results from formation of inactivating disulfide bonds promoted by air oxidation (Ortega et al., 1991) and, perhaps, catalyzed by trace metals (Linemeyer et al., 1990). The protein's half-life may be greatly increased by replacement of one of the three buried cysteines with a serine residue (S^{117}) (Linemeyer et al., 1990). This single S-to-O atom substitution does not alter either the conformational unfolding temperature or mitogenic potency of FGF-1 (Ortega et al., 1991) and, because of its lack of exposure, should not present a distinct immunological surface epitope. Thus altered, S^{117}-FGF-1 has an activity half-life of 1.4 hours (Ortega et al., 1991) compared to a half-life of only 15 minutes for the wild-type protein at 37°C, apparently reflecting a diminished rate of disulfide bond formation. Wild-type FGF-1 binds tightly to heparin, which increases its thermal stability to approximately 60°C (Volkin et al., 1993) and its mitogenic half-life at 37°C by nearly 100-fold to 24 hours (Ortega et al., 1991). However, even a 1-day half-life can lead to a nearly complete loss of activity well before the end of long duration needed for slow-release dosing. In the presence of heparin, the S^{117} mutant exhibits a 10-fold greater 240-hour activity half-life (Ortega et al., 1991).

The therapeutic efficacy of the S^{117}-FGF-1 preparation was tested by incorporating 10 μg of the mutant protein into ethylene-vinyl acetate copolymer (EVAc) matrices that were then applied to the ameroid-compromised myocardium of a pig (Lopez et al., 1998a). Comparison of

FGF-1-treated and control animals demonstrated significant improvement of myocardial flow in the treated territory that was accompanied by improvement in global and regional left ventricular function. Analysis of microvascular responses demonstrated normalization of abnormal responses to β-adrenergic and endothelium-dependent vasodilation by FGF-1 treatment in the ischemic myocardium (Sellke et al., 1996a). Thus, the S^{117}-FGF-1 mutant form of FGF-1 demonstrates significant therapeutic potential in a pig chronic ischemia model.

Clinical Studies

A clinical trial of FGF-1 injections into the left ventricular wall myocardium immediately distal to the internal mammary artery anastamosis demonstrated somewhat increased vessel density at the site of injections as assessed by digital angiography (Schumacher et al., 1998).

Fibroblast Growth Factor-5

Animal Studies

A single study has examined the efficacy of an adenoviral infection of an FGF-5 construct into ischemic myocardium in a pig ameroid model (Giordano et al., 1996). Two intracoronary injections of 2×10^{11} viral particles of recombinant adenovirus carrying full-length cDNA encoding human FGF-5 gene into the left main and right coronary arteries were performed 3 weeks following ameroid implantation. Contrast echocardiographic analysis of coronary perfusion 2 weeks following the adenoviral injections demonstrated improved perfusion in FGF-5 but not control (Lac-Z-treated) mice, compared to preinjection baseline that was associated with an improvement in the regional left ventricular function. Further analysis demonstrated that FGF-5 treatment was associated with increased bromodeoxyuridine (marker of DNA synthesis) incorporation as well as higher number of capillaries per myofiber. Interestingly, increased capillary numbers were seen both in ischemic and nonischemic territories. Microscopic examination did not demonstrate any significant inflammation associated with Adv-FGF-5-injections (Giordano et al., 1996). Thus, adenoviral therapy with FGF-5 based vectors may provide another means of angiogenic therapy in chronic myocardial ischemia.

Vascular Endothelial Growth Factor

Animal Studies

Four major forms of VEGF are generated as a result of alternative splicing of a single gene: $VEGF_{121}$, $VEGF_{165}$, $VEGF_{189}$, and $VEGF_{206}$. Most of the studies have been performed with a $VEGF_{165}$ isoform although recently $VEGF_{121}$ has been receiving increasing attention.

While the work of Isner and colleagues has demonstrated considerable therapeutic efficacy of VEGF administration either in protein or gene therapy form in patients with ischemic limb disease (see Chapter 14), experience with VEGF administration in the setting of myocardial ischemia has been more controversial. A study carried out in a dog ameroid model suggested that daily intracoronary injections of 45 μg of VEGF delivered distal to the occluder over an 28-day period (total dose 900 μg) result in faster restoration of collateral zone flow than did similar injections of normal saline (Banai et al., 1994). Morphological analysis demonstrated a significantly higher number of small vessels (>20 μm diameter) but no capillaries (<20 μm vessels) in VEGF-treated compared to control animals. A subsequent study by the same group of investigators using an identical model, however, failed to show any beneficial effect of a 7-day course of VEGF infusions (total dose 720 μg) (Lazarous et al., 1996). It is not clear why there was such a dramatic difference between the two studies; the reduction in total dose and a shorter duration of infusion in the second study may have played a role.

The therapeutic efficacy of VEGF in porcine circulation was tested using an implantable minipump primed with 2 μg of VEGF and 50 U of heparin delivered over 4 weeks periadventitially to the circumflex coronary artery distal to the ameroid occluder (Harada et al., 1996). Comparison of VEGF/heparin-and heparin-only-treated animals demonstrated that while coronary flow in the ischemic territory at rest was no different between the two groups, VEGF treatment was associated with better coronary flow during pacing. Assessment of myocardial perfusion using magnetic resonance imaging demonstrated not only significantly better perfusion of the compromised territory in VEGF-treated animals but also a reduction in size of this territory (Fig. 13.7) (Pearlman et al., 1995; Lopez, 1998b). Morphometric analysis found nearly a four-fold increase in the number of collateral vessels in VEGF-treated animals that was limited to the ischemic zone (Harada et al., 1996).

Development of myocardial ischemia is associated with a decrease in the subendocardial-to-subepicardial blood flow ratio (Q_{endo}/Q_{epi}). To determine the effect of perivascular delivery of VEGF on the transmyocardial distribution of blood flow, the subendocardial and subepicardial flows in VEGF-treated and control animals were examined under resting and pacing conditions. While at rest there was no difference in the subendocardial or subepicardial flows or transmyocardial blood flow distribution (Q_{endo}/Q_{epi}) between VEGF-treated and control animals in the compromised myocardium, during pacing subendocardial flow in the control group became significantly lower compared to the VEGF group. No statistically significant differences in subepicardial flows between the groups were found, resulting in a significantly higher Q_{endo}/Q_{epi} flow ratio in the VEGF group (Fig 13.8). Thus, epicardial administration of the growth factor resulted in a significantly better preservation of transmyocardial flow distribution during pacing stress (Harada et al., 1996).

Analysis of microvascular function demonstrated significantly better res-

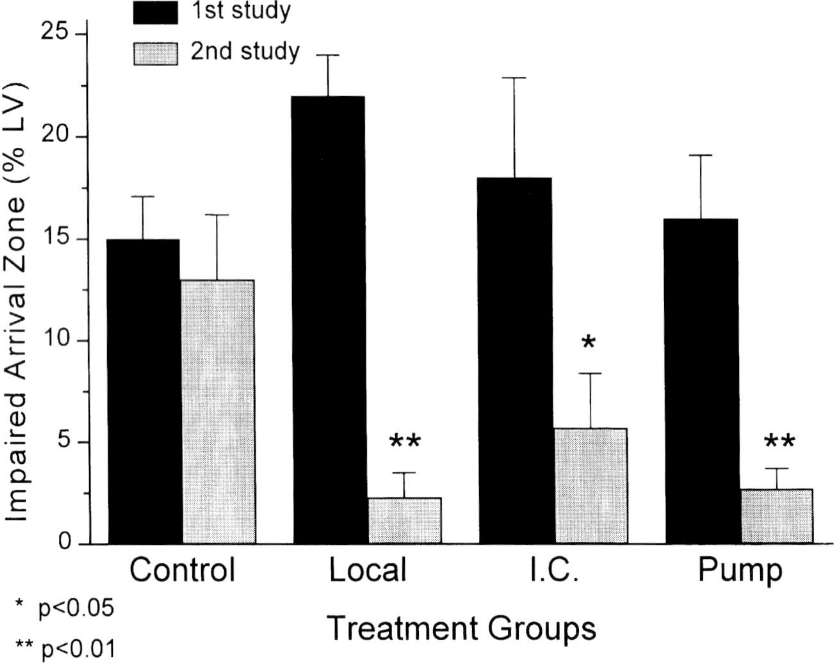

Figure 13.7. Forty ameroid constrictor pigs were randomized to receive VEGF (20 mg, by a single intracoronary (i.c.) or local delivery, or by an infusion pump) or saline. The extent of the impaired arrival zone (zone of delayed contrast arrival by perfusion magnetic resonance imaging) decreased significantly in VEGF treated animals compared to controls. (Lopez et al., 1998).

toration of endothelium-mediated, receptor-dependent relaxation in VEGF-treated animals. These improvements in coronary flow and microvascular function were reflected in enhanced left ventricular performance in VEGF-treated animals, as demonstrated by higher ejection fraction and better preservation of regional wall shortening during pacing stress (Harada et al., 1996).

Thus, VEGF administration in this porcine ameroid model of myocardial ischemia resulted in significant improvement of a number of endpoints, including increased capillary density, improved coronary blood flow and myocardial perfusion, restoration of microcirculatory function, and recovery of global and regional left ventricular function. The fundamental differences between this study and the dog studies described above include the use of perivascular rather than intravascular delivery, concomitant use of heparin (that could potentially stabilize VEGF), and differences between porcine and canine models of chronic ischemia.

While perivascular sustained release delivery is appealing because of a number of theoretical considerations (see Chapter 12), single-bolus intracoronary delivery is much more practical. The feasibility of such an ap-

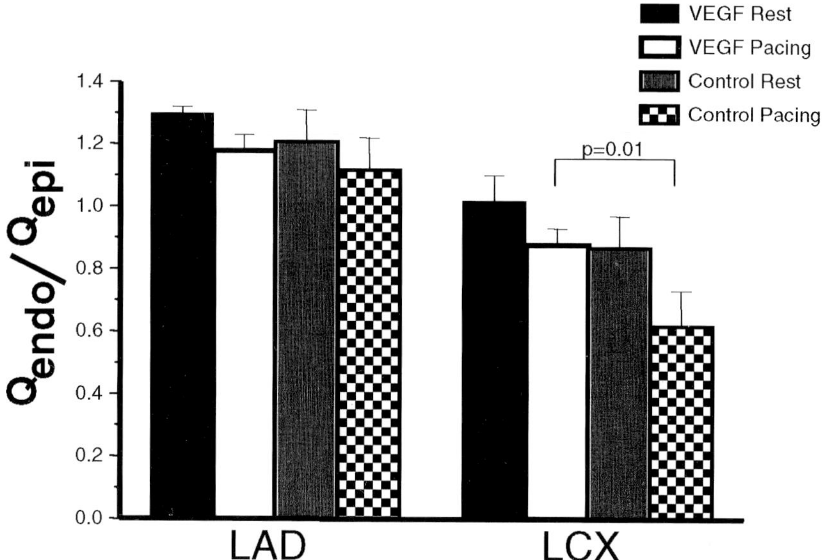

Figure 13.8. Transmyocardial coronary flow distribution in VEGF-treated (infusion pump) and control animals. Regional coronary blood flow (Q) was measured in the epicardial (Q_{epi}) and endocardial (Q_{endo}) segments of the LAD (left anterior descending) and occluded LCX (left circumflex artery) under resting conditions and with pacing. VEGF treated animals (solid bar: rest, open bar: pacing) and control animals (hatched bar: rest, crosshatched bar: pacing). During pacing, LCX Q_{endo}/Q_{epi} was significantly higher in VEGF treated animals. From Harada et al., 1996.)

proach was tested by Hariawala et al., who injected 2 mg of rhVEGF$_{165}$ into the left coronary artery of eight pigs. Four of the eight animals survived the injection (with four animals dying acutely of refractory hypotension); however, 30 days later, the remaining animals demonstrated improved coronary flow compared to the control group (Hariawala et al., 1996). Given 50% mortality of high dose single-bolus VEGF therapy, the efficacy of a lower-dose (20 μg) single-bolus intracoronary injection was compared to the same amount of VEGF delivered either perivascularly or locally using an InfusaSleeve™ catheter. The studies conducted in a porcine model demonstrated that both intracoronary bolus injection and local delivery resulted in significant increase in angiographically visible left-to-left, but not right-to-left, collaterals, and improvement in myocardial blood flow and regional left ventricular function. Although there was a trend toward better results with local compared to intracoronary bolus delivery, both methods appeared equally efficacious (Fig 13.9). There was no significant hemodynamic compromise associated with any of these delivery approaches (Lopez et al., 1998b).

Thus, VEGF, delivered by either intracoronary or periadventitial meth-

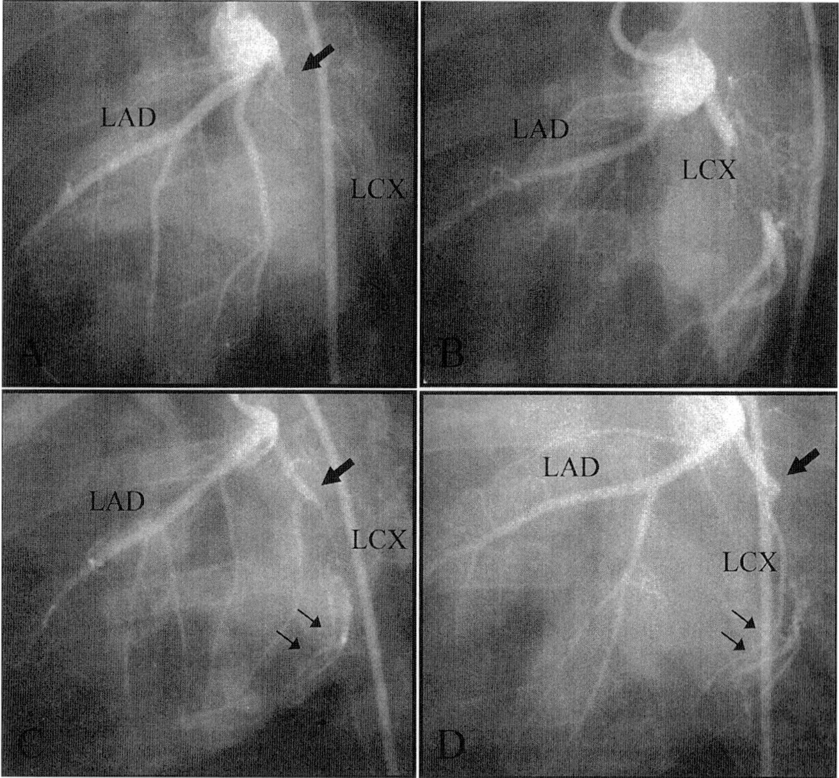

Figure 13.9. Left coronary angiography in ameroid constricted animals treated with VEGF. *Wide black arrow* refers to the LCX occlusion. *Narrow arrows* point to the reconstituted distal vessel (by left-to-left collaterals). **(A)** Control animals, **(B)** animals treated with locally delivered VEGF (20 μg). **(A)** Intracoronary VEGF (20 μg). **(A)** VEGF pump (20 μg). Note the abundance of collaterals and reconstitution of distal LCX in VEGF treated animals particularly in the local delivery group. (From Lopez et al., 1998b.)

ods, appears to be an effective angiogenic agent. The cytokine seems to induce both tissue angiogenesis (as documented by increased vessel counts) in the ischemic territory and neoarteriogenesis as suggested by coronary angiography.

Clinical Studies

The success of animal studies prompted clinical evaluation of VEGF in patients with chronic myocardial ischemia. To date, Phase I studies evaluating the effect of intracoronary and intravenous administration have been completed (Henry et al., 1998) and the Phase II studies have been initiated. In addition, a gene therapy trial using adenoviral constructs with $VEGF_{121}$ is currently in progress.

ACUTE MYOCARDIAL ISCHEMIA

Although studies of therapeutic angiogenesis are based on the premise that the growth-factor-dependent neovascularization is responsible for therapeutic benefit, the first study of FGF-2 administration in a dog ischemia model suggested that neovascularization may not be the only mode of benefit. In this study, Yanagisawa-Miwa and colleagues injected 20μg of FGF-2 by intracoronary route in dogs with acute myocardial infarction and observed not only an increase in the number of capillaries and arterioles in FGF-2-treated compared to control animal but also a reduction in infarct size and improvement in left ventricular function (Yanagisawa-Miwa et al., 1992). These findings were confirmed in a larger study in which intrapericardial injection of 30 μg of FGF-2 in dogs with acute myocardial infarction resulted in significant reduction of the size of myocardial infarction as well as improvement in left ventricular function, both of which were augmented by a simultaneous administration of heparan sulfate (Uchida et al., 1995). Similar findings were obtained in an acute ischemia/reperfusion study in which administration of 10μg of FGF-2 10 minutes after initiation of coronary occlusion and again immediately before reperfusion resulted in significant salvage of myocardium at risk compared to control animals (Horrigan et al., 1996).

Since new vessel growth could not have been fast enough to account for reduction in infarct size in the setting of acute coronary occlusion, the observed effect must have resulted from FGF-2-facilitated recruitment of preexisting collaterals or from myocardial tissue "protection" by the growth factor. The former is clearly a possibility since FGF-2 can induce significant vasodilation (Cuevas et al., 1991) and since dogs possess a rich network of preexisting collaterals. In addition, collateral vessels appear to be more sensitive than are normal vessels to this effect of the growth factor.

It is also possible that the myocardial "protective" effects of FGF-2 are responsible for observed myocardial salvage. The ability of FGF-2 to ameliorate ischemic injury independent of its effects on blood flow has been shown in a stroke model in mice. In these studies, FGF-2-induced reduction of stroke size resulting from acute arterial occlusion was similar in wild-type and "eNOS knockout" mice even though the FGF-2-induced increase in cerebral blood flow seen in wild-type mice was absent in animals missing the eNOS gene (Huang et al., 1996). Additional evidence for the cardioprotective effects of FGF-2 comes from studies of ischemia/reperfusion in isolated rat heart in which growth factor's administration reduced the magnitude of ischemic damage and improved functional recovery (Padua et al., 1995). One possible mechanism for FGF-2-mediated myocardial protection is its ability to stimulate nitric oxide release that in turn may exert a protective effect on the myocardium.

HEMODYNAMIC EFFECTS OF GROWTH FACTOR ADMINISTRATION

Early experience with both FGF-2 and VEGF suggested that both cytokines are potent vasodilators. Injections of intravenous FGF-2 and FGF-1 in rats led to profound, albeit transient, hypotension that could largely be prevented by injection of l-NNA (Cuevas et al., 1991). Interestingly, a hypertensive rebound following the transient period of hypotension was characterized by increased heart rate variability that may have implications for electrical stability of the myocardium (Boussairi and Sassard, 1994).

Similar effects on blood pressure have been observed in larger animals with either cytokine cytokines, both of which induced dose-dependent hypotension. In studies in dogs, the onset of hypotension occurred within 1 minute following left atrial injection of FGF-2, with a peak at 5 minutes. The blood pressure recovered within 20–30 minutes of injection. Long-term administration of FGF-2 did not alter this hemodynamic response even after several weeks of daily injections. There also were no significant changes in the heart rate or the contractile state (as assessed by dP/dt) of the left ventricle (Lazarous et al., 1995). Pharmacokinetic studies of plasma FGF-2 levels following left atrial administration demonstrated an elimination half-time of about 50 minutes (Lazarous et al., 1995). In contrast to significant hypotension following systemic administration of FGF-2, local extravascular delivery using the heparin-alginate polymer resulted in no significant changes in systemic blood pressure or heart rate (Lopez et al., 1996).

Administration of VEGF results in hemodynamic alterations even more profound than those seen with FGF-2, both in rats (Yang et al., 1996) and in larger animals. In dog studies, left atrial injection of 720 μg reduced mean arterial blood pressure by 50% within 5 minutes of injection, with pressure returning to baseline by 90 minutes (Lazarous et al., 1996). Intracoronary injections of 500 μg of VEGF in pigs resulted in 50% mortality from refractory hypotension (Hariawala et al., 1996). In another study of hemodynamic response to VEGF administration in normal pigs, growth factor injections produced a dose-dependent increase in coronary blood flow and reduction in left ventricular filling and mean arterial pressures. Furthermore, VEGF-induced increase in coronary blood flow equaled the maximal responses obtained with intracoronary injections of adenosine and significantly exceeded increases in coronary blood flow induced by injections of nitroglycerine or serotonin. Pretreatment of animals with the NO synthase inhibitor L-NNA almost completely suppressed VEGF-induced increases in coronary blood flow (Lopez et al., 1997b). This observation, which suggests that VEGF-induced vasodilation is at least in part NO-dependent, has been confirmed in in vitro studies of arterial (Ku et al., 1993) and microvascular responses to VEGF and FGF-2 (Sellke et al., 1996c).

An interesting feature of repeat exposure to VEGF is the development of tachyphylaxis to cytokine's vasodilatory effects. In in vivo studies, administration of 10 μg of the growth factor completely prevents a further increase in coronary flow following administration of the same or tenfold higher amounts of VEGF when given within 2 hours of initial injection. The coronary bed remained responsive to the vasodilating effects of adenosine and nitroglycerine but not those of serotonin, suggesting that development of tachyphylaxis resulted from impaired endothelial production of NO rather than a defective response of vascular smooth muscle (Lopez et al., 1997b). The observed increase in coronary flow following intracoronary VEGF administration occurred in the absence of significant changes in the epicardial coronary artery diameter. In contrast, intracoronary injections of nitroglycerine, while resulting in far smaller overall changes in coronary blood flow, produced significant increase in epicardial coronary diameter. These observations suggest that the predominate effect of VEGF is small-vessel vasodilation (Laham et al., 1997b).

As already mentioned, the sensitivity of the microvasculature to vasodilating effects of VEGF and FGF-2 is higher in ischemic than in normal tissues (Sellke et al., 1996c). This heightened sensitivity does not appear to result from changes in eNOS expression, which is similar in ischemic and normal microvessels (Laham et al., 1997a), but may perhaps be explained by higher FGF and VEGF receptor expression in the ischemic myocardium (Sellke et al., 1996c). Although it produces profound effects on blood pressure and coronary flow, VEGF does not appear to possess any direct inotropic or chronotropic effects (Lopez et al., 1997b; Yang et al., 1996).

SIDE EFFECTS OF GROWTH FACTOR ADMINISTRATION

Administration of pluripotent agents such as the FGFs and VEGF is likely to produced unwanted side effects, in addition to hemodynamic effects. Diabetic retinopathy is associated with the presence of VEGF in the vitreous humor (Aiello et al., 1994) and administration of VEGF-neutralizing antibodies arrests the process in experimental animals; thus it is possible that this process could be worsened. Furthermore, VEGF, by virtue of its effect on vessel permeability, may lead to development of edema and inflammatory reactions. As already noted, because of the cytokine's prominent vasoactive properties, substantial systemic hypotension may represent a dose-limiting toxicity. To date, in limited clinical experience, plasmid-mediated VEGF gene transfer in a clinical trial has led to development of extensive extremity edema and telangiectasia in a patient to whom the expression construct was administered intraarterially in the leg (Isner et al., 1996). Administration of FGF-2 in high dosages is also associated with a number of side effects, including anemia, thrombocytopenia, membranous nephropathy with morphologic evidence of glomerular damage including fusion of foot processes and changes in Bowman's capsule and podocytes, as well as hyperostosis (Mazue et al., 1991).

An important theoretical concern regarding growth factor therapy is that plaque angiogenesis might be exacerbated, perhaps stimulating progression of coronary disease or inducing plaque instability. In particular, VEGF-mediated enhancement of permeability could facilitate plaque expansion or rupture, since intraplaque vessels tend to be quite permeable even without exogenous VEGF. In addition, one might imagine that these growth factors could accelerate progression of coronary atherosclerotic lesions by stimulating growth of fibroblasts and medial smooth muscle cells. For instance, dogs were subjected to ameroid-induced occlusion of the left circumflex coronary artery and randomized to 1.74 mg FGF-2 (n=9), VEGF 0.72 mg (n=9), or saline (n=10) as a daily left atrial bolus (days 10–16). Additional dogs were randomized to VEGF 0.72 mg (n=6) or saline (n=5); however, treatment was delayed by 1 week. Coincident with the institution of treatment, all dogs underwent balloon denudation injury of the iliofemoral artery. FGF-2 markedly increased maximal collateral flow but did not exacerbate neointimal accumulation. VEGF had no discernible effect on maximal collateral flow, but it exacerbated neointimal thickening after vascular injury (Lazarous et al., 1996). The same group found no significant structural or vasoproliferative effect of chronic systemic (left atrial) administration of FGF-2, at a dose sufficient to enhance collateral vessel formation, on the nonischemic retina of dogs with myocardial ischemia (Jacot et al., 1996)

MECHANISMS OF ANGIOGENIC EFFECT

While a number of animal studies have clearly shown beneficial physiologic effect of growth factor administration in myocardial ischemia, as reviewed above, a number of unanswered questions (Table 13.3) remain regarding the mechanisms of the observed improvements. As expected, administration of cytokines such as FGF-2 increases the rate of cell proliferation in treated animals (Unger et al., 1994). Interestingly, this increased proliferation rate is largely limited to the ischemic zone even during systemic (or nonselective coronary) growth factor administration. Similarly, a preponderance of evidence suggests that the increases in vascularity seen following either FGF-2 or VEGF administration are largely limited to the ischemic zone. Thus, it is possible that potent local factors, including perhaps both angiogenesis promoters and inhibitors, control the local angiogenic response. Factors in the latter category may include recently described angiogenesis inhibitors such as angiostatin (O'Reilly et al., 1994, 1996; Wu et al., 1997) and endostatin (O'Reilly et al., 1997), the endothelial proliferation inhibitor *btg* 1 (Westernacher and Schaper, 1995), and matrix proteins capable of angiogenesis suppression, such as

Table 13.3 Unanswered Questions in Therapeutic Angiogenesis

UNRESOLVED BIOLOGICAL ISSUES

Why is administration of a small amount of exogenous growth factor so beneficial?
Why does the effect appear to be limited to the ischemic zone?
What is the role of high-affinity receptors and extracellular matrix in the regulation of angiogenesis?
What process controls angiogenesis in mature tissue?
What is the role of inflammation in angiogenesis?
What is the mechanism of action of various heparin-binding growth factors with regard to angiogenesis?
What is the role of nitric oxide in the process of ischemia and growth-factor-induced angiogenesis?

UNRESOLVED DELIVERY ISSUES

Single Bolus versus Repeated Administration versus Sustained Delivery

Local versus Systemic Delivery
Myocardial delivery
Coronary vessel wall deposition
Pericardial administration
Intravenous infusion
Combination delivery techniques (TMR/PMR with growth factor delivery, CABG with growth factor delivery, cardiomyoplasty with growth factor delivery)

Protein versus Gene Therapy

TMR: Laser Trans Myocardial Revascularization.
PMR: Laser Percutaneous Myocardial Revascularization.
CABG: Coronary Artery Bypass Surgery.

thrombospondin 1 (Bertin et al., 1997; Panetti et al., 1997; Patel et al., 1996), and thrombospondin 2 (Bertin et al., 1997; Kyriakides et al., 1998; Panetti et al., 1997; Volpert et al., 1995). In addition, the absence or low level of appropriate high-affinity receptors (FGF R1, flk-1, flt-1, etc.) may limit the angiogenic potency of these cytokines in normal tissues. Finally, changes in the composition of the extracellular matrix, including expression of matrix-digesting enzymes such as matrix metalloproteinases and collagenases, as well as their inhibitors, such as TIMP 1, in addition to changes in endothelial cell expression of integral matrix proteins, such as $\alpha v\beta 3$ and $\alpha v\beta 5$ integrins and heparan-sulfate-carrying proteoglycans such as syndecans, may regulate the ability of tissues to respond to angiogenic signaling.

Therapeutic administration of either FGFs or VEGF results in both intramyocardial and epicardial neovascularization. The relative importance of those events is not clear, however. While increased intramyocardial vessel growth clearly may promote better distribution of flow throughout the ischemic myocardium, epicardial collateral development may well be necessary to provide the source of blood flow to intramyocardial vessels that is impaired by obstruction of native epicardial vessels. It is not known whether both of these processes respond to the same stimuli, although it seems clear that ischemia is far more important in stimulation of intramyocardial than of epicardial collateral development (see Chapter 9). Furthermore, while angiographic and morphometric studies show that both

FGFs and VEGF augment both the presence of epicardial collaterals and intramyocardial neovascularization, it is not clear if these modes of new vessel growth are in any way growth-factor specific. Although on theoretical grounds, as discussed in Chapter 9, FGF may be more likely to induce neoarteriogenesis and VEGF angiogenesis, the crosstalk between various components of angiogenic response and the ability of FGF-2 to induce VEGF expression (Stavri et al., 1995) suggests that there may be little difference in the final result.

In addition to promoting neovascularization, therapy with growth factor is associated with improved microvascular vasodilation that may itself lead to significant improvement in myocardial performance. The relative contribution of this effect, especially in light of far greater sensitivity of ischemic tissue to VEGF-and FGF-2-mediated vasomotion, to the overall improvement in myocardial blood flow and function is not well understood.

While a number of studies have documented the therapeutic benefit of prolonged infusions or sustained-release delivery, other investigators have reported similar benefits from single-dose administration. With the short half-life of these cytokines and their rapid washout from the systemic circulation, the effectiveness of a single dose raises the possibility of a local positive feedback circuit that is established and then maintained in the absence of continued presence of the growth factor. Moreover, serum and/or tissue levels of some of the growth factor doses used in animal studies were low (or even undetectable), suggesting that very little cytokine is required to initiate such a circuit. The nature of the circuit, if it exists, is not understood at present.

Chronic ischemia results in appreciable induction of expression of VEGF and FGF-2 as well their receptors. Yet, exogenous administration of even small amounts of the same growth factor leads to significant augmentation of angiogenesis. This observation raises again the question of a controlling circuit that propagates and maintains the angiogenic response following a growth factor delivery, as well as the relative importance of epicardial versus intramyocardial collaterals. The latter question may be particularly relevant in light of the observation that endogenous growth factor expression is augmented in the myocardial, and not in the epicardial, coronaries.

Finally, thus far essentially all animal studies of angiogenesis have been carried out in normocholesterolemic animals. Since hyperlipidemia is known to induce a number of alterations in both vascular smooth muscle and endothelial cells as well as extracellular matrix including alterations in NO-dependent responses(Chinellato et al., 1997), it can possibly modify angiogenic response to growth factor administration.

In summary, animal studies have conclusively shown the therapeutic benefit of angiogenic growth factor administration. While there are many unanswered questions relating to the biology of these therapeutic effects, it is clear that a new chapter in therapy of ischemic heart disease may be opened shortly.

REFERENCES

Aiello, L. P., Avery, R. L., Arrigg, P. G., Keyt, B. A., Jampel, H. D., Shah, S. T., Pasquale, L. R., Thieme, H., Iwamoto, M. A., and Park, J. E. (1994). Vascular endothelial growth factor in ocular fluid of patients with diabetic retinopathy and other retinal disorders [see comments]. N. Engl. J. Med. 331: 1480–1487.

Aird, W. C., Jahroudi, N., Weiler-Guettler, H., Rayburn, H. B., and Rosenberg, R. D. (1995). Human von Willebrand factor gene sequences target expression to a subpopulation of endothelial cells in transgenic mice. Proc. Natl. Acad. Sci. USA 92: 4567–4571.

Banai, S., Jaklitsch, M. T., Casscells, W., Shou, M., Shrivastav, S., Correa, R., Epstein, S. E., and Unger, E. F. (1991). Effects of acidic fibroblast growth factor on normal and ischemic myocardium. Circ. Res. 69: 76–85.

Banai, S., Jaklitsch, M. T., Shou, M., Lazarous, D. F., Scheinowitz, M., Biro, S., Epstein, S. E., and Unger, E. F. (1994). Angiogenic-induced enhancement of collateral blood flow to ischemic myocardium by vascular endothelial growth factor in dogs. Circulation 89: 2183–2189.

Bart, B. A., Shaw, L. K., McCants, C. B., Jr., Fortin, D. F., Lee, K. L., Califf, R. M., and O'Connor, (1997). Clinical determinants of mortality in patients with angiographically diagnosed ischemic or nonischemic cardiomyopathy. J. Am. Coll. Cardiol. 30: 1002–1008.

Battler, A., Scheinowitz, M., Bor, A., Hasdai, D., Vered, Z., Di Segni, E., Varda-Bloom, N., Nass, D., Engelberg, S., Eldar, M., and et al. (1993). Intracoronary injection of basic fibroblast growth factor enhances angiogenesis in infarcted swine myocardium. J. Am. Coll. Cardiol. 22: 2001–2006.

Bertin, N., Clezardin, P., Kubiak, R., and Frappart, L. (1997). Thrombospondin-1 and 1-2 messenger RNA expression in normal, benign, and neoplastic human breast tissues: correlation with prognostic factors, tumor angiogenesis, and fibroblastic desmoplasia. Cancer Res. 57: 396–399.

Bjornsson, T. D., Dryjski, M., Tluczek, J., Mennie, R., Ronan, J., Mellin, T. N., and Thomas, K. A. (1991). Acidic fibroblast growth factor promotes vascular repair. Proc. Natl. Acad. Sci. USA 88: 8651–8655.

Boussairi, E. H. P. and Sassard, J. P. (1994). Cardiovascular effects of basic fibroblast growth factor in rats. J. Cardiovasc. Pharmacol. 23: 99–102.

Chinellato, A., Ragazzi, E., Pandolfo, L., Froldi, G., Caparrotta, L., Amore, B., and Sartore, S. (1997). Prolonged inhibition of nitric oxide synthesis in Yoshida hyperlipidemic rat: aorta functional and structural properties. Life Sci. 60: 1249–1262.

Cuevas, P., Carceller, F., Ortega, S., Zazo, M., Nieto, I., and Gimenez-Gallego, G. (1991). Hypotensive activity of fibroblast growth factor. Science 254: 1208–1210.

Edelberg, J., Aird, W., and Rosenberg, R. (1997). Cardiac myocyte regulation of cardiac microvascular endothelial cell gene expression: a critical role for PDGF. Circulation 96: I–414.

Edelman, E. R., Nugent, M. A., and Karnovsky, M. J. (1993). Perivascular and intravenous administration of basic fibroblast growth factor: vascular and solid organ deposition. Proc. Natl. Acad. Sci. USA 90: 1513–1517.

Giordano, F. J., Ping, P., McKirnan, M. D., Nozaki, S., DeMaria, A. N., Dillmann, W. H., Mathieu-Costello, O., and Hammond, H. K. (1996). Intracoronary transfer of fibroblast growth factor-5 increases blood flow and contractile function in an ischemic region of the heart. Nat. Med. 2: 534–539.

Harada, K., Grossman, W., Friedman, M., Edelman, E. R., Prasad, P. V., Keighley, C. S., Manning, W. J., Sellke, F. W., and Simons, M. (1994). Basic fibroblast growth factor improves myocardial function in chronically ischemic porcine hearts. J. Clin. Invest. 94: 623–630.

Harada, K., Friedman, M., Lopez, J. J., Wang, S. Y., Li, J., Prasad, P. V., Pearlman, J. D., Edelman, E. R., Sellke, F. W., and Simons, M. (1996). Vascular endothelial growth factor administration in chronic myocardial ischemia. Am. J. Physiol. 270: H1791–H1802.

Hariawala, M. D., Horowitz, J. J., Esakof, D., Sheriff, D. D., Walter, D. H., Keyt, B., Isner, J. M., and Symes, J. F. (1996). VEGF improves myocardial blood flow but produces EDRF-mediated hypotension in porcine hearts. J. Surg. Res. 63: 77–82.

Henry, T., Rocha_Singh, K., Isner, J., Kereiakes, D. J., Giordano, F., Simons, M., Losordo, D., Hendel, R., Bonow, R., Rothman, J., Borbas, E., and McCluskey, E. (1998). Results of intracoronary recombinant human vascular endothelial growth factor (rhVEGF) administration trial. J. Am. Coll. Cardiol. 31: 65A.

Horrigan, M., MacIsaac, A., Nicolini, F., Vince, D., Lee, P., Ellis, S., and Topol, E. (1996). Reduction in myocardial infarct size by basic fibroblast growth factor after temporary coronary occlusion in a canine model. Circulation 94: 1927–33.

Huang, Z., Chen, K., Huang, P., Finkelstein, S., and Moskowitz, M. (1996). bFGF ameliorates focal ischemic injury by blood flow-independent mechanism in eNOS mutant mice. Am. J. Physiol. 272: H1401–H1405.

Isner, J. M., Pieczek, A., Schainfeld, R., Blair, R., Haley, L., Asahara, T., Rosenfield, K., Razvi, S., Walsh, K., and Symes, J. F. (1996). Clinical evidence of angiogenesis after arterial gene transfer of phVEGF165 in patient with ischaemic limb. Lancet 348: 370–374.

Jacot, J. L., Laver, N. M., Glover, J. P., Lazarous, D. F., Unger, E. F., and Robison, W. G., Jr. (1996). Histological evaluation of the canine retinal vasculature following chronic systemic administration of basic fibroblast growth factor. J. Anat. 188: 349–354.

Kelly, R. A., Balligand, J. L., and Smith, T. W. (1996). Nitric oxide and cardiac function. Circ. Res. 79: 363–380.

Ku, D. D., Zaleski, J. K., Liu, S., and Brock, T. A. (1993). Vascular endothelial growth factor induces EDRF-dependent relaxation in coronary arteries. Am. J. Physiol. 265: H586–H592.

Kyriakides, T., Zhu, Y.-H., Smith, L., Bain, S., Yang, Z., Lin, M., Danielson, K., Iozzo, R., LaMarca, M., McKinney, C., Ginns, E., and Bornstein, P. (1998). Mice that lack thrombospondin 2 display connective tissue abnormalities that are associated with disordered collagen fibrillogenesis, an increased vascular density, and a bleeding diathesis. J. Cell Biol. 140: 419–430.

Laham, R., Mehrdad, R., Li, J., Post, M., Tofukuji, M., Sellke, F., and Simons, M. (1997a). Adaptive responses of ischemic microvessels: increased expression of inducible nitric oxide synthase (iNOS) but not endothelial NOS (eNOS). Circulation 96: I–355.

Laham, R., Tofukuji, M., Sellke, F., and Simons, M. (1997b). Vascular endothelial growth factor (VEGF) affects microvessels but not epicardial coronary arteries and veins. Circulation 96: I–551.

Laham, R., Sellke, F., Edelman, E., Pearlman, J., and Simons, M. (1998a). Local perivascular basic fibroblast growth factor (bFGF) treatment in patients with ischemic heart disease. J. Am. Coll. Cardiol. 31: 394A.

Laham, R., Tofukuji, M., Simons, M., Hung, D., and Sellke, F. (1998b). Modulation of myocardial perfusion and vascular reactivity by pericardial bFGF: implications in the treatment of inoperable coronary artery disease. J. Thorac. Cardiovasc. Surg. In Press

Landau, C., Jacobs, A. K., and Haudenschild, C. C. (1995). Intrapericardial basic fibroblast growth factor induces myocardial angiogenesis in a rabbit model of chronic ischemia. Am. Heart J. 129: 924–931.

Lazarous, D. F., Scheinowitz, M., Shou, M., Hodge, E., Rajanayagam, S., Hunsberger, S., Robison, W. G., Jr., Stiber, J. A., Correa, R., Epstein, S. E., and et al. (1995). Effects of chronic systemic administration of basic fibroblast growth factor on collateral development in the canine heart. Circulation 91: 145–153.

Lazarous, D. F., Shou, M., Scheinowitz, M., Hodge, E., Thirumurti, V., Kitsiou, A. N., Stiber, J. A., Lobo, A. D., Hunsberger, S., Guetta, E., Epstein, S. E., and Unger, E. F. (1996). Comparative effects of basic fibroblast growth factor and vascular endothelial growth factor on coronary collateral development and the arterial response to injury. Circulation 94: 1074–1082.

Li, J., Brown, L. F., Hibberd, M. G., Grossman, J. D., Morgan, J. P., and Simons, M. (1996). VEGF, flk-1, and flt-1 expression in a rat myocardial infarction model of angiogenesis. Am. J. Physiol. 270: H1803–H1811.

Linemeyer, D. L., Menke, J. G., Kelly, L. J., DiSalvo, J., Soderman, D., Schaeffer, M. T., Ortega, S., Gimenez-Gallego, G., and Thomas, K. A. (1990). Disulfide bonds are neither required, present, nor compatible with full activity of human recombinant acidic fibroblast growth factor. Growth Factors 3: 287–298.

Lopez, J., Edelman, E., Stamler, A., Morgan, J., Sellke, F., and Simons, M. (1996). Local perivascular administration of basic fibroblast growth factor: drug delivery and toxicological evaluation. Drug Metab. Dispos. 24: 922–924.

Lopez, J., Laham, R. J., Carrozza, J. C., Tofukuji, M., Sellke, F. W., Bunting, S., and Simons, M. (1997b). Hemodynamic effects of intracoronary VEGF delivery: evidence of tachyphylaxis and NO dependence of response. Am. J. Physiol. 273: H1317–H1323.

Lopez, J. J., Edelman, E. R., Stamler, A., Hibberd, M. G., Prasad, P., Caputo, R. P., Carrozza, J. C., Douglas, P. S., Sellke, F. W., and Simons, M. (1997c). Basic fibroblast growth factor in a porcine model of chronic myocardial ischemia: a comparison of angiographic, echocardiographic and coronary flow parameters. J. Pharmacol. Exp. Ther. 282: 385–390.

Lopez, J., Edelman, E., Stamler, A., Thomas, K., DiSalvo, J., Hibberd, M., Caputo, R., Carrozza, J., Douglas, P., Sellke, F., and Simons, M. (1998a). Angiogenic potential of perivascularly delivered acidic FGF in a porcine model of chronic myocardial ischemia. Am. J. Physiol., 274: H930–H936

Lopez, J. J., Laham, R. J., Stamler, A., Pearlman, J. D., Bunting, S., Kaplan, A., Carrozza, J. P., Sellke, F. W., and Simons, M. (1998b). VEGF administration in chronic myocardial ischemia in pigs. Cardiovasc. Res. (in press).

Mazue, G., Bertolero, F., Jacob, C., Sarmientos, P., and Roncucci, R. (1991). Preclinical and clinical studies with recombinant human basic fibroblast growth factor. Ann. N.Y. Acad. Sci. 638: 329–340.

Mellin, T. N., Mennie, R. J., Cashen, D. E., Ronan, J. J., Capparella, J., James, M. L.,

Disalvo, J., Frank, J., Linemeyer, D., Gimenez-Gallego, G., and et al. (1992). Acidic fibroblast growth factor accelerates dermal wound healing. Growth Factors 7: 1–14.

O'Reilly, M., Holmgren, L., Shing, Y., Chen, C., Rosenthal, R. A., Moses, M., Lane, W. S., Cao, Y., Sage, E. H., and Folkman, J. (1994). Angiostatin: a novel angiogenesis inhibitor that mediates the suppression of metastases by a Lewis lung carcinoma [see comments]. Cell 79: 315–328.

O'Reilly, M., Holmgren, L., Chen, C., and Folkman, J. (1996). Angiostatin induces and sustains dormancy of human primary tumors in mice. Nat. Med. 2: 689–692.

O'Reilly, M., Boehm, T., Shing, Y., Fukai, N., Vasios, G., Lane, W. S., Flynn, E., Birkhead, J. R., Olsen, B. R., and Folkman, J. (1997). Endostatin: an endogenous inhibitor of angiogenesis and tumor growth. Cell 88: 277–285.

Ortega, S., Schaeffer, M. T., Soderman, D., DiSalvo, J., Linemeyer, D. L., Gimenez-Gallego, G., and Thomas, K. A. (1991). Conversion of cysteine to serine residues alters the activity, stability, and heparin dependence of acidic fibroblast growth factor. J. Biol. Chem. 266: 5842–5846.

Padua, R. R., Sethi, R., Dhalla, N. S., and Kardami, E. (1995). Basic fibroblast growth factor is cardioprotective in ischemia-reperfusion injury. Mol. Cell. Biochem. 143: 129–135.

Panetti, T. S., Chen, H., Misenheimer, T. M., Getzler, S. B., and Mosher, D. F. (1997). Endothelial cell mitogenesis induced by LPA: inhibition by thrombospondin-1 and thrombospondin-2. J. Lab. Clin. Med. 129: 208–216.

Patel, V. A., Hill, D. J., Eggo, M. C., Sheppard, M. C., Becks, G. P., and Logan, A. (1996). Changes in the immunohistochemical localisation of fibroblast growth factor-2, transforming growth factor-beta 1 and thrombospondin-1 are associated with early angiogenic events in the hyperplastic rat thyroid. J. Endocrinol. 148: 485–499.

Pearlman, J. D., Hibberd, M. G., Chuang, M. L., Harada, K., Lopez, J. J., Gladstone, S. R., Friedman, M., Sellke, F. W., and Simons, M. (1995). Magnetic resonance mapping demonstrates benefits of VEGF-induced myocardial angiogenesis. Nat. Med. 1: 1085–1089.

Schlaudraff, K., Schumacher, B., Specht, B. U., Seitelberger, R., Schlosser, V., and Fasol, R. (1993). Growth of new coronary vascular structures by angiogenic growth factors. Eur. J. Cardiothorac Surg. 7: 637–641.

Schumacher, B., Pecher, P., von Specht, B., and Stegmann, T. (1998). Induction of neoangiogenesis in ischemic myocardium by human growth factors. Circulation 97: 645–650.

Sellke, F. W., Quillen, J. E., Brooks, L. A., and Harrison, D. G. (1990). Endothelial modulation of the coronary vasculature in vessels perfused via mature collaterals. Circulation 81: 1938–1947.

Sellke, F. W., Wang, S. Y., Friedman, M., Harada, K., Edelman, E. R., Grossman, W., and Simons, M. (1994). Basic FGF enhances endothelium-dependent relaxation of the collateral-perfused coronary microcirculation. Am. J. Physiol. 267: H1303–H1311.

Sellke, F. W., Li, J., Stamler, A., Lopez, J. J., Thomas, K. A., and Simons, M. (1996a). Angiogenesis induced by acidic fibroblast growth factor as an alternative method of revascularization for chronic myocardial ischemia. Surgery 120: 182–188.

Sellke, F., Wang, S., Harada, K., Lopez, J., and Simons, M. (1996b). VEGF-induced angiogenesis as an alternate method of revascularization for chronic myocardial ischemia: improved perfusion and vascular reactivity. J. Am. Coll. Cardiol. 96: 92A.

Sellke, F. W., Wang, S. Y., Stamler, A., Lopez, J. J., Li, J., Li, J., and Simons, M. (1996c). Enhanced microvascular relaxations to VEGF and bFGF in chronically ischemic porcine myocardium. Am. J. Physiol. 271: H713–H720.

Sellke, F. W., Laham, R. J., Edelman, E. R., Pearlman, J. D., and Simons, M. (1998). Therapeutic angiogenesis with basic fibroblast growth factor: technique and early results. Ann. Thorac. Surg. 65: 1540–1544.

Shou, M., Thirumurti, V., Rajanayagam, S., Lazarous, D. F., Hodge, E., Stiber, J. A., Pettiford, M., Elliott, E., Shah, S. M., and Unger, E. F. (1997). Effect of basic fibroblast growth factor on myocardial angiogenesis in dogs with mature collateral vessels [see comments]. J. Am. Coll. Cardiol. 29: 1102–1106.

Shreeniwas, R., Ogawa, S., Cozzolino, F., Torcia, G., Braunstein, N., Butura, C., Brett, J., Lieberman, H. B., Furie, M. B., Joseph-Silverstein, J., and et al. (1991). Macrovascular and microvascular endothelium during long-term hypoxia: alterations in cell growth, monolayer permeability, and cell surface coagulant properties. J. Cell. Physiol. 146: 8–17.

Stavri, G. T., Zachary, I. C., Baskerville, P. A., Martin, J. F., and Erusalimsky, J. D. (1995). Basic fibroblast growth factor upregulates the expression of vascular endothelial growth factor in vascular smooth muscle cells. Synergistic interaction with hypoxia. Circulation 92: 11–14.

Thomas, K. A. (1992). Biochemistry and molecular biology of fibroblast growth factors. In "Neurotropic Factors" (J. H. Fallon and S. E. Loughlin, eds.) pp. 285–312. Academic Press, Orlando, FL.

Uchida, Y., Yanagisawa-Miwa, A., Nakamura, F., Yamada, K., Tomaru, T., Kimura, K., and Morita, T. (1995). Angiogenic therapy of acute myocardial infarction by intrapericardial injection of basic fibroblast growth factor and heparan sulfate: an experimental study. Am. Heart J. 130: 1182–1188.

Unger, E. F., Banai, S., Shou, M., Jaklitsch, M., Hodge, E., Correa, R., Jaye, M., and Epstein, S. E. (1993a). A model to assess interventions to improve collateral blood flow: continuous administration of agents into the left coronary artery in dogs. Cardiovasc. Res. 27: 785–791.

Unger, E. F., Shou, M., Sheffield, C. D., Hodge, E., Jaye, M., and Epstein, S. E. (1993). Extracardiac to coronary anastomoses support regional left ventricular function in dogs. Am. J. Physiol. 264: H1567–H1574.

Unger, E. F., Banai, S., Shou, M., Lazarous, D. F., Jaklitsch, M. T., Scheinowitz, M., Correa, R., Klingbeil, C., and Epstein, S. E. (1994). Basic fibroblast growth factor enhances myocardial collateral flow in a canine model. Am. J. Physiol. 266: H1588–H1595.

Vandormael, M., Deligonul, U., Taussig, S., and Kern, M. J. (1991). Predictors of long-term cardiac survival in patients with multivessel coronary artery disease undergoing percutaneous transluminal coronary angioplasty. Am. J. Cardiol. 67: 1–6.

Volkin, D. B., Tsai, P. K., Dabora, J. M., Gress, J. O., Burke, C. J., Linhardt, R. J., and Middaugh, C. R. (1993). Physical stabilization of acidic fibroblast growth factor by polyanions. Arch. Biochem. Biophys. 300: 30–41.

Volpert, O. V., Tolsma, S. S., Pellerin, S., Feige, J. J., Chen, H., Mosher, D. F., and Bouck, N. (1995). Inhibition of angiogenesis by thrombospondin-2. Biochem. Biophys. Res. Commun. 217: 326–332.

Ware, J. A., and Simons, M. (1997). Angiogenesis in ischemic heart disease. Nat. Med. 3: 158–164.

Weiner, H. L. and Swain, J. L. (1989). Acidic fibroblast growth factor mRNA is expressed by cardiac myocytes in culture and the protein is localized to the extracellular matrix. Proc. Natl. Acad. Sci. USA 86: 2683–2687.

Westernacher, D. and Schaper, W. (1995). A novel heart derived inhibitor of vascular cell proliferation. Purification and biological activity. J. Mol. Cell. Cardiol. 27: 1535–1543.

Wu, Z., MS, O. R., Folkman, J., and Shing, Y. (1997). Suppression of tumor growth with recombinant murine angiostatin. Biochem. Biophys. Res. Commun. 236: 651–654.

Yanagisawa-Miwa, A., Uchida, Y., Nakamura, F., Tomaru, T., Kido, H., Kamijo, T., Sugimoto, T., Kaji, K., Utsuyama, M., and Kurashima, C. (1992). Salvage of infarcted myocardium by angiogenic action of basic fibroblast growth factor. Science 257: 1401–1403.

Yang, R., Thomas, G., Bunting, S., Ko, A., Ferrara, N., Keyt, B., Ross, J., and Jin, H. (1996). Effects of vascular endothelial growth factor on hemodynamic and cardiac performance. J. Cardiovasc. Pharmacol. 27: 838–844.

14

Therapeutic Angiogenesis in Peripheral Limb Ischemia

JEFFREY M. ISNER, ANN PIECZEK, ROBERT SCHAINFELD, RICHARD BLAIR, LAURA HALEY, AND TAKAYUKI ASAHARA

The prognosis for patients with chronic critical leg ischemia, i.e., rest pain and/or established lesions that jeopardize the integrity of the lower limbs, is often poor. Psychological testing of such patients has typically disclosed quality-of-life indices similar to those of patients with cancer in critical or even terminal phases of their illness (Albers et al., 1992). It has been estimated that 150,000 patients (Dormandy and Thomas, 1988) require lower limb amputations for ischemic disease in the United States per year. Their prognosis after amputation is even worse (European Working Group on Critical Leg Ischemia, 1991): The perioperative mortality for below-knee amputation in most series is 5%–10% and for above-knee amputation 15%–20%. Even when they survive, nearly 40% will have died within 2 years of their first major amputation; a major amputation is required in 30% of cases; and full mobility is achieved in only 50% of below-knee and 25% of above-knee amputees.

These grim statistics are compounded by the lack of efficacious drug therapy. As concluded in the Consensus Document of the European Working Group on Critical Leg Ischemia (European Working Group on Critical Leg Ischemia, 1991), "there presently is inadequate evidence from published studies to support the routine use of primary pharmacological treatment in patients with critical leg ischemia." Evidence for the utility of medical therapy in the treatment of claudication is no better (Isner and Rosenfield, 1993; Pentecost et al., 1994). Consequently, the need for alternative treatment strategies in such patients is compelling.

The therapeutic implications of angiogenic growth factors were identified by the pioneering work of Folkman and colleagues over two decades ago (Folkman et al., 1971; Folkman, 1971, 1972). More recent investigations have established the feasibility of using recombinant formulations of such angiogenic growth factors to expedite and/or augment collateral artery development in animal models of myocardial and hindlimb ischemia (Banai et al., 1991, 1994; Baffour et al., 1988; Yanagisawa-Miwa et al., 1992; Takeshita et al., 1994c; Pearlman et al., 1995; Pu et al., 1993b). This novel strategy for the treatment of vascular insufficiency has been termed *therapeutic angiogenesis* (Höckel et al., 1993).

Among the various growth factors which have been shown to promote angiogenesis (Folkman and Klagsbrun, 1987; Folkman and Shing, 1992), vascular endothelial growth factor (VEGF) (Ferrara and Henzel, 1989), also known as vascular permeability factor (VPF) (Keck et al., 1989) and vasculotropin (VAS) (Plouet et al., 1989), is an endothelial-cell-specific mitogen (See Chapter 5 for more details.) Because endothelial cells represent the critical cell type responsible for new vessel formation (D'Amore and Thompson, 1987; Folkman and Haudenschild, 1980; Vernon and Sage, 1995), and because smooth muscle cells—one of the critical cell types responsible for the development of certain vascular lesions (Ross, 1993; Clowes et al., 1983; Pickering et al., 1993)—would not be directly activated by VEGF, cell-type specificity has been considered to represent an important advantage of this cytokine for therapeutic angiogenesis over those with more pleotropic actions.

VEGF is further distinguished from other angiogenic cytokines by the fact that the first exon of the VEGF gene includes a secretory signal sequence that permits the protein to be naturally secreted from intact cells (Tischer et al., 1991). Previous studies from our laboratory (Takeshita et al., 1994b; Losordo et al., 1994) had shown that arterial gene transfer of cDNA encoding for a secreted protein could yield meaningful biological outcomes despite a low transfection efficiency. We therefore performed preclinical animal studies to establish the feasibility of site-specific gene transfer of $phVEGF_{165}$, encoding the 165-amino-acid isoform of VEGF, applied to the hydrogel polymer coating of an angioplasty balloon (Riessen et al., 1993) and delivered percutaneously to the iliac artery of rabbits in which the femoral artery had been excised to cause unilateral hindlimb ischemia (Pu et al., 1993a). Analysis of the transfected internal iliac arteries using reverse transcription-polymerase chain reaction (RT-PCR) confirmed reproducible gene expression at the mRNA level for up to 21 days post gene transfer. Augmented development of collateral vessels was documented by serial angiograms in vivo, and increased capillary density at necropsy (Takeshita et al., 1993). Consequent amelioration of the hemodynamic deficit in the ischemic limb was documented by improvement in the calf blood pressure ratio (ischemic/normal limb), as well as increased resting and maximum vasodilator-induced blood flow (Takeshita et al., 1994a) in the VEGF-transfected animals versus controls transfected with a reporter gene. These findings formed the basis for the current clinical investigation.

Based on these preclinical studies, we developed clinically applicable strategies for therapeutic angiogenesis employing either recombinant human VEGF protein (rhVEGF) (Takeshita et al., 1994c) or the gene encoding VEGF (phVEGF) (Takeshita et al., 1996). Because the protein is not yet available for human application, we initiated clinical trials of human gene therapy involving percutaneous arterial gene transfer of phVEGF for patients with critical limb ischemia in December 1994. The gene encoding VEGF is delivered as so-called "naked DNA," i.e., DNA unassociated with other vectors, including viruses or liposomes. The solution of plasmid DNA is applied to the hydrogel coating of an angioplasty balloon; the polymer acts as a "sponge" to retain DNA until the balloon is inflated at the site of gene transfer, at which time the DNA is transferred to the arterial wall.

CLINICAL COURSE

The first eight patients to receive $phVEGF_{165}$ arterial gene transfer included five men and three women ranging in age from 54 to 92 years (M+SEM=71.9±12.6) (Table 14.1).

Four patients presented with ischemic ulcers of the foot and/or toes. In these four patients, the size of the ulcers at the time of presentation ranged from 1 cm × 1 cm, to 7 cm × 3 cm; the depth ranged from 2 (two patients) to 3 (two patients) cm. During the time required to complete screen tests prescribed by the protocol prior to gene therapy, tissue loss continued to progress in all four patients, despite optimized foot care. By the time of gene transfer, the ulcers ranged in size from 1 cm × 1 cm to 5 cm × 8 cm.

In one of the two patients with an ulcer (Pt. #3, Table 14.1) who received 1,000 μg of $phVEGF_{165}$, the size and depth of the ulcer appeared to stabilize for a period of approximately 2 months following arterial gene transfer; the progressive increase in the size of this ulcer pre gene therapy versus the apparent plateau observed for 2 months post gene therapy suggest that the VEGF had a therapeutic effect. During these 2 months, the patient experienced a reduction in rest pain, sufficient to allow him to proceed with a 2-week trip to Germany for a reunion of former U.S. and German generals who fought in the Battle of the Bulge. Near the end of this trip, which involved extensive walking across previous battlefields, the patient experienced an increase in rest pain, and the ulceration of the great toe became gangrenous. Subsequently, the patient was referred back to his physician for amputation of his left great toe and distal bypass surgery using a composite graft. Two weeks following surgery, the patient returned for a transmetatarsal amputation. Pt. 8 had a similar course; despite developing angiographic evidence of new collateral vessels (vide infra), she ultimately underwent a below-knee amputation.

Three patients presented with claudication and rest pain unassociated

Table 14.1 Clinical Features of Patients Treated with phVEGF$_{145}$[a]

								Rest Pain		
Pt.	*Sex*	*Age*	*Cigs*	*DM*	*Rutherford Class*	*ABI*	*Prev. Rx*	*+/0*	*Dur'n*	*Meds*
1	M	54	+	O	5	0.43	Fem-Fem BP; Fem-pop BP[b]; PTA of Fem-pop BP[b]	+	7 mo	Percocet Fentanyl patch
2	M	60	+	+	5	0.00	PF, EA, & Fem-pop BP; Revision of BP; PTA of BP×2[b]	+	6 mo	Percocet
3	M	81	O	O	5	0.39	Fem-pop BP; SFA/pop PTA[b]	+	6 mo	E-S Tylenol
4	M	92	O	O	5	0.28	Recommended for AKA	+	5 mo	Percocet Fentanyl patch Morphine sulfate
5	F	72	O	O	4	0.31	Fem-pop BP	+	17 mo	Vicoden
6	F	71	+	O	4	0.31	Fem-pop PTA; Fem-per BP; PTA of Fem-per BP; Iliac PTA; Repeat PTA of Fem-per BP	+	6 mo	Vicoden Percocet Codeine
7	M	73	+	O	4	0.47	Fem-pop BP; Fem-AT BP; CABG CEA (bilateral)	+	6 mo	Percocet
8	F	70	+	O	5	0.26	None	+	15 mo	Percocet Fentanyl patch Vicoden

Ulcer							Vacular Occlusion in Affected Limb					
+/0	*Dur'n.*	*Loc'n.*	*Size*	*Depth*[c]	*Other*	*DF*	*SFA*	*Pop*	*AT*	*PT*	*Per*	*BP*
+	7 mo	foot	8cm×5cm	3	Pitting edema	O	TO	TO	TO	TO	TO	TO
+	6 mo	foot	1cm×1cm to 2cm×2cm	3	O	O	TO	TO	TO	TO	TO	TO
+	6 mo	toe	3cm×3cm	2	O	O	TO	TO	TO	TO	TO	TO
+	4 mo	toes	1cm×1cm	2	Pitting edema	O	O	O	TO	TO	TO	NA

(continued)

Table 14.1—Continued

Ulcer							Vacular Occlusion in Affected Limb						
+/0	*Dur'n.*	*Loc'n.*	*Size*	*Depth*[c]	*Other*	*DF*	*SFA*	*Pop*	*AT*	*PT*	*Per*	*BP*
O	NA	NA	NA	NA	O	O	TO	TO	O	TO	O	TO
O	NA	NA	NA	NA	O	O	TO	TO	TO	O	O	TO
O	NA	NA	NA	NA	O	O	TO	O	O	TO	TO	TO
+	7 mo	toes	3cmx3cm	3	O	O	O	O	TO	TO	TO	NA

[a]Abbreviations: (+)=yes; (O)=no; ABI=ankle-brachial index; AKA=above-knee amputation; AT= anterior tibial; BP=bypass surgery of lower extremity; CABG=coronary artery bypass graft; CEA=carotid endarterectomy; Cigs=cigarette smoker; DF=deep femoral; DM=diabetes mellitus; Dur'n.=duration; EA=endarterectomy; F=female; Fem-fem=femoral-femoral; Fem-pop=femoral-popliteal; Loc'n.=location; Meds=analgesic medications; mo=months; NA=not applicable; PF=profundaplasty; Pop=popliteal; Per=peroneal; Prev. Rx=previous angioplasty or surgery in affected limb; Pt.=patient; PT=posterior tibial; R=right; SFA=superficial femoral artery; TO=total occlusion.

[b]Performed following development of ulcer.

[c]1=superficial; 2=involves subcutaneous tissue; 3=exposure of tendon or bone; 4=necrosis of tendon or bone.

with loss of tissue integrity. Rest pain in each of these patients was manifested principally by nocturnal episodes of forefoot pain waking the patients from sleep; the pain was typically relieved by placing the affected limb in a dependent position. At 3 months post gene therapy, all three patients remain free of rest pain. Prior to gene therapy, all three patients had also complained of claudication at less than 100 yards on a level surface. At 3-month follow-up, Pt. 5 was walking ≥ 0.5 miles/day without pain; in Pts. 6 and 7 the extent of pain-free walking was unchanged.

Ankle-Brachial Index (ABI)

The ABI measured prior to gene therapy ranged from 0 to 0.47 (0.31 ± 0.15). Compared to the ABI measured prior to gene therapy, the mean value of measurements recorded for each patient at weekly intervals up to 3 months post gene therapy did not improve by >0.1, the increment suggested to represent a significant change following angioplasty or reconstructive surgery (Guo et al., 1996).

Magnetic Resonance Angiography (MRA)

One patient (Pt. 4) with a permanent cardiac pacemaker was not studied by MRA. In three patients (Pts. 1–3), no significant change was apparent on serial assessment of MRA scans. In the last three patients to receive the 1,000 μg dose, however, MRA performed subsequent to gene transfer demonstrated improved perfusion of the infrapopliteal circulation. In Pt. 5 (Fig. 14.1), optimization of signal intensity was noted by 6 weeks, involving a large corkscrew-appearing collateral and the peroneal artery subserved by this collateral artery. In Pt. 6 (Fig. 14.2), improvement in flow, inferred from an increase in signal intensity in the posterior tibial and peroneal arteries, was observed by 3 weeks follow-up. In Pt. 7 (Fig. 14.3), improved flow involving all three major infrapopliteal arteries, but most prominent in the peroneal and posterior tibial, was optimal by 4 weeks post gene transfer; geniculate collateral vessels reconstituting the distal popliteal artery also showed increased flow in comparison to the MRA-recorded pre gene transfer. In Pt. 8, improved flow was documented at the ankle level.

Intravascular Ultrasound (IVUS)

IVUS examination performed in preparation for gene transfer identified accessible arterial segments for arterial gene transfer that were free of atherosclerotic narrowing in 6/8 patients; the arterial wall at the site of gene transfer in these six patients had a clearly recognizable three-layer appearance, indicating minimal to absent intimal thickening (Rosenfield and Isner, 1993). In two patients (Pts. 2 and 3), no site could be identified in either the superficial femoral artery (SFA) or deep femoral artery that was similarly pristine; the site least narrowed by atheroslcerotic plaque was therefore selected for arterial gene transfer.

IVUS inspection of the site of arterial gene transfer was repeated at 4 weeks (Pts. 1, 2, 8) or 12 weeks (Pts. 3, 5, 6, 7, and 8) post gene transfer. In Pt. 4, as described above, gene transfer performed immediately proximal to the site of occlusion in the popliteal artery resulted in retrograde propagation of the original occlusion for approximately 2 cm, occluding the gene transfer site. In the remaining six patients, arterial gene transfer to a normal (four patients) or mildly atherosclerotic (two patients) artery did not compromise vessel patency; specifically, subsequent IVUS examinations disclosed no new intimal thickening up to 3 months post gene transfer (Fig. 14.4).

Intravascular Doppler flow Analysis

Intraarterial blood flow was measured in the ischemic limb at the time of 3-month follow-up angiography in Pts. 3, 5, 6, 7, and 8. In comparison to flow measured immediately prior to arterial gene transfer, no improve-

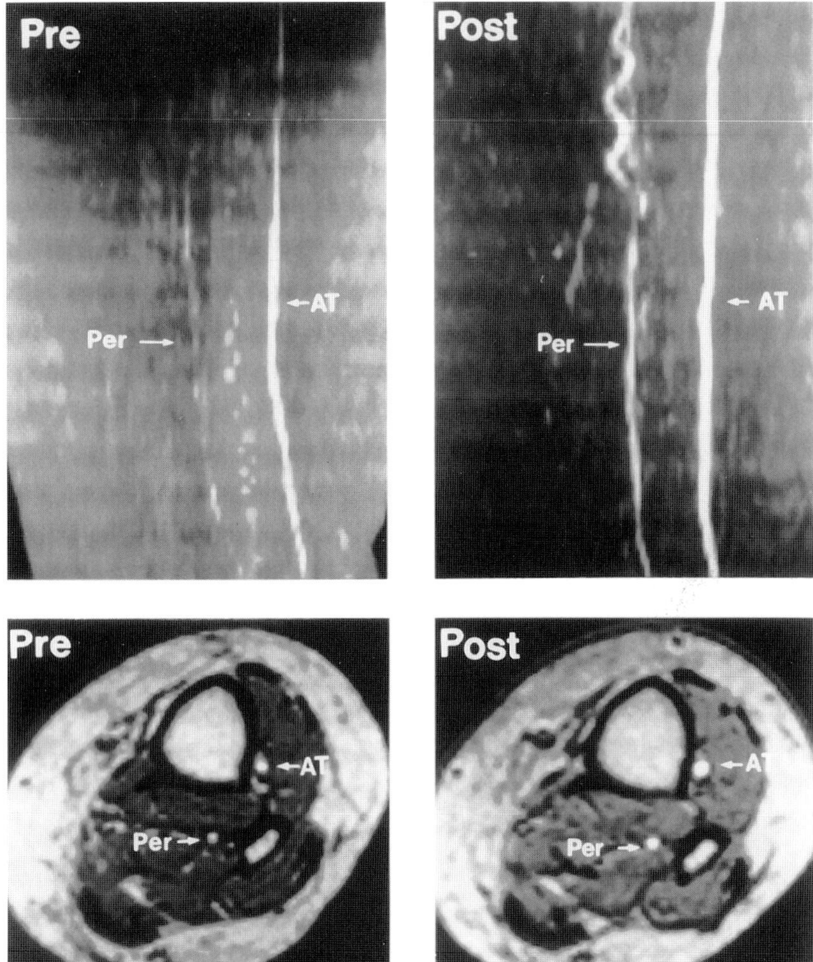

Figure 14.1. Magnetic resonance angiography (MRA, performed without contrast media) pre and post gene therapy in Pt. 5. In comparison to the longitudinal reconstruction (top) and tomographic view of the infrapopliteal vessels recorded pre gene therapy, the study recording post gene therapy shows enhanced flow via a tortuous collateral (arrow) to the peroneal (Per) artery distally; flow into the anterior (AT) artery is improved as well.

ment in flow was observed in Pt. 3. In the remaining four patients, however, including all three patients (Pts. 5, 6, 7) in whom evidence of clinical improvement was observed, improved flow was documented at 3 months post gene transfer (Fig. 14.5). The improvement in flow included both flow measured at rest (132.3% to 188.5% of baseline), as well as that recorded 30 to 90 seconds following administration of the endothelium-independent vasodilator nitroglycerine (120.0% to 158.6% of baseline).

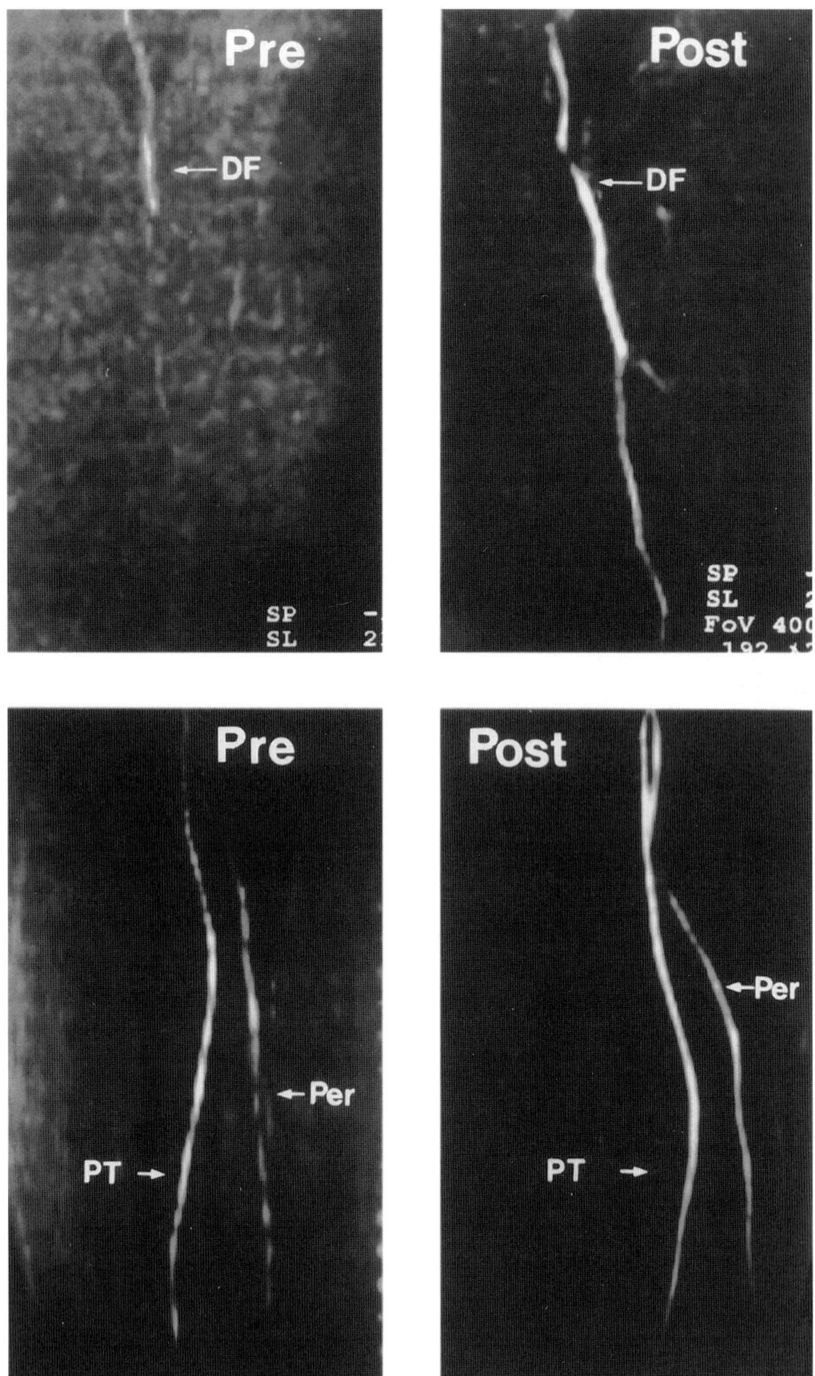

Figure 14.2. MRA pre and post gene therapy in Pt. 6: Post gene therapy there is improved flow in the deep femoral (DF) artery, as well as the posterior tibial (PT) and peroneal (Per) arteries.

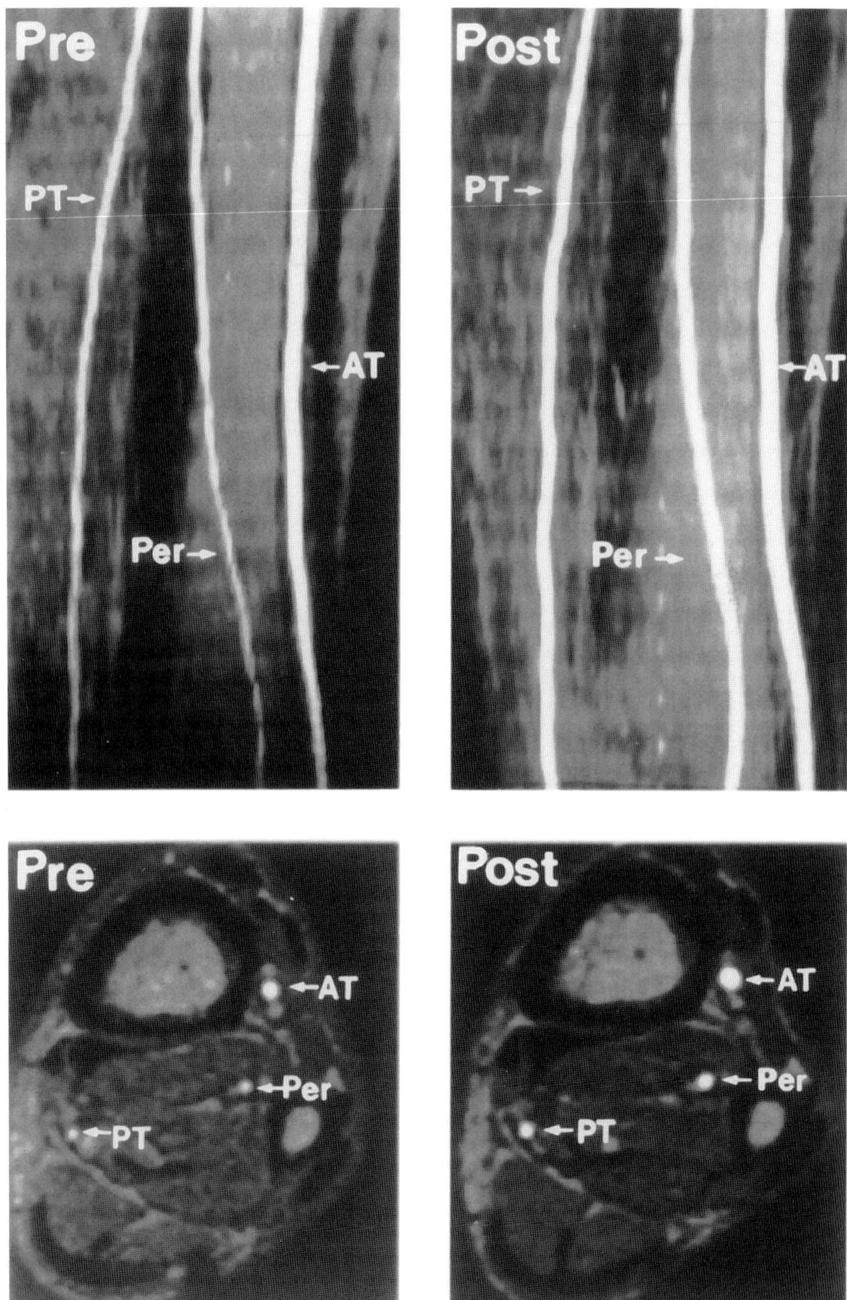

Figure 14.3. MRA pre and post gene therapy in Pt. 7: post gene therapy, markedly improved flow is seen in the posterior tibial (PT) and peroneal (Per) arteries, and, to a lesser degree, in the anterior tibial (AT) artery as well.

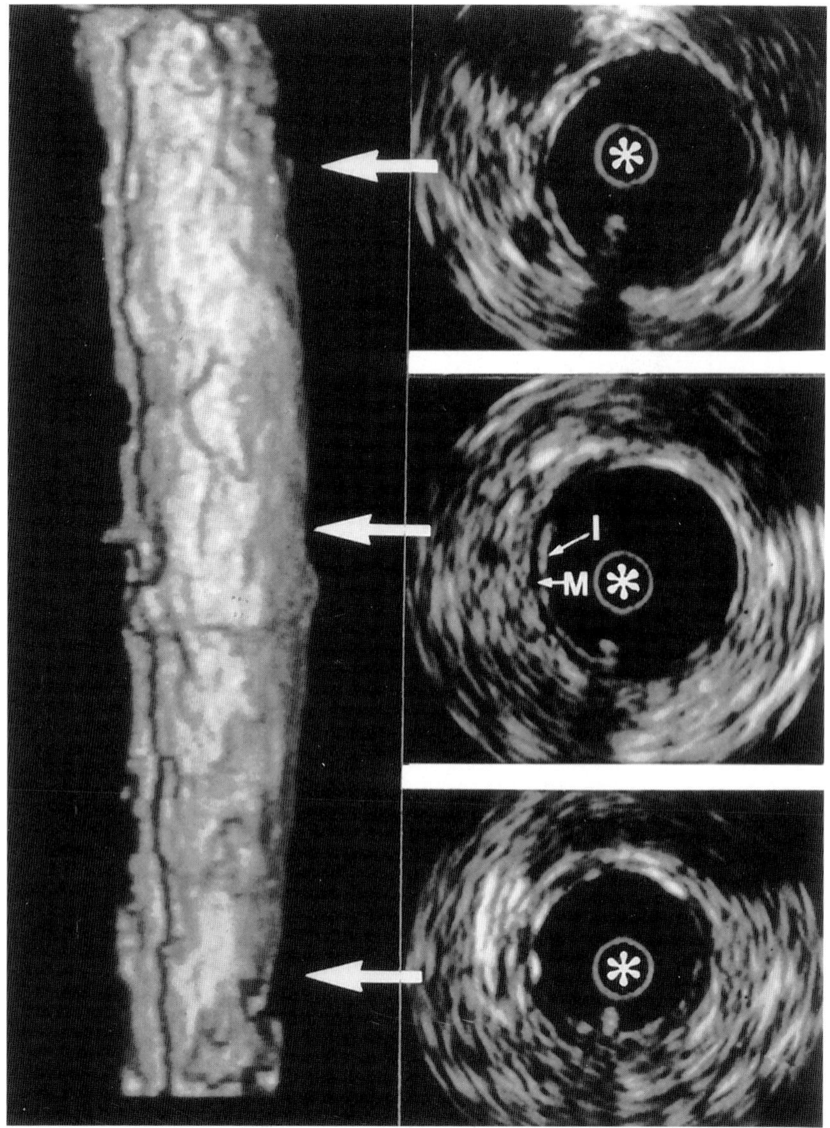

Figure 14.4. Three-dimensional reconstruction and representative tomographic views of entire length of gene transfer site in Pt. 5. Uniform luminal caliber is preserved, and tomographic views confirm preserved three-layer appearance of arterial wall with no new intimal thickening at any site.

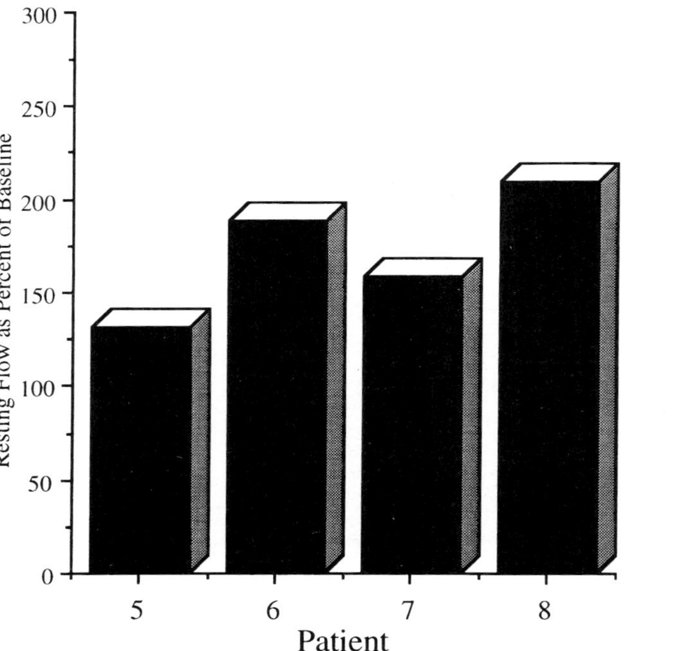

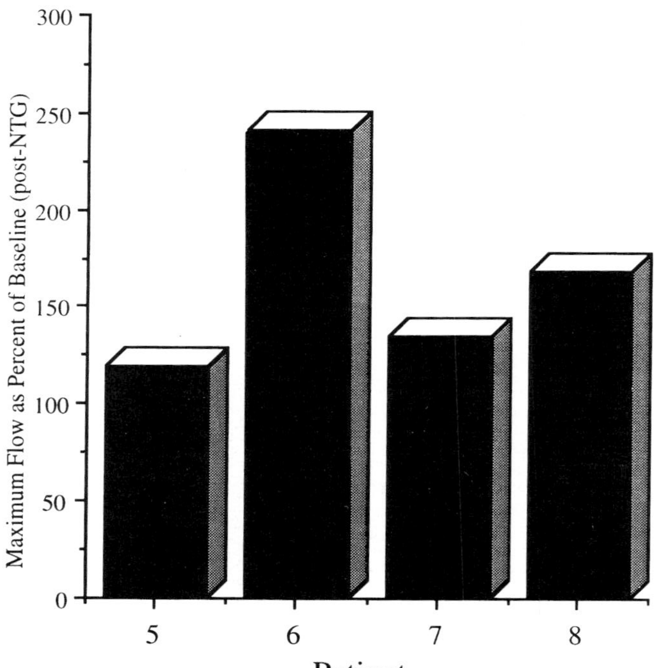

Figure 14.5. Resting and maximum (postnitroglycerine) blood flow in ischemic limb measured by intravascular Doppler flow wire pre versus 3 months post gene therapy in Pts. 5, 6, 7, and 8. In Pts. 5, 6, 7, and 8, resting flow was increased by 32.3%, 88.5%, 59.0%, and 109%; maximum flow was increased by 20.0%, 142.0%, 35.5%, and 68%.

Digital Subtraction Angiography (DSA)

In the first seven patients, serial DSA examinations disclosed no gain or loss of collateral vessels. In Pt. 8, however, the first patient to be treated with the 2000 μg dose, DSA performed 4 weeks post gene therapy disclosed a marked increase in collateral vessels in the ischemic limb at the knee, midtibial, and ankle levels (Fig. 14.6). These persisted unchanged at the time of a subsequent angiogram recorded 8 weeks later.

Other Findings

In Pt. 8, evidence of angiogenesis consequent to arterial gene transfer was also apparent on inspection of the integument of the distal portion of the

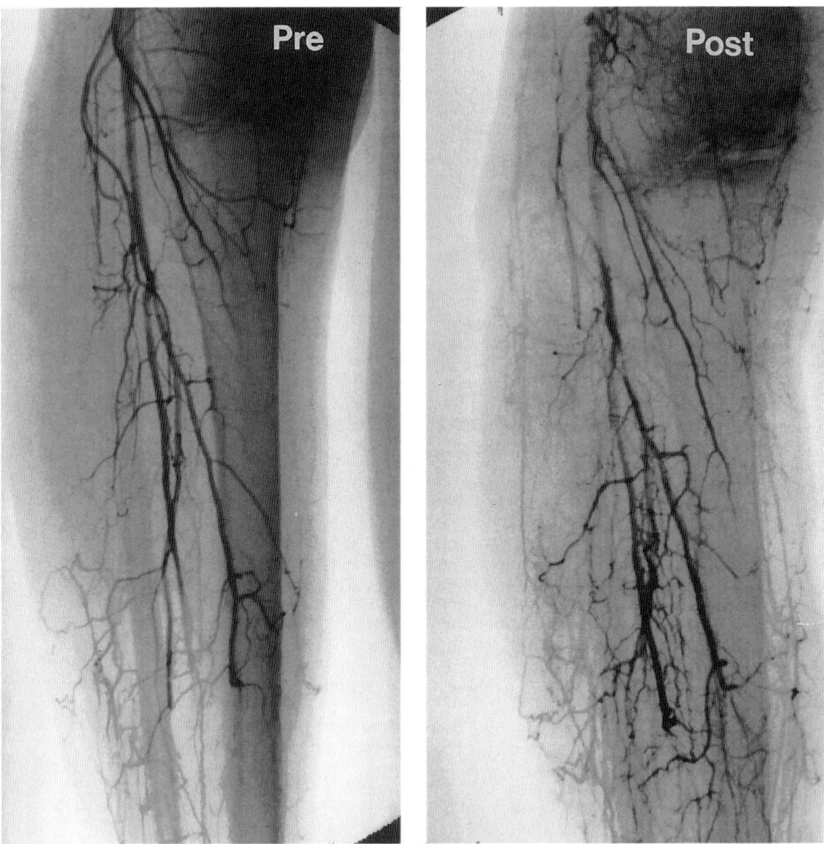

Figure 14.6. Selective digital subtraction angiography performed immediately prior to (left) and 1 month post (right) gene therapy disclosed plethora of new collateral vessels in ischemic limb. Reproduced from Isner et al. (1996) with permission.

ischemic limb. Three separate telangiectasia developed over the medial ankle (1) and dorsal forefoot (2) approximately 1 week following gene transfer (Plate 10). Excisional biopsy and light microscopic examination (Plate 10) of one of these lesions disclosed markedly positive staining for CD31, identifying endothelial cells comprising vessels within this lesion; the proliferative nature of these endothelial cells was shown by immunostaining of adjacent sections with an antibody to proliferating cell nuclear antigen (PCNA). The two lesions not removed by surgical biopsy underwent spontaneous regression by 8 weeks post gene transfer.

ADDITIONAL TESTING

Ophthalmologic Examination

In no patient were changes noted in funduscopic examination performed at 3-month follow-up.

COMPLICATIONS

One patient (Pt. 3) developed a pseudoaneurysm at the site of antegrade cannulation for arterial gene transfer. This was treated successfully by ultrasound-guided compression and resolved without sequelae.

Our preliminary experience with arterial gene transfer in the treatment of peripheral vascular disease extends previous studies performed in live animals to human subjects. No adverse consequences attributable to the recombinant protein encoded by phVEGF$_{165}$ were observed. The absence of these complications is consistent with site-specific activity observed in preclinical animal studies of VEGF, administered either as plasmid DNA or the recombinant protein (Bauters et al., 1995); such site-specific angiogenesis appears to be mediated by paracrine induction of VEGF receptors in endothelial cells exposed to factors secreted by hypoxic myocytes (Brogi et al., 1996). IVUS examinations disclosed no new intimal thickening up to 1 year post gene transfer. It is indeed likely that phVEGF$_{165}$ gene transfer accelerates reendothelialization and thereby obviates luminal compromise of the transfected segment (Asahara et al., 1995).

Because the current investigation is a Phase 1 trial, evidence of bioactivity was considered a secondary objective. Furthermore, a dose-escalating strategy was mandated for this trial due to the fact that VEGF, either as a recombinant protein or otherwise, had not been previously administered to human subjects. In contrast to the dose employed in preclinical animal studies (500 μg, or 0.114 mg/kg for 3.5 kg rabbits), the dose of plasmid DNA for the first two patients was limited to 100 and 500 μg (0.001 and 0.007 mg/kg), respectively. The subsequent five patients were approved for 1,000 μg (0.014 mg/kg). At what may still be considered to be a relatively low dose (the dose will ultimately escalate to 4,000 μg for the final seven patients of the total 22 approved for this Phase 1 trial), evidence of bioactivity was nevertheless observed. In three of the four patients treated with 1,000 μg of plasmid DNA in whom the gene transfer site remained patent, evidence of augmented flow to the distal portion of the ischemic limb was documented by three independent modalities. In these three patients, intravascular Doppler analysis disclosed an increase in both resting flow (132.3% to 188.5% of baseline) and maximum flow (120.0% to 158.6%) provoked by intraarterial nitroglycerine; these results compare favorably with the mean increase in rest (140%) and maximum (173%) flow documented in the rabbit model of limb ischemia 30 days following administration of $VEGF_{165}$ recombinant protein (Bauters et al., 1994). Contrast-negative MRA graphically confirmed the increased infrapopliteal blood flow in these three patients, and contrast angiography documented accelerated delivery of contrast media from the common femoral artery to the pedal arch vessels in these three patients as well. Moreover, these latter three patients, each of whom presented with several (6 to 17) months of ischemic rest pain, remain free of rest pain at 3-month follow-up. In the fourth patient, in whom rest pain was associated with aggressive growth in the size of an ischemic ulcer during the 3 months prior to gene therapy, further extension of the ulcer was blunted for 2 months post gene therapy.

Recently reported clincial trials of human gene therapy for cystic fibrosis (Knowles et al., 1995) and Duchenne's muscular dystrophy (Meddell et al., 1995) yielded somewhat disappointing results, perhaps in part related to the challenge of expressing the gene product—which in both of these cases remains intracellular—among a large proportion of airway epithelia or skeletal myocytes, respectively. In the current protocol, the requirement for a higher transfection efficiency may be obviated by the fact that VEGF protein includes a leader sequence which permits active secretion from intact cells; thus, even if VEGF gene expression is limited to a small number of cells, the paracrine effects of the secreted gene product may be sufficient to achieve a meaningful biologic effect. The question, however, as to whether naked plasmid DNA (Wolff et al., 1990; Lin et al., 1990; Buttrick et al., 1992; Chapman et al., 1992; Gal et al., 1993; Conry et al., 1994) will suffice, or whether, in spite of the secreted feature of the gene product, the magnitude of gene expression required will demand the use of adjunctive, including viral, vectors (Ohno et al., 1994; Schulick et al., 1995; Chang et al., 1995; Zwiebel et al., 1989; Mulligan, 1993; von der Leyen et al., 1995; Willard et al., 1994; Guzman et al., 1994; Grossman et al., 1994; Lemarchand et al., 1993), remains to be addressed. If naked plasmid DNA alone is to be used, then the optimal dose of plasmid DNA remains to be established. Other critical issues which remain to be clarified include the optimal frequency of administration; if the gene product is limited to a 30-day window—as suggested by preclinical studies—then the time interval required for full maturation of a lengthy collateral network might benefit from repeated administration, 3 weeks, for example, after the first dose. The extent to which a favorable response is affected by the proximity of the site of gene transfer to the ischemic focus in the affected limb also remains uncertain.

The broader issue regarding the relative merits of gene therapy versus administration of the recombinant protein for achieving therapeutic angiogenesis also remains uncertain. When VEGF recombinant protein can be compared to gene transfer, it will be intriguing to see whether the "slow-release depot" aspect of gene therapy (Riessen and Isner, 1994), administered in a site-specific fashion and targeted to local pathology, will yield outcomes that are superior to that which can be achieved with bolus and/or continuous administration of the protein.

Certain limitations of the current study must be explicitly underscored. With regard to safety, these findings are preliminary and do not establish the long-term safety of VEGF, administered either as a gene or gene product. Likewise, the preliminary nature of the results dictates that evidence of bioactivity, while encouraging, must be viewed cautiously. This is particularly so given that this first phase of clinical investigation was nonrandomized. While consideration was given to the issue of a control group, the FDA concurred that there was limited justification for undertaking catheter manipulation in patients with marginal limb perfusion and extensive atherosclerosis solely for the purpose of performing a sham transfection. For the patient undergoing gene transfer, the procedural risks were offset by the potential for relief from unremitting rest pain or healing of refractory ulcers; for the patient undergoing a sham transfection, the risks would not be offset by any potential benefit. To minimize the likelihood of spontaneous improvement in either rest pain and/or the appearance of an established ulcer, inclusion criteria required, in the case of rest pain alone, a minimum duration of 4 weeks of rest pain with dependence on narcotics without improvement; and, in the case of nonhealing ulcerations, a minimum of 4 weeks of conservative therapy without evidence of healing. While rest pain and/or ulcerations of this nature may precipitously deteriorate, the potential for spontaneous improvement under these circumstances is remote (European Working Group on Critical Leg Ischemia, 1991). The short-term nature of the follow-up obtained to date also leaves undetermined the durability of apparent clinical improvement observed in selected patients.

The precise mechanism responsible for the salutary effects observed in patients who received the 1,000 μg dose of DNA remains uncertain. What we have observed, by three independent examinations, is evidence of increased flow to the distal extremities—specifically, distal to the preexisting occluded vessels. This was most graphically illustrated by MRA performed pre and post gene therapy. In Pt. 5, for example, striking reconstitution of the distal peroneal artery developed in association with a similarly lengthy occlusion of the SFA/popliteal artery. In Pt. 6, flow was improved to both the peroneal and posterior tibial. In Pt. 7, flow appeared substantially increased in the posterior tibial, peroneal, and to a lesser degree, in the anterior tibial—all distal to the SFA/popliteal, which was occluded over its entire length. In each of these patients, measurement of increased blood flow using an intravascular Doppler wire and accelerated transit of angiographic contrast media supported the results of MRA.

These findings are consistent with experimental observations described recently by Pearlman et al., who used magnetic resonance imaging (MRI) to study the time delay in delivery of contrast media to the collateral-dependent myocardium of pigs in which the circumflex coronary artery was occluded by an ameroid constrictor (Pearlman et al., 1995). Following 6 weeks of treatment with VEGF (recombinant protein), contrast arrival time in the myocardium subserved by the occluded circumflex was markedly accelerated. Because survival and function of this ischemic myocardial zone is dependent upon collateral flow, the observed improvement in contrast delivery was inferred to represent augmented neovascularity, although direct demonstration of same was not shown. Previous DNA labeling studies in this swine model (White et al., 1992), a similar canine model (Unger et al., 1994), and the ischemic rabbit hind limb (Takeshita et al., 1995) have established that improvements in flow associated with collateral development are typically associated with proliferation of new vessels <180 μm in diameter, including a statistically significant increase in capillary density. We presume that among the three patients described above, flow from the profunda to the infrapopliteal vessels was improved via an augmented network of collaterals. Direct evidence of new blood vessel formation, however, remains pending, either because the size of the new vascular structures is beyond the resolution of conventional angiography, or because of other as yet undisclosed reasons.

We have also considered the alternate possibility that the increase in distal-extremity blood flow might be the result of vasodilation. VEGF has been shown in vivo to produce endothelium-dependent hypotension that can be blocked and/or reversed by administration of N^G-monomethyl-L-arginine (L-NMMA), an inhibitor of nitric oxide synthase (Horowitz et al., 1995). Moreover, in vitro studies have demonstrated VEGF-induced relaxation of canine coronary arteries that was abolished by endothelial denudation or pretreatment with L-NMMA (Ku et al., 1993), and recent studies in our laboratory have directly documented VEGF-induced release of nitric oxide from isolated rings of enothelium-intact (but not endothelium-denuded) rabbit aorta (R. van der Zee, unpublished data). It is our current feeling, however, that relief of rest pain at 12 weeks accompanied by evidence of augmented flow in the ischemic limb is unlikely to represent a vasodilator effect of VEGF, given that preclinical animal studies have consistently demonstrated cessation of gene expression (and, by inference, synthesis of recombinant VEGF protein) between 21 and 30 days post gene transfer (Minutes Recombinant DNA Advisory Committee, 1994).

These findings have thus established proof of principle for two concepts. The first is the potential for the administration of angiogenic growth factors to promote development of new collateral blood vessels in human patients. While not yet sufficient to prevent distal limb amputation in patients with advanced gangrene, use of higher doses, multiple applications, and/or alternative delivery routes, *viz.* intramuscular injection, of the gene or protein may yield sufficient neovascularity to make this goal a reality.

The second concept is the feasibility of arterial gene transfer of naked DNA. The use of naked DNA is admittedly inefficient, permitting successful transfection of <1% of target smooth muscle cells. In the case of VEGF, there are several aspects of the gene, protein, and target tissue which may have contributed to modulation of the host phenotype (increased vascularity and flow) despite a low transfection efficiency. VEGF, as noted above, is actively secreted by intact cells; previous studies in our laboratory (Losordo et al., 1994) have documented that genes that encode for secreted proteins—as opposed to proteins that remain intracellular—may yield meaningful biological outcomes due to paracrine effects of the secreted gene product.

REFERENCES

Minutes Recombinant DNA Advisory Committee (RAC) of National Institutes of Health, Sept 13, 1994. RAC #9409-088 approved in final form 11/15/94.

Albers, M., Fratezi, A. C., and DeLuccia, N. (1992). Assessment of quality of life of patients with severe ischemia as a result of infrainguinal arterial occlusive disease. J. Vasc. Surg. 16: 54–59.

Asahara, T., Bauters, C., Pastore, C. J., Kearney, M., Rossow, S., Bunting, S., Ferrara, N., Symes, J. F., and Isner, J. M. (1995). Local delivery of vascular endothelial growth factor accelerates reendothelialization and attenuates intimal hyperplasia in balloon-injured rat carotid artery. Circulation 91: 2793–2801.

Baffour, R., Danylewick, R., and Burdon, T. (1988). An angiographic study of ischemia as a determinant of neovascularization in arteriovenous reversal. Surg. Gynecol. Obstet. 166: 28–32.

Banai, S., Jaklitsch, M. T., Casscells, W., Shou, M., Shrivastav, S., Correa, R., Epstein, S. E., and Unger, E. F. (1991). Effects of acidic fibroblast growth factor on normal and ischemic myocardium. Circ. Res. 69: 76–85.

Banai, S., Jaklitsch, M. T., Shou, M., Lazarous, D. F., Scheinowitz, M., Biro, S., Epstein, S. E., and Unger, E. F. (1994). Angiogenic-induced enhancement of collateral blood flow to ischemic myocardium by vascular endothelial growth factor in dogs. Circulation 89: 2183–2189.

Bauters, C., Asahara, T., Zheng, L. P., Takeshita, S., Bunting, S., Ferrara, N., Symes, J. F., and Isner, J. M. (1994). Physiologic assessment of augmented vascularity induced by VEGF in ischemic rabbit hindlimb. Am. J. Physiol. 267: H1263–H1271.

Bauters, C., Asahara, T., Zheng, L. P., Takeshita, S., Bunting, S., Ferrara, N., Symes,

J. F., and Isner, J. M. (1995). Site-specific therapeutic angiogenesis following systemic administration of vascular endothelial growth factor. J. Vasc. Surg. 21: 314–325.

Brogi, E., Schatteman, G., Wu, T., Kim, E. A., Varticovski, L., Keyt, B., and Isner, J. M. (1996). Hypoxia-induced paracrine regulation of VEGF receptor expression. J. Clin. Invest. 97: 469–476.

Buttrick, P. M., Kass, A., Kitsis, R. N., Kaplan, M. L., and Leinwand, L. A. (1992). Behavior of genes directly injected into the rat heart in vivo. Circ. Res. 70: 193–198.

Chang, M. W., Barr, E., Jonathan, S., Jiang, Y. Q., Nabel, G. J., Nabel, E. G., Parmacek, M. S., and Leiden, J. M. (1995). Cytostatic gene therapy for vascular proliferative disorders with a constitutively active form of the retinoblastoma gene product. Science 267: 518–522.

Chapman, G. D., Lim, C. S., Gammon, R. S., Culp, S. C., Desper, J. S., Bauman, R. P., Swain, J. L., and Stack, R. S. (1992). Gene transfer into coronary arteries of intact animals with a percutaneous balloon catheter. Circ. Res. 71: 27–33.

Clowes, A. W., Reidy, M. A., and Clowes, M. M. (1983). Kinetics of cellular proliferation after arterial injury. I. Smooth muscle growth in the absence of endothelium. Lab. Invest. 49: 327–333.

Conry, R. M., LoBuglio, A. F., Kantor, J., Schlom, J., Loechel, F., Moore, S. E., Sumerel, L. A., Barlow, D. L., Abrams, S., and Curiel, D. T. (1994). Immune response to a carcinoembryonic antigen polynucleotide vaccine. Cancer Res. 54: 1164–1168.

D'Amore, P. A. and Thompson, R. W. (1987). Mechanisms of angiogenesis. Annu. Rev. Physiol. 49: 453–464.

Dormandy, J. A. and Thomas, P. R. S. (1988). What is the natural history of a critically ischemic patient with and without his leg? In *"Limb Salvage and Amputation for Vascular Disease"* (R. M. Greenhalgh, C. W. Jamieson, and A. N. Nicolaides, eds.) pp. 11–26. WB Saunders, Philadelphia.

European Working Group on Critical Leg Ischemia (1991). Second European consensus document on chronic critical leg ischemia. Circulation 84: IV–1–IV–26.

Ferrara, N. and Henzel, W. J. (1989). Pituitary follicular cells secrete a novel heparin-binding growth factor specific for vascular endothelial cells. Biochem. Biophys. Res. Commun. 161: 851–855.

Folkman, J. (1971). Tumor angiogenesis: therapeutic implications. N. Engl. J. Med. 285: 1182–1186.

Folkman, J. (1972). Anti-angiogenesis: new concept for therapy of solid tumors. Ann. Surg. 175: 409–416.

Folkman, J. and Haudenschild, C. (1980). Angiogenesis in vitro. Nature 288: 551–556.

Folkman, J. and Klagsbrun, M. (1987). Angiogenic factors. Science 235: 442–447.

Folkman, J. and Shing, Y. (1992). Angiogenesis. J. Biol. Chem. 267: 10931–10934.

Folkman, J., Merler, E., Abernathy, C., and Williams, G. (1971). Isolation of a tumor factor responsible for angiogenesis. J. Exp. Med. 133: 275–288.

Gal, D., Weir, L., Leclerc, G., Pickering, J. G., Hogan, J., and Isner, J. M. (1993). Direct myocardial transfection in two animal models: evaluation of parameters affecting gene expression and percutaneous gene delivery. Lab. Invest. 68: 18–25.

Grossman, M., Raper, S. E., Kozarsky, K., Stein, E. A., Engelhardt, J. F., Muller, D., Lupien, P. J., and Wilson, J. M. (1994). Successful ex vivo gene therapy directed to liver in a patient with familial hypercholesterolaemia. Nat. Genet. 6: 335–341.

Guo, Z. S., Wang, L.-H., Eisensmith, R. C., and Woo, S. L. C. (1996). Evaluation of promoter strength for hepatic gene expression in vivo following adenovirus-mediated gene transfer. Gene Ther. 3: 802–810.

Guzman, R. J., Hirschowitz, E. A., Brody, S. L., Crystal, R. G., Epstein, S. E., and Finkel, T. (1994). In vivo suppression of injury-induced vascular smooth muscle cell accumulation using adenovirus-mediated transfer of the herpes simplex virus thymidine kinase gene. Proc. Natl. Acad. Sci. USA 91: 10732–10736.

Horowitz, J., Hariawala, M., Sheriff, D. D., Keyt, B., and Symes, J. F. (1995). In vivo administration of vascular endothelial growth factor is associated with EDRF-dependent systemic hypotension in porcine and rabbit animal models [abstract]. Circulation 92: I–630–I–631.

Höckel, M., Schlenger, K., Doctrow, S., Kissel, T., and Vaupel, P. (1993). Therapeutic angiogenesis. Arch. Surg. 128: 423–429.

Isner, J. M. and Rosenfield, K. (1993). Redefining the treatment of peripheral artery disease: role of percutaneous revascularization. Circulation 88: 1534–1557.

Isner, J. M., Pieczek, A., Schainfeld, R., Blair, R., Haley, L., Asahara, T., Rosenfield, K., Razvi, S., Walsh, K., and Symes, J. (1996). Clinical evidence of angiogenesis following arterial gene transfer of phVEGF$_{165}$. Lancet 348: 370–374.

Keck, P. J., Hauser, S. D., Krivi, G., Sanzo, K., Warren, T., Feder, J., and Connolly, D. T. (1989). Vascular permeability factor, an endothelial cell mitogen related to PDGF. Science 246: 1309–1312.

Knowles, M. R., Hohneker, K. W., Shou, Z., Olsen, J. C., Noah, T. L., Hu, P-C., Leigh, M. W., Engelhardt, J. F., Edwards, L. J., Jones, K. R., Grossman, M., Wilson, J. M., Johnson, L. G., and Boucher, R. C. (1995). A controlled study of adenoviral-vector-mediated gene transfer in the nasal epithelium of patients with cystic fibrosis. N. Engl. J. Med. 333: 823–831.

Ku, D. D., Zaleski, J. K., Liu, S., and Brock, T. A. (1993). Vascular endothelial growth factor induces EDRF-dependent relaxation in coronary arteries. Am. J. Physiol. 265: H586–H592.

Lemarchand, P., Jones, M., Yamada, I., and Crystal, R. G. (1993). In vivo gene transfer and expression in normal uninjured blood vessels using replication-deficient recombinant adenovirus vectors. Circ. Res. 72: 1132–1138.

Lin, H., Parmacek, M. S., Morle, G., Bolling, S., and Leiden, J. M. (1990). Expression of recombinant genes in myocardium in vivo after direct injection of DNA. Circulation 82: 2217–2221.

Losordo, D. W., Pickering, J. G., Takeshita, S., Leclerc, G., Gal, D., Weir, L., Kearney, M., Jekanowski, J., and Isner, J. M. (1994). Use of the rabbit ear artery to serially assess foreign protein secretion after site specific arterial gene transfer in vivo: evidence that anatomic identification of successful gene transfer may underestimate the potential magnitude of transgene expression. Circulation 89: 785–792.

Meddell, J. R., Kissel, J. T., Amato, A. A., King, W., Signore, L., Prior, T. W., Sahenk, Z., Benson, S., McAndrew, P. E., Rice, R., Nagaraja, H., Stephens, R., Lantry, L., Morris, G. E., and Burghes, A. H. M. (1995). Myoblast transfer in the treatment of Duchenne's muscular dystrophy. N. Engl. J. Med. 333: 832–838.

Mulligan, R. C. (1993). The basic science of gene therapy. Science 260: 926–932.

Ohno, T., Gordon, D., San, H., Pompili, V. J., Imperiale, M. J., Nabel, G. J., and

Nabel, E. G. (1994). Gene therapy for vascular smooth muscle cell proliferation after arterial injury. Science 265: 781–784.

Pearlman, J. D., Hibberd, M. G., Chuang, M. L., Harada, K., Lopez, J. J., Gladston, S. R., Friedman, M., Sellke, F. W., and Simons, M. (1995). Magnetic resonance mapping demonstrates benefits of VEGF-induced myocardial angiogenesis. Nat. Med. 1: 1085–1089.

Pentecost, M. J., Criqui, M. H., Dorros, G., Goldstone, J., Johnston, K. W., Martin, E. C., Ring, E. J., and Spies, J. B. (1994). Guidelines for peripheral percutaneous transluminal angioplasty of the abdominal aorta and lower extremity vessels: a statement for health professionals from a special writing group of the Councils on Cardiovascular Radiology, Arteriosclerosis, Cardio-Thoracic and Vascular Surgery, Clinical Cardiology, and Epidemiology and Prevention, the American Heart Association. Circulation 89: 511–531.

Pickering, J. G., Weir, L., Jekanowski, J., Kearney, M. A., and Isner, J. M. (1993). Proliferative activity in peripheral and coronary atherosclerotic plaque among patients undergoing percutaneous revascularization. J. Clin. Invest. 91: 1469–1480.

Plouet, J., Schilling, J., and Gospodarowicz, D. (1989). Isolation and characterization of a newly identified endothelial cell mitogen produced by AtT-20 cells. EMBO J. 8: 3801–3806.

Pu, L. Q., Sniderman, A. D., Arekat, Z., Graham, A. M., Brassard, R., and Symes, J. F. (1993a). Angiogenic growth factor and revascularization of the ischemic limb: evaluation in a rabbit model. J. Surg. Res. 54: 575–583.

Pu, L. Q., Sniderman, A. D., Brassard, R., Lachapelle, K. J., Graham, A. M., Lisbona, R., and Symes, J. F. (1993b). Enhanced revascularization of the ischemic limb by means of angiogenic therapy. Circulation 88: 208–215.

Riessen, R. and Isner, J. M. (1994). Prospects for site-specific delivery of pharmacologic and molecular therapies. J. Am. Coll. Cardiol. 23: 1234–1244.

Riessen, R., Rahimizadeh, H., Blessing, E., Takeshita, S., Barry, J. J., and Isner, J. M. (1993). Arterial gene transfer using pure DNA applied directly to a hydrogel-coated angioplasty balloon. Hum. Gene. Ther. 4: 749–758.

Rosenfield, K. and Isner, J. M. (1993). Intravascular ultrasound in patients undergoing coronary and peripheral arterial revascularization. In *"Interventional Cardiology, Second Edition,"* (E. Topol, ed.) pp. 1153–1185. W. B. Saunders, Philadelphia.

Ross, R. (1993). The pathogenesis of atherosclerosis: a perspective for the 1990s. Nature 362: 801–805.

Schulick, A. H., Newman, K. D., Virmani, R., and Dichek, D. A. (1995). In vivo gene transfer into injured carotid arteries: optimization and evaluation of acute toxicity. Circulation 91: 2407–2414.

Takeshita, S., Zheng, L. P., Asahara, T., Riessen, R., Brogi, E., Ferrara, N., Symes, J. F., and Isner, J. M. (1993). In vivo evidence of enhanced angiogenesis following direct arterial gene transfer of the plasmid encoding vascular endothelial growth factor [abstract]. Circulation 88: I–476.

Takeshita, S., Bauters, C., Asahara, T., Zheng, L. P., Rossow, S. T., Kearney, M., Barry, J. J., Ferrara, N., Symes, J. F., and Isner, J. M. (1994a). Physiologic assessment of angiogenesis by arterial gene therapy with vascular endothelial growth factor [abstract]. Circulation 90: I–90.

Takeshita, S., Losordo, D. W., Kearney, M., and Isner, J. M. (1994b). Time course of recombinant protein secretion following liposome-mediated gene transfer in a rabbit arterial organ culture model. Lab. Invest. 71: 387–391.

Takeshita, S., Zheng, L. P., Brogi, E., Kearney, M., Pu, L. Q., Bunting, S., Ferrara, N., Symes, J. F., and Isner, J. M. (1994c). Therapeutic angiogenesis: a single intra-arterial bolus of vascular endothelial growth factor augments revascularization in a rabbit ischemic hindlimb model. J. Clin. Invest. 93: 662–670.

Takeshita, S., Rossow, S. T., Kearney, M., Zheng, L. P., Bauters, C., Bunting, S., Ferrara, N., Symes, J. F., and Isner, J. M. (1995). Time course of increased cellular proliferation in collateral arteries following administration of vascular endothelial growth factor in a rabbit model of lower limb vascular insufficiency. Am. J. Pathol. 147: 1649–1660.

Takeshita, S., Tsurumi, Y., Couffinhal, T., Asahara, T., Bauters, C., Symes, J. F., Ferrara, N., and Isner, J. M. (1996). Gene transfer of naked DNA encoding for three isoforms of vascular endothelial growth factor stimulates collateral development in vivo. Lab. Invest. 75: 487–502.

Tischer, E., Mitchell, R., Hartmann, T., Silva, M., Gospodarowicz, D., Fiddes, J., and Abraham, J. (1991). The human gene for vascular endothelial growth factor: multiple protein forms are encoded through alternative exon splicing. J. Biol. Chem. 266: 11947–11954.

Unger, E. F., Banai, S., Shou, M., Lazarous, D. F., Jaklitsch, M. T., Scheinowitz, M., Klingbeil, C., and Epstein, S. E. (1994). Basic fibroblast growth factor enhances myocardial collateral flow in a canine model. Am. J. Physiol. 266: H1588–H1595.

Vernon, R. B. and Sage, E. H. (1995). Between molecules and morphology. Extracellular matrix and creation of vascular form. Am. J. Pathol. 147: 873–883.

von der Leyen, H. E., Leyen, V. D., Gibbons, G. H., Morishita, R., Lewis, N. P., Zhang, L., Nakajima, M., Kaneda, Y., Coole, J. P. and Dzau, V. J. (1995). Gene therapy inhibiting neointimal vascular lesion: in vivo transfer of endothelial cell nitric oxide synthase gene. Proc. Natl. Acad. Sci. USA 92: 1137–1141.

White, F. C., Carroll, S. M., Magnet, A. and Bloor, C. M. (1992). Coronary collateral development in swine after coronary artery occlusion. Circ. Res. 71: 1490–1500.

Willard, J. E., Landau, C., Glamann, B., Burns, D., Jessen, M. E., Pirwitz, M. J., Gerard, R. D., and Meidell, R. S. (1994). Genetic modification of the vessel wall: comparison of surgical and catheter-based techniques for delivery of recombinant adenovirus. Circulation 89: 2190–2197.

Wolff, J. A., Malone, R. W., Williams, P., Chong, W., Acsadi, G., Jani, A., and Felgner, P. L. (1990). Direct gene transfer into mouse muscle in vivo. Science 247: 1465–1468.

Yanagisawa-Miwa, A., Uchida, Y., Nakamura, F., Tomaru, T., Kido, H., Kamijo, T., Sugimoto, T., Kaji, K., Utsuyama, M., Kurashima, C., and Ito H. (1992). Salvage of infarcted myocardium by angiogenic action of basic fibroblast growth factor. Science 257: 1401–1403.

Zwiebel, J., Freeman, S., Kantoff, P., Cornetta, K., Ryan, U., and Anderson, W. (1989). High-level of recombinant gene expression in rabbit endothelial cells transduced by retroviral vectors. Science 243: 220–243.

Index